ENCYCLOPAEDIA OF HOSPITAL ADMINISTRATION AND DEVELOPMENT

ENCYCLOPAEDIA
OF
HOSPITAL ADMINISTRATION
AND
DEVELOPMENT

VOLUME - 2

Hospital Management

Editor-in-Chief

Arun Kumar

INSTITUTE FOR SUSTAINABLE DEVELOPMENT
LUCKNOW

&

ANMOL PUBLICATIONS PVT. LTD.
NEW DELHI - 110 002 (INDIA)

ANMOL PUBLICATIONS PVT. LTD.
4374/4B, Ansari Road, Daryaganj
New Delhi - 110 002

Encyclopaedia of Hospital Administration and Development

First Edition, 2000

ISBN 81-261-0538-0 (Vol. 2)
ISBN 81-261-0489-9 (Set)

PRINTED IN INDIA

Published by J.L. Kumar for Anmol Publications Pvt. Ltd., New Delhi and Printed at Mehra Offset Press, Delhi.

Contents

	Preface	*vii*
1.	Indian Hospitals in the Context of Health for All-by 2000 A.D.	1
2.	Administration of Hospital Services	8
3.	Administration, Finance and Implementation	46
4.	Issues Related to Health and Hospital	55
5.	X-Ray Department	64
6.	The Outpatient Department	69
7.	The Architecture of Hospitals and Health Centres	79
8.	Medical Records	92
9.	Doctor-Patient Relationship: A Conversational Approach	106
10.	Administration of Primary Health Centre	114
11.	Administration of A Primary Health Centre	134
12.	Management of Primary Health Care	151
13.	The Health Centre	171
14.	The Cross-Cultural Outlook in Medicine	183
15.	Administration of the Indigenous System of Medicine	190
16.	Voluntary Health Agencies & Health Care Administration	205
17.	Modernising Health Administration	227
18.	The Particulars of Health Care Delivery	263
19.	Providing for Immediate felt Health Needs	329
20.	Maternal and Child Health	342
21.	Requirement of Paediatricians by 2000 A.D.	392
22.	Role Structure and Job Satisfaction Among Allied Health Professional in Hospitals	406
23.	Health Services in Tribal Areas	420
	Annexures	429

Preface

'Health is wealth' as the saying goes on, Health facilities are indicator of the development stage/ status of a country.

Health, according to the constitution of India is a state subject, the main responsibility of providng health services to all people lies with the State Health Department with the assistance of local health organisations wherever these exist, e.g. Corporation, Municipalities, Panchayati Raj, and adhoc statutory bodies.

This encyclopaedia is first effort to bring together authoritative information on Hospital Management and administration.

Details of the Volumes:

- Health Administration
- Hospital Management

We are deeply beholden to all the scholars in field whose learned writings are cited or substantially made use of in this work. Our intention is to disseminate the fruits of the erudition of those scholars, which will be shared by a large readership. However we are solely responsible for any shortcomings in presentation or other way.

We are also grateful to Mr. J.L. Kumar, Managing Director, Anmol Publications Pvt. Ltd., New Delhi, for timely publication of this work despite his tight schedule of publications.

—Arun Kumar

1

Indian Hospitals in the Context of Health for All—By 2000 A.D.

Introduction

Establishment of hospitals and other institutions providing mostly curative services represents an interesting facets of the various cultural, social, economic and political faces which have influenced the making of the health services in India today. Historically, these services were developed to cater mostly to the needs of certain special strata of the population and because of this, they were located in urban areas.

Hospitals in India is one of the culture technical diffusions from the west which in a period of time changed itself in very many ways but always keeping an eye on the west. Hospitals of modern India act as the index of development both in scientific and technological sense of the term.

Health For All By A.D. 2000

Free health care treatment for Indian citizens and health as subject under "directive principles of our Constitution" have by and large remained rhetoric than reality.

It is a challenge which we accepted during our Independence in 1947 still lies in a sorry state of affairs and we are yet grappling with it in a very little hope of getting any success in near future.

This dismal situation is not a product of one or two wrong planning mismanagement, mishandling of certain sectors of health but there are gross defects lying in almost all the sectors which are directly or indirectly related with health.

This article is an endeavour to scrutinise one of the areas of health care viz, institutional health care, and an effort will be made to think a viable alternative of the present system.

Institutional health care pertains to the hospital or similar organisational health care systems in general. As the caption of the article denotes that hospital health care will be the subject matter of the paper so it is necessary to know little history, development and the existing hospital situation to give a real operational alternative which is long due in this country.

Modern hospital is a welcome diffusion of cultural innovation from the west to India. So it becomes essential to know about the beginning of it in the west and then in India.

Development of Hospital in India

The Indian hospitals were very few and scanty, these were the citadels of charity and magnanimity of popular rulers. The ancient documents and chronicles by different scholars and travellers mentioned of *"bhagisyya graha"*, *"tiggichya chikitsasala"*, *"arogyasala"* etc. Those were popular during the reign of Emperor Ashok. And after his death there are very few mentions of such infirmities till the Muslim invasion in India which gave slight philip to the stagnant medical system and crippled infermities and destitute homes. But it is true that hospitals in India were nowhere near to the present mark till the Portugese invasion on India. Francisco-de Almadia had built the first Western type of hospital in India in the year 1506. It was built at Cochin. And this was built exclusively for the Portugese.

Real development of western hospitals in India started with the entry of East India Company. It had built the first hospital in Madras in 1664, in Bombay in 1676 and in Calcutta 1707-08, which were built exclusively for the Company staffs and limited number of Europeans who were staying in India. It is in the year of 1792 when these hospitals were open for the native Indians besides the English and Europeans.

Until 1835 there were no medical colleges and schools in India eventually there were no native doctors and medical students of native origin in those existing hospitals, the first medical college for the natives came up in 1835. And by 1847 all the three presidencies had its medical colleges. It is important to note here that these were installed and guided at the instructions of Royal British Medical Councils.

It was difficult for a commoner or a poor to go for medical education and the treatment as well. As it is clear from the writings that the basic aim of these institutions were primarily the maintenance of these British forces and civilians (of English origin) in India or other words it was meant to keep the British rule hail and hearty on Indian soil. In pursuance of that policy a few well to do natives also got a little share of the exclusive British profession. And those natives were the "Brown Sahibs", who could exercise their power mainly over the natives only. So there grew a bunch of native practitioners who enjoyed high status and prestige amongst their native brothers and sisters.

As these kinds of policies and activities continued the members of medical colleges and schools grew from 3 to 14 within a period of half a century (1846-1900).

The doctor-patient ratio was far below to the ratio of 1:30000 uptil 1900. The patient-bed ratio was less than 0.24 beds per 1000 (Bhore Committee, 1946). By 1947 there were 15 medical colleges and schools in India. The annual rate of admission was 1000 students.

As Bhore Committee found the following, which clearly states the tailspin of Indian health status up to 1947. There were 7400 hospitals and dispensaries the ration (person is to organisation) was 1:4000. Number of beds 113000 which is 0.24 per 1000. Doctors 47524, the ratio was 1: 6300, Nurses 7000 which is 1: 43000. And there were no Primary Health Centres (PHCs) in British India.

Independent India

After the Independence it was felt that there should be a sound health care policy for the newly formed nations. So, the implementation of the Bhore Committee suggestions became the guideline of national health care pattern. With acceptance of that report establishment of Primary Health Centres in each block, the district hospital and finally the State capital's hospital came up in a big way. But it so unfortunate that detailed operational guideline in reference to that vast socio-cultural variation of the country remained unnoticed in the committee report, rather it became structurally Indian but spiritually Anglo-American model of health care dispensation.

As a matter of fact, the Bhore Committee and successive Committees became the reference model of health care delivery in India. A perusal of those committee reports will make the situation more clear.

The Bhore Committee of 1946 and the Mudaliar Committee of 1962 recommended very many things for the face-lift of rusted health care status of India.

The Bhore Committee estimated the following up to 1960, 12000 hospitals and dispensaries so as to make the ratio 1: 35800. Beds 18500 so that it can be 0.40 per 1000, 88000 doctors to make the ratio 1: 4850, Nurses 30000 that is 1: 14300, 2800 PHCs that is 1: 70000. Unfortunately, these targets were never met. In 1962, Mudaliar Committee again recommended the long term and short term programmes (Bhore Committee) with sight modifications for their implementations. Mudaliar Committee highlighted the shortcomings and inability of our Independent India to cope with health issues up to 1961. It also expressed the incapability of implementing Bhore's, one bed per 1000. Though the PHC grew but these remained non-coordinated with the hospitals contrary to the Committee recommendations. The referral system inadequate and scanty. And number of hospitals, doctors and nurses did not grow as recommended.

By 1966, there were 81 medical colleges with an annual rate of admission of 11000 students. By 1977-78, it became 12500 per annum and by 1981, 13000 per annum. The doctor-population ratio became 1: 5150 in 1968 and 1: 3600 in 1979-80, unfortunately which could not yet reach the target envisaged by Bhore Committee.

The most tragic part of the episode is the distribution of rural and urban doctor-population ratio highly imbalanced.

There are 80 per cent doctors serving 25 per cent people who are all urban and 20 per cent doctors serving 75 per cent population who are all rural.

The allocations of health budget comprises of 3 per cent to 4 per cent of the total national budget and out of that nominal share of 6 per cent to 7 per cent goes for hospitals, dispensaries and PHCs out of which the largest share is definitely of hospitals.

The rate of hospital development in relation to PHC is a clear marker of lopsided development of hospital versus PHCs.

The number of health care institutions in 1950 and 1983 are as follows:

Years	*Hospitals*	*Dispensaries*	*PHCs*
1950	30	—	—
1983	6690	15970	5570

Modern Hospitals: A Critical Review

It is quite clear to have a sociological view of hospitals after serutinising the above facts. Hospital in India is a replica of the Western hospitals in almost all the aspects. The misappropriate grafting of hospital in India has eventually given rise to many ambiguities in the medical as well as in the socio-cultural fields.

The hospitals in India is the apex-body of modern medical system which is subserved by dispensaries, PHCs and subcentres all over the country. Hospitals in India are welcome diffusion for a handful of urban patients but for many rurals it is no less then a bugaboo.

The hospital culture is very much lopsided and are governed mainly by the doctors and echelons of staffs. The patient culture is of no great importance because he is a passive recipient of partial help. The hospitals are getting more and more technocratised and non-patient oriented.

As a scholar puts it, ". . . . modernisation of hospital in India are that they may be moving in the direction of increased responsiveness. . . to international knowledge, standards communication and consultation with reduced responsiveness to local demands" (John Bell, 1969).

A patient who is not accustomed to undergo "sick role" and that too in a totally new atmosphere, cannot be the real beneficiary of the hospital (this is the case of most of the villagers). The bureaucrative set-up of the hospital has been spoiled by the preferential treatments. The hospitals in India are running with below average staffs, doctors and other medical requirements, in other words the managerial administrative atmosphere is sick. The hospitals are not taking other smaller medical institutions as complementary to the comprehensive health care process rather these act more as subservient to the hospitals.

The general hospitals are following the super institutes (AIIMS & PGI) though which is ideally good but bad in practice, that is to say the high institutions in India are mainly research-oriented and less patient focal, the doctors in these institutes get specialisation in different fields and go abroad for super specialisation and if possible, stay back over there (T. N. Madan).

The recent studies show that once the hospitals are becoming unable to reach their goal and are not being penalised (penalisation of staffs, including doctors) they are becoming more and more lax and non-productive. The hospitals are under utilising their staffs due to improper management, policies and planning. There is a constant latent and manifest fight evinced between the staffs of different levels. Even there are tussles which are conspicuous within the staff of the same category, in which case doctor is no exception. And unfortunately the patient becomes the scape-goat in most of the cases many a times. For seventy-five per cent of the population it is the last resort when every hope is lost where one has to do (mostly) unhappy compromise with the alien hitherto unappreciable body of institutional health care in the name of the alleviation of ailment.

This type of attitude clearly shows that had the institutional health care been a healthy and comprehensive alternative for the villagers they would have preferred the hospital first than anything else. The system is yet urban-oriented, alien, non-comprehensive mystical and highly technocratised which acts detrimental to the very objective of hospital health care (it is meant to care, to the health needs of the community is most comprehensive, conclusive, adequate and economical manner).

To overcome such unwelcome situation there is a necessity to rehash the total situation by doing amendments and changes in medical education and by understanding the health culture of the majority instead of compelling to a forceful compromise of the majorities health culture and hospital culture. The hospital health care can only be popular and highly taken advantage of when there will be a perfect understanding of hospitals management and administration on one hand and patients socio-cultural dimensions on the other.

To bring about such a change in the hospital health care social scientists must not act, mere mouth piece of authorities rather should help make a true alternative which is long overdue to get rid of the inter-phase situation.

Hospitals thus become closely integrated with the entire health service system even while they may be at the apex. Even beyond this, the approach or Health for All -AD 2000 envisages that the entire pyramid of the health service system is specifically subordinated to the interests and requirements of the community as a whole.

In the context of hospitals, translation of such a perspective into concrete programmes of action involves the following processes :

1. An epidemiological approach to define the role of hospitals as community institutions;

2. Having defined the entire range of Community Health problems, one has also to define the health culture of the community, including the felt needs that are generated by various health problems;

3. Determination of community felt need for health services of various kinds makes it possible to define the areas of an overlap between epidemiologically defined needs and community felt needs;

4. Participation of the community in the decision making process. The degree of democratisation with a population determining the degree of success in subordinating health services to the people.

As has been pointed out above, changes in the relationship between a hospital and the community it services forms the most dominant feature of the changing role of hospitals in the context of Health for All—AD 2000.

Conclusion

By and large one can say that in India as in many other developing countries the development of health services did not keep pace with the changing need of the population either in quantity or in quality. There was no improvement from the point of view of the consumer, among the people there is widespread dissatisfaction with the existing health services to provide and adequate level of national coverage to meet the stated demand of different communities and groups, the expectations of the population as while still remains a far cry.

One can see a marked gap in our different levels of health care delivery. As a matter of fact the gap is prominent even within a particular area itself. A feeling of helplessness is evident amongst the consumers particularly in the rural and periurban or semiurban areas. It is felt that the health services and personnel developing uncontrolled along lines that may be satisfying to the medical profession but not to those in need of health care. Despite technical advances including advances in medical sciences the industrial revolution coupled with green revolution with the far reaching impact on Indian society there has been no change in the health development needs of the majority.

Hospital being a living symbol of organised institutional health care enjoying an unequivocal status and not only that it enjoys the largest share of health budget outlay. So it is quite clear that hospital is largely responsible for the appalling reality of health care status of India today. Keeping these things in mind one must obviously demand for an institute which would be more people oriented and much democratic in practice rather than being an institute of alien nature. And it has to be more meaningful and purposive for the *hoi polloi*.

It has to be an institute where the workers including of doctors to have certain degree of institutional commitment over and above the individual objectives. Moreover there is a necessity of a regular periodical assessment of the situation time and again in this field. The gross neglect of the hospital health care demands instead a sound énough model to make this much more accessible to people rather than keeping it merely available one.

The present hospital and health culture is a legacy of colonial heritage so it can only do justice of those who still happen to be the people of *"sahib"* cult. An alternative would be only possible when the training imbibed to the medical students are people-oriented and not a profession meant to serve the rich few. So long there is no attention is paid to the present lopsided equation of health care delivery there is definitely going to be a large interphase between the community and the institution of health care between the larger society and the hospital of which it is a part. And it is necessary to bridge that gap if the hospital has to survive more meaningfully and adequately in our society.

References

Banerji, D., *Poverty Class and Health Culture in India*, Vol. I, Prachi Prakashan, New Delhi, 1982.

Banerji, D., *Family Planning in India: A Critique and Perspective*, Peoples Publishing House, New Delhi, 1971.

Bhore, J., *et al.*, *National Health Survey and Development Committee*, Ministry of Health, Government of India, New Delhi, Vols. 1-4, 1946.

Borkar, G., *Health in Independent India*, Ministry of Health, Government of India, New Delhi, 1957.

Candill, W., "Applied Anthropology in Medicine", *Anthropology today* (Ed. Krocber A.L.) University of Chicago Press, Chicago, 1953.

Chattopadhyay, D., *Science and Society in Ancient India*, Research India Publication, CAlcutta, 1979.

Coc. R.M., *Medical Sociology*, McGraw Hill Book Co., 1970.

Friedson, E., *Profession of Medicine: A study of the society of Applied knowledge,* Harper and Row, New York, 1970.

Gladstone, G., *Medicine in Transition*, Chicago University Press, Chicago, 1965.

Green, S., *The Hospital: An Organisational Analysis*, Blackie, London, 1974.

Mumford, E. (Jr.) and Skipper, J.K. (Jr.), *Sociology in Hospital Care*, Harper and Row, New York, 1967.

Mathur, Indu, *Human Organisation of a Hospital*, Alekh Publications, Jaipur, 1975.

Seal, S.C., *Health Administration in India,* Dawn Books, Calcutta, 1975.

Rosengren, W. *Sociology of Medicine* Harper and Row, New York, *1980.*

Venkataraman, R., *Medical Sociology in an Indian Setting*, Macmillan, Madras, 1979.

2

Administration of Hospital Services

A. Nature, Classification and Indices for the Measurement of the Efficiency of Hospital

Nature

Since many health problems require a level of medical treatment and personal care that extends beyond the range of services normally available in the patient's home or in the office of the physician, modern society has developed formal institutions for patient care intended to help meet the more complex health needs of its members. The hospital, the major social institution for the delivery of health care in the modern world, offers considerable advantages to both patient and society. From the standpoint of individual, the sick or injured person has access to centralized medical knowledge and technology so as to render treatment much more thorough and efficient. From the standpoint of society, hospitalization both protects the family from many of the disruptive effects of caring for the ill in the home and operates as a means of guiding the sick and injured into medically supervised institutions where their problems are less disruptive for society as a whole.

Today, a hospital is a place for the definition and treatment of human ills and restoration of health and well-beings of those temporarily deprives of these. A large number or professionally and technically skilled people apply their knowledge and skill with the help of complicated equipment and appliances to produce quality care for patient. The excellence of the product — the *raison d'etre* for a hospital, therefore, depends on how well the human and material resources are applied to promote patient care.

Functions

(a) Patient Care: The first and foremost function of a hospital is to give care to the sick and injured and restore the health of diseased persons. Ethically, this care should be given to all without discrimination of social, economic or racial nature. However, the hospitals as national investments in people's health and as centres for scientific practice of medicine, must do many more things than 'produce' medical care. The success with which a hospital contributes towards meeting the patient's need can be measured by the fullness of the life he is able to lead on leaving it.

(b) Training: The education and training of doctors and nurses have traditionally been carried out in hospitals. It is a workshop wherein the student learns by seeing what his superiors and peers do Radiology, laboratory, radiotherapy, highly advanced surgical techniques demand a variety of skills and knowledge, all of which cannot be mastered by the doctor specialist. These activities have created the need for a large number of skilled technicians who are today the vital support to the specialist whether he is the surgeon, physician, diagnostician or therapeutist.. These people are indispensable for the all round excellence of all specialist work. To develop these technical skill a programme should be organized by the hospital under the direction of people who have the required experience, knowledge and aptitude to teach others. The purpose of inservice education and training programme is to develop such knowledge and skills in all categories of para-medical personnel as are required to make them fit for the job they hold and keep them attuned to the growing needs of their jobs.

(c) Medical Research: The third important function of hospital is to give support to medical research. A good hospital, where the quality of professional work is excellent, is an ideal ground for medical research. As a matter of fact, excellent professional care of patients largely results from the fruits of research into new problems. An aptitude of enquiry and investigation should permeate through the day-to-day care of patients. The hospital can develop facilities for research with comparative ease and speed if the staff and administration are properly motivated. True, elaborate research is expensive. There, nevertheless, remain clinical investigations of applied nature that call for little capital investment. Responsibility for creation of new knowledge is that of any enlightened profession. It is in a hospital that opportunities exist, if not abound, for organized as well as individual initiative for research.

(d) Health Education: The fourth and final object is to support and assist all activities carried out by various public health and voluntary agencies to prevent disease and promote positive health attitudes in the community through health education. Health education, immunization, social and economic rehabilitation are some of the many activities for which the hospital may provide assistance in terms of physical facilities and advisory services to staff. As a matter of fact, in the western countries, this aspect of the hospital as a community health centre is being emphasized more and more. Many ways are being devised to integrate the hospital with the activities of community health agencies.

The main function of a hospital is to promote the health of the community which it serves. Hospitals in the past were set up primarily as charity institutions for poor and weaker sections of society. These were considered as alms houses. The only function of such institutions was the care of the sick and the poor. The hospital was considered only a shelter for the society unfit. Hospitals are being re-oriented from just the centres for medical care and treatment to hospitals which are supposed to provide comprehensive system of preventive and curative medicine and rehabilitation services. It has been stated in a WHO document that the hospital is an integral part of a social and medical organisation, the function of which is to provide for the population, complete health care, both curative and preventive, and whose out-patient services reach out to the family in its home environment; the hospital is also a centre for the training of health workers and for bio-social research"[1] and "an institution that provides in-patient accommodation for medical and nursing care." The hospital has a noble purpose expressed in the phrase "Promotion of health and welfare of the people." Hospitals have now become indispensable to the proper care of the broad spectrum of health problems.

In the dunamic society, the hospital occupies a unique place to accommodate explosion of science into medicine and the whole galaxy of new treatment techniques, new equipment and proliferation of services which have made a profound impact on the provision of care facilities and services. Besides this, the development of socio-politico, cultural and educational systems have made the people conscious of their rights and they demand that modern and best means of medical and health care be made available to them; not only within the four walls of the hospital but at their doorstep or in the vicinity of living places. These impacts and made a hospital a complex organisation.

Administration of such a complex organisation requires blending of technical and administrative competence in the right quantity, at the right time, at the right place, by the right man and in the right way or process. Each hospital is a distinct entity and as such each has to be tailored to the specific aims to be accomplished, the specific tasks to be performed, the volume of services to be rendered and the type of the community to be served. The basic purpose of the hospital is "better patient care" and return the patient back to the community as a productive unit of that community. Hospital administration is an activity to secure better output through optimum utilisation of inputs.

Classification of Hospitals

Each hospital is distinct in its characteristics as it differs in structure, functions, performance and the community it serves. However, we can classify the hospitals into different types depending upon different criteria.

According to the objectives, hospitals can be classified into three categories:

1. *Teaching-Cum-Research Hospitals.* The main objective of these hospitals is teaching based on research and the provision of health care is secondary, e.g., All-India Institute of Medical Sciences, New Delhi, Post-Graduate Medical Education and Research Institute, Chandigarh.

2. *General Hospitals.* The main objective of these hospitals is to provide medical care to the people while teaching and research is secondary and incidental, e.g., district or taluka hospital, PHCs.

3. *Special Hospitals.* These hospitals concentrate on a particular aspect or organ of the body and provide medical care in that field e.g., Cancer, Dental, Psychiatry Hospitals, T.B. Hospitals, etc.

On the basis of *ownership*, hospitals can be classified into four categories.

1. Government Hospitals
2. Semi-Government Hospitals
3. Voluntary Agencies' Hospitals
4. Private/Charitable Hospitals.

According to the system of medicine we can have the following categories:

1. Allopathic Hospitals
2. Ayurvedic Hospitals
3. Homoeopathic Hospitals
4. Unani Hospitals
5. Hospitals of other systems of medicine.

Classification According to the Size

One of the major recommendations of the Health Survey and Development Committee (Bhore Committee) was the setting up of Peripheral Health Centres catering to a population of 40,000 each, which were to be linked up with secondary health centres and hospitals for purposes of referral services. In 1962, the Mudaliar Committee went further into this problem. The infrastructure for the delivery of health and medical care has closely followed the recommendations of these committees. However, the Government felt it necessary to set up a study group on hospitals in 1966. This group submitted its report in 1968.

The group found that out of 335 districts in the country, only 125 had more than 200-bed hospitals, and out of 3,000 taluks, only 2,053 had hospitals. However, out of 5,080 primary health centres planned for the country, 4,973 were found to be established. It also found that there was unequal distribution of hospitals in various areas of the country. It recommended that the following pattern of development for hospitals be adopted:

Teaching Hospitals	500 (to be increased according to the number of students).
District Hospitals	200 (may be raised up 300 beds depending on population).
Tehsil/Taluk Hospitals	50(may be raised depending on population).
Primary Health Centres	6 (may be increased to 10 depending on needs).

The bed strength of 125 districts which have at least one 200-bed hospital may bed raised to 300 depending on the population served. In the remaining 210 districts, hospitals having less than 200 beds, the strength should be raised to a minimum of 200 beds. Ordinarily, the distribution of these beds should be as under:

Medical	60
Surgical	40
Gynaecology and Obstetrics including Maternity	35
Paediatrics	15
Orthopaedics	5
Eye	10
ENT	10
Skin	5
Emergency	5
Isolation	10
Psychiatry	5
	200

Since the district hospital is to serve as a referral centre it should provide specialist services in Medicine, Surgery, Obstetrics, Gyneacology, Eye, ENT, Paediatrics, Dentistry, Psychiatry, VD, T.B. Clinic etc.

The staff norms as fixed by the Government for the different kinds of hospitals in India are as under:[3]

Sr. No.	*Name of the Post*	*No. of Posts (norms)*
	50-BED HOSPITAL	
1.	Medical Officer PCMS I	1
2.	Medical Officer PCMS II (including one Female)	2
3.	PJMS	—
4.	Dental Surgeon	1
5.	Pharmacists	3
6.	Nursing Sister	1
7.	Staff Nurses\ANMS	8
8.	Lab. Technician (Grade I) Lab. Technician (Grade II)	1
9.	Radiographer	1
10.	Clerk-cum-Storekeeper	1
11.	Cooks	2
12.	Mali	1
13.	Dhobi	2
14.	Class IV including Sweepers	17

Contd./-

100-BED HOSPITAL

1.	Medical Officer PCMS I	1
2.	Medical Officers PCMS II	3
3.	Dental Surgeon	1
4.	Anaesthetist	1
5.	Radiologist	1
6.	Pathologist	1
7.	Casualty Medical Officers	3
8.	House Surgeons	5
9.	Matron	1
10	Nursing Sisters	4
11.	Staff Nurses	20
12.	Pharmacists	5
13.	Storekeepers	2
14.	Clerks	4
15.	Accountant	1
16	Lab. Technician Grade I	2
17.	Lab. Technician Grade II	—
18.	Lab. Attendant	1
19.	Cooks	2
20.	Helper	2
21.	Radiographer	1
22.	Carpenter\Painter	1
23.	Chowkidar	3
24.	Class IV including Sweepers	50
25.	Biochemist	—
26.	Operation Room Asstt.	2
27.	Cashier	1
28.	Head Clerk	1
29.	Electrician	1
30.	Plumber	1

Contd./-

200-BED HOSPITAL

1.	Medical Officer PCMS I	2
2.	Medical Officer PCMS II	4
3.	Anaesthetist	1
4.	Pathologist	1
5.	Radiologist	1
6.	Biochemist	1
7.	Dental Surgeon	1
8.	Casualty Medical Officers	3
9.	House Surgeons	10
10.	Matron	1
11.	Nursing Sisters	10
12.	Staff Nurses	32
13.	Radiographer	1
14.	Pharmacists	5
15.	Lab. Asstt. Grade I	4
16.	Lab. Asstt. Grade II	—
17.	Lab. Attendants	2
18.	Dietician	1
19.	Cooks	4
20.	Head Cook	1
21.	Stenographer	1
22.	Accountant	1
23.	Storekeepers	3
24.	Clerks	2
25.	Dental Mechanic	1
26.	Carpenter/Painter	1
27.	Caretaker/Steward	1
28.	Chowkidar	3

Contd./-

29.	Mali	2
30.	Other Class IV posts including Sweeners	81
31.	Registrar	—
32.	Hawaldar	
33.	Assistant Matron	1
34.	Cashier	1
35.	Head Clerk	1
36.	Operation Room Assistants	2
37.	Electrician	1
38.	Barber	—
39.	Plumber	1

Indices for Measuring the Efficiency of a Hospital

It is very difficult to measure the efficiency of a hospital because of the complex nature of problems that it entails. There are many indices which can help us in evaluation of its quantitative performance. But, what about quality? It can be ascertained only through specially designed surveys. These surveys may be conducted both by persons inside the organisation and outside the organisation to locate the problems and suggest remedies for its future performance. Very few studies are available which have been conducted in this field. The studies carried out by NIHFW on different aspects of hospital administration throw light on various issues. Besides, the Committees of Parliament have done a useful work in analysing the performance of the All-India Institute of Medical Sciences and the three hospitals of Delhi. Research institutions and the universities should take interest and help the hospital management to improve their services. We mention below some of the indices which are commonly used to measure the efficiency of hospitals.

1. *Bed occupancy ratio* $= \dfrac{\text{Number of patient-days during the year} \times 100}{\text{Number of bed-days during the year}}$

This ratio tells us to how far the available bed capacity has been utilised

2. *Average duration of illness* $= \dfrac{\text{The number of in-patient days during the year}}{\text{Total number of in-patient admissions during the year}}$

The index is complementary to the other index 'average turnover interval'. This is more useful if computed for individual diseases.

3. *Turn-over interval* = $\frac{\text{The total vacant bed-days during the year}}{\text{The number of in-patients admission during the year}}$

The index indicates the number of days on an average per patient for which a bed has been remained unused.

4. *The average out-patient admission* = $\frac{\text{The total number of out-patients during the year}}{\text{The total number of out-patient admissions during the year}}$

5. *Average daily out-patient admissions* = $\frac{\text{The total number of new out-patients admissions during the year}}{\text{The number of working days during the year}}$

The index tells the average work load on OPD

6. *Cost of daily diet* = $\frac{\text{Total expenditure on diet during the year}}{\text{Total number of in-patient days}}$

7. *Average cost of medicine* = $\frac{\text{Total cost of medicines for in-patients for the year}}{\text{Total number of in-patients admissions}}$

8. *Fatality rate* = $\frac{\text{No. of in-patients deaths during a specified period} \times 100}{\text{No. of discharges during the same period}}$

9. *Autopsy rate* = $\frac{\text{No. of autopsies performed} \times 100}{\text{No. of in-patients deaths}}$

B. Aspects of Hospital Services

The services provided in a hospital differ from one hospital to another. It is very difficult to discuss all these services here. We can classify these services into three categories e.g., Line services. Staff services and Auxiliary services. These are explained with the help of a chart (Fig. 2.1). Let us discuss some of these services to understand the mechanics of hospital administration.

PROCEDURE IN AN EMERGENCY SERVICE

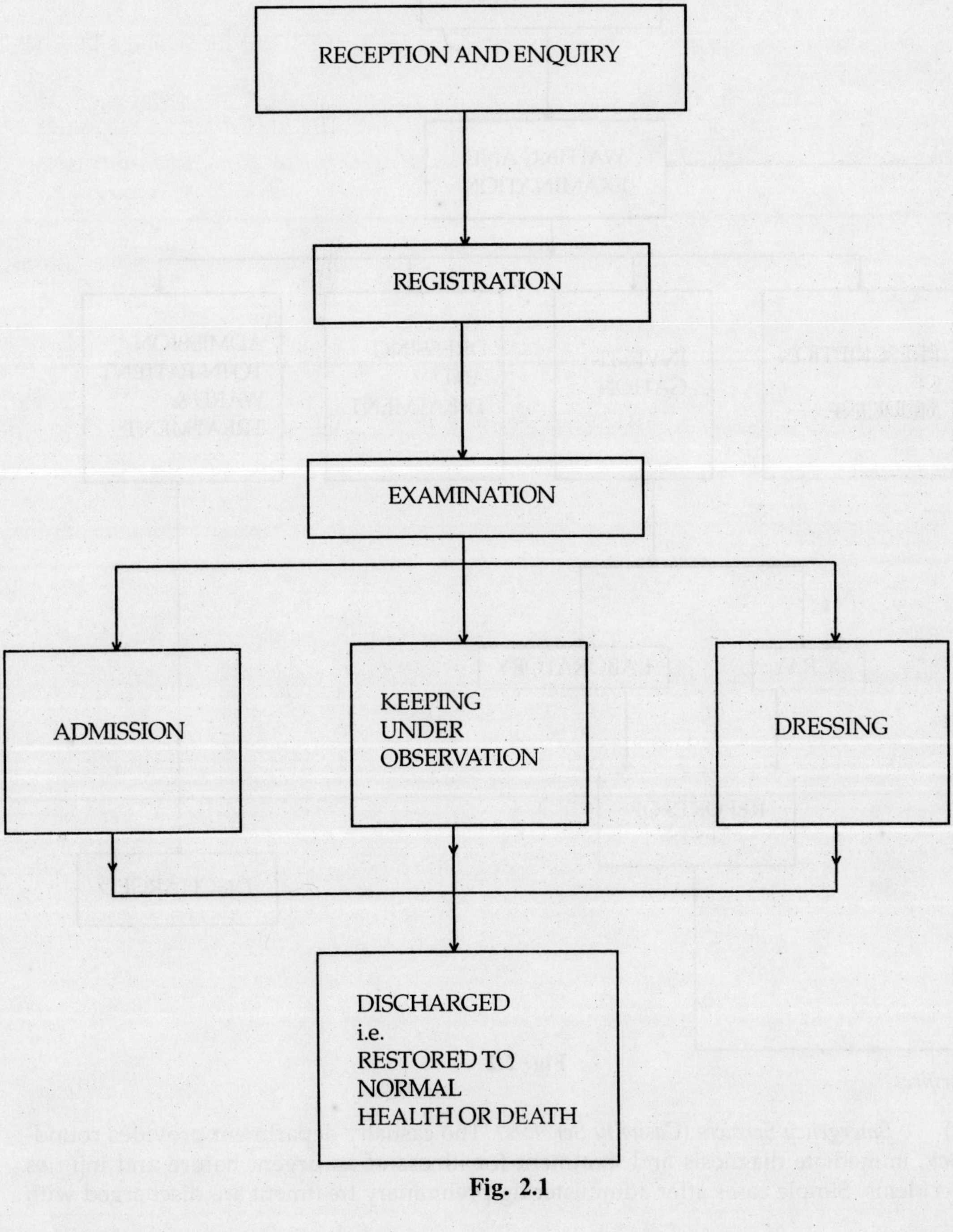

Fig. 2.1

PROCEDURE OF AN O.P.D.

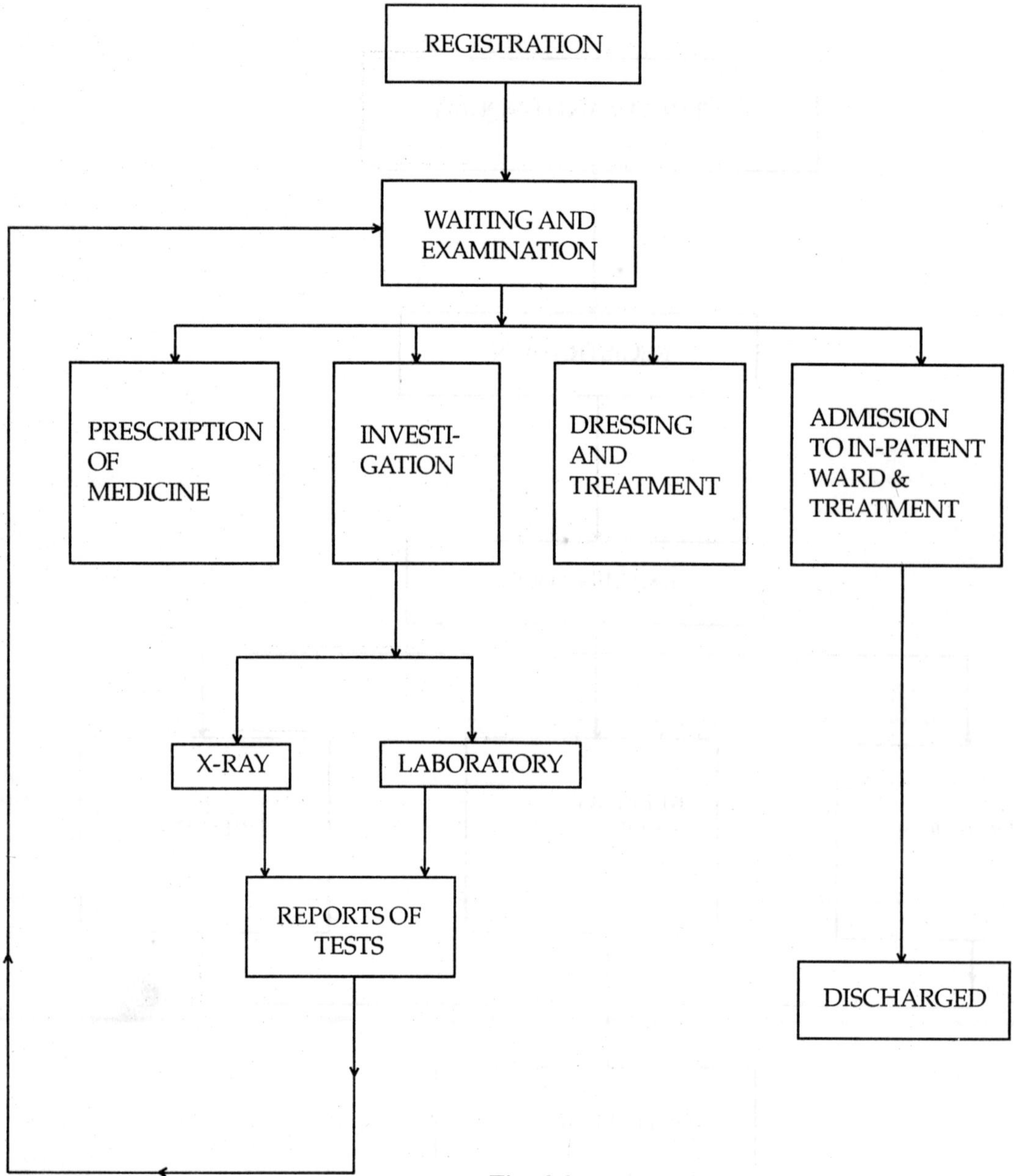

Fig. 2.2

Line Services

(a) *Emergency Services (Casualty Services)*. The casualty department provides round-the-clock, immediate diagnosis and treatment for illness of an urgent nature and injuries from accidents. Simple cases after administering preliminary treatment are discharged with instructions to attend OPD as a follow-up measure. Cases of serious nature are admitted in emergency wards to provide immediate medical care. Such patients are either discharged after 2-3 days or are transferred to permanent in-patient wards. Emergency service is acquiring increasing importance due to modern problems arising out of urbanisation and mechanisation. The best services must be provided to the patients in the Emergency wards as the patients and their relatives are under emotional strain and surcharged with suspense and anxiety about the consequences of the disease or calamity that has come up suddenly. Such an approach would alleviate a large part of sufferings born out of fear and suspicion of the unknown. The Public Accounts Committee (1977-78) suggested that.

> In order that the emergencies are attended to quickly and effectively, it is necessary to have an efficient set-up, well-knit with other departments of the hospitals with well laid-out procedure and work distribution.

(b) *Out-Patient Services.* The Out-Patient department is one of the most important departments. All the patients suffering from diseases of minor, serious, acute and chronic nature are examined. It should be designed to provide services to one per cent of the population of the area. It should be large enough to avoid congestion. The functions of the out-patient services are—provision of diagnostic, curative, preventive and rehabilitative services on an ambulatory basis. We can explain the whole process with the help of a flow diagram (fig. 2.2).

Out-patient department should be so planned that the building is separate from the indoor area. It should be well connected to the laboratories, X-ray department and other supportive services. It should have enough accommodation to avoid congestion. Depending upon size of the hospital and resources available separate areas of examination for the specialists should be provided.

(c) *In-Patient Services (Wards).* After the patient has been examined in the OPD or the emergency area, he may be advised admission in the wards. Wards are of different types—open general wards, (rows of beds in a big ward area), 4-5 bed units, and private wards for paying patients. Each ward has generally a doctor's duty room, dressing room, central Nursing Staff Station and other essential items needed for patient care. The departments to which direct patient access should be provided are the operating theatre suite, X-ray and physical medicine departments. the pharmacy and pathology departments should also be readily accessible from the wards for the convenience of the staff.

(d) *Intensive-Care Unit:* Some of the patients admitted to hospitals require acute, multi-disciplinary and intensive observation and treatment, e.g., patients of shock, coma, heart attack, lung, kidney, brain diseases, etc. It is desirable to have an intensive-care unit for such patients. Like the emergency services, this requires much better staffing pattern—one nurse for 1 ½ beds per shift. The staff needs to be specially trained to work in this area. This is very costly and should be set up only at the apex-hospitals.

(e) *Operation Theatres:* Each operating room set should have a pre-anaesthesia room and sterilisation room and a scrub room for nurses and doctors. There is a trend to provide simple laboratory facilities within the operating area to serve the purpose during emergency.

Supportive Services

(a) *Central Sterile Supply Services Management:* The Central Sterile Supply department is supposed to store, sterilise, maintain and issue those instruments, materials and garments which are required to be sterile. This requirement may steadily decrease as the use of disposable items becomes more economical.The Central Sterile Supply department should have direct lines of communication with all wards, operation theatres, out-patient and casualty departments, and to a lesser extent, with X-ray and pathology departments. Air control in this department is essential to check contamination through air. Proper control with indicators for sterilisation procedures essential.

(b) *Diet Management;* The catering department, which comprises the kitchen, bulk-food stores and dinning rooms, supplies all meals throughout the hospital. Direct and easy access is required from the main kitchen to the wards. The food should be transported in heated trolleys. This department is required to provide (i) general diet, (b) special diet for patients suffering from certain diseases. Food served in an attractive manner provides an incentive for the patients to eat.

(c) *Pharmaceutical Services Management:* The pharmaceutical services in most of the hospitals in India today represent the functions of procurement and distribution of medicaments by medical store and compounding and dispensing of medicine on doctor's prescriptions by persons hitherto known as compounders, generally under the control of Medical Officers.

In OPD, drugs are distributed on prescription while in wards the drugs are sent either on indents collecting for all patients; or indents for individual patient. Besides, every good hospital has a manufacturing section for various formulations and intravenous fluids.

(d) *Laundary:* There is a need for an efficient mechanical laundry to ensure the availability of bacteria-free washed linen. The small hospitals may get the cleaning done from washermen with due care and supervision. The aim is to make available to the patients clean and disinfected linen.

(e) *Laboratory and X-Ray Facilities*: For proper diagnosis of ailments of patients it is necessary to have diagnostic laboratory facility properly manned. The success of medical prescription would depend upon proper laboratory diagnosis. Laboratories for routine blood, urine, microbiology, X-Ray, etc., should provide round the clock service. It is desirable to locate the laboratory block and X-ray block in between the OPD and indoor area to be able to serve both the areas.

We must ensure that the technicians are really doing the job because a minor mistake on their part may ruin the life the patients. There is a need for constant supervision over the functioning of these laboratory services.

(f) *Nursing Services* : Nursing services should be managed by a matron who is assisted by a sister in-charge of the wards and staff nurses. Nursing sisters control the ward and arrange the leave day off of nurses. The accepted norms by Indian Nursing Council for a general ward is one staff nurse per five beds. The norm is never achieved in practice resulting in poor service. Besides, nurses are engaged in non-nursing activities which results in poor service to the patients. The Public Accounts Committee was critical of Nursing Services in three hospitals of Delhi. The Committee remarked.

> In view of the fact that the nurse-patient ratio excluding the specialised departments, is 1:33 in the Safdarjung Hospital and 1:19 in the Willingdon Hospital as against the ideal ratio of 1:5, the Committee feels that there is considerable shortage of nurses for manning the emergency and casualty services in the three hospitals.

The same situation prevails in most of the hospitals.

Auxiliary Services

(a) *Registration and Indoor Case Records*: Registration is a must for a hospital to enroll new patients with proper entry in OPD cards and keep track of the revisits of the patients. Medical records help in regulating admission of patients. It helps in codifying the record according to internal disease index. It also collects statistics of hospital stay of patients, i.e., admission, discharge, average stay, etc., for future planning and management. According to Calender. The hospital's admission procedure should be such that the patient is made to feel welcome and secure. Every employee who comes in contact with the patient should make him feel that each one is genuinely interested in his welfare. This experience is the patient's first introduction to the hospital and should be a pleasant one.[4]

(b) *Stores*: The Central Store receives, stores and issues bulk items which can, with advantage, be stored centrally. Stores are of different types—Pharmacy Stores, Chemical Stores, Linen Stores Surgical Stores, Glassware Stores, Stock policy should be devised in such a way that vital and essential items are always available. It should be managed by a competent stores officer.

(c) *Transport* : Transport requirements for the carriage of supplies and patients are:

* Trolleys;
* Stretchers; and
* Wheel chairs.

It is preferable to have a central transport gang to shift the patients. Supplies should also be distributed to all wards by the central areas.

(d) *Mortuary*: Each hospital should have a cold storage area or mortuary where dead bodies are kept before they are claimed by the relations. Sometimes post-motems need to be done for medico-legal reasons. Unclaimed bodies should be disposed off according to rules.

ASPECTS OF HOSPITAL SERVICES

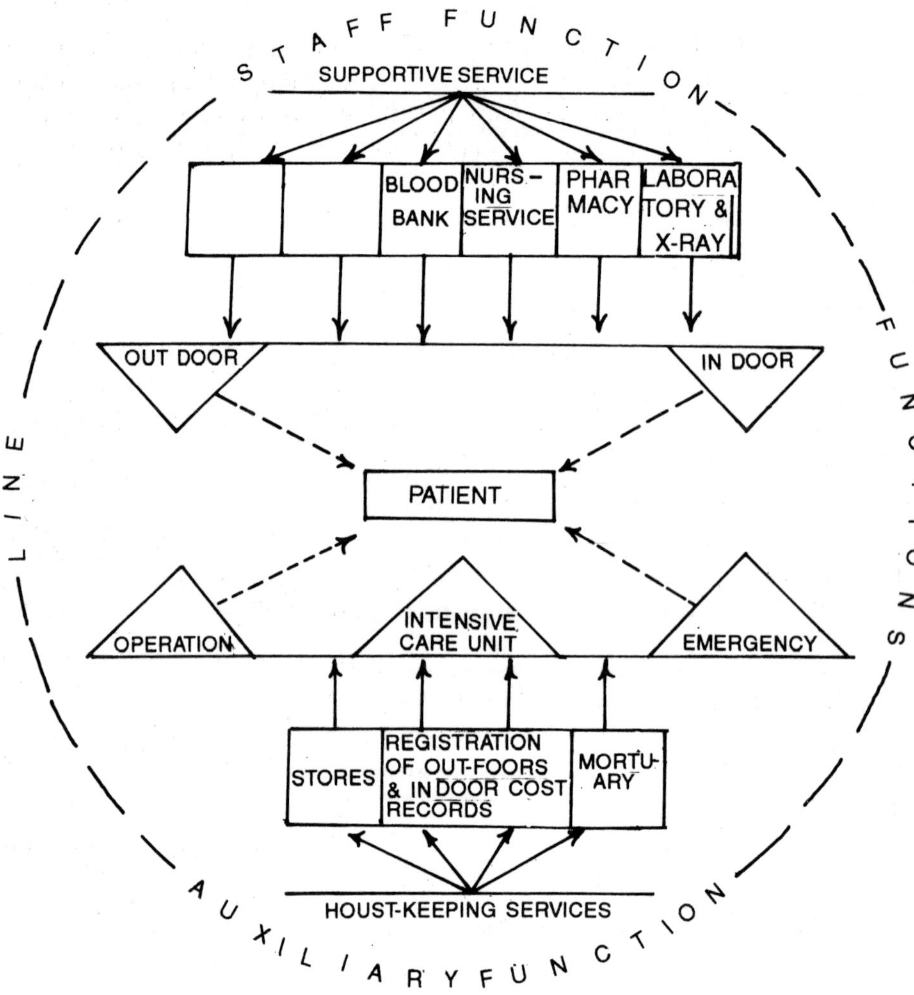

Fig. 2.3

C. Brief Descriptions of Some Hospitals of Different Kinds and Systems

(i) *Teaching-cum-Research Hospitals*

Every teaching institution has an attached hospital which provides clinical material for teaching and training of the students. Such hospitals also provide facilities for research both for the teachers and the taught.

The method of treating a patient in a teaching-cum-research hospital varies from that available in a general hospital. In the case of the former, apart from treatment, the patient is used for teaching and research. Here the patient is first handled by a trainee who examines him thoroughly, records his detailed history and suggests the diagnosis and treatment. The case is then presented by the trainee to the teacher (called consultant) who goes through the history recorded by the trainee and also examines the patient. The treatment is prescribed only by the consultant. In this way the patient, besides receiving treatment also acts as 'material' for teaching. He is used for research by the teachers and the taught. It has to be accepted that the treatment in a teaching-cum-research institute takes more time than in a general hospital.

Let us describe briefly Post-Graduate Institute of Medical Education and Research, Chandigarh, to understand the organisation and working of such hospitals.

The Post-Graduate Institute of Medical Education and Research, Chandigarh, was established by the Government of Punjab in 1962. It was declared an institution of national importance by an Act of Parliament with effect from April 1967.

The PGIMER Chandigarh offers 68 different courses leading to the award of degrees of B.Sc., M.Sc., M.D., M.S., M.Ch., D.M., M.D.S. and Ph.D., etc. As on 31 March 1982, a total of 1,671 residents completed their training and obtained their post-graduate qualifications. The Nehru Hospital attached to the institute has a bed strength of 774. During the year 1981-82, the registration of in-patients and out-patients was 25,403 and 5,67,726 respectively.

The administration of the institute including the Nehru Hospital is under the control of a Director, who is assisted by the Dean (for teaching purposes) and the Medical Superintendent (administrative purposes).

(ii) *General Hospital*

The main function of the general hospital is to provide treatment to the patient. No detailed history of the illness of the patient is recorded. Here the medical officer hears a verbal account of the illness of the patient, examines him and prescribes the treatment. The treatment is quick and less time consuming. The only disadvantage of this system of treatment is that sometimes the serious illness may go undiagnosed properly.

Let us describe a Government General Hospital with reference to Civil Hospital, Ropar (Punjab). It is a 100-bed hospital (56 male and 44 female) with a provision for 10 extra beds. It provides the following special services :

Speciality	*Bed strength*
Medical	30
Surgery	30
Eye	10
Paediatrics	10
Obstetrics and Gynaecology	20

It has been provided will all the facilities which can serve the patients.

STRUCTURE OF CIVIL HOSPITAL ROPAR

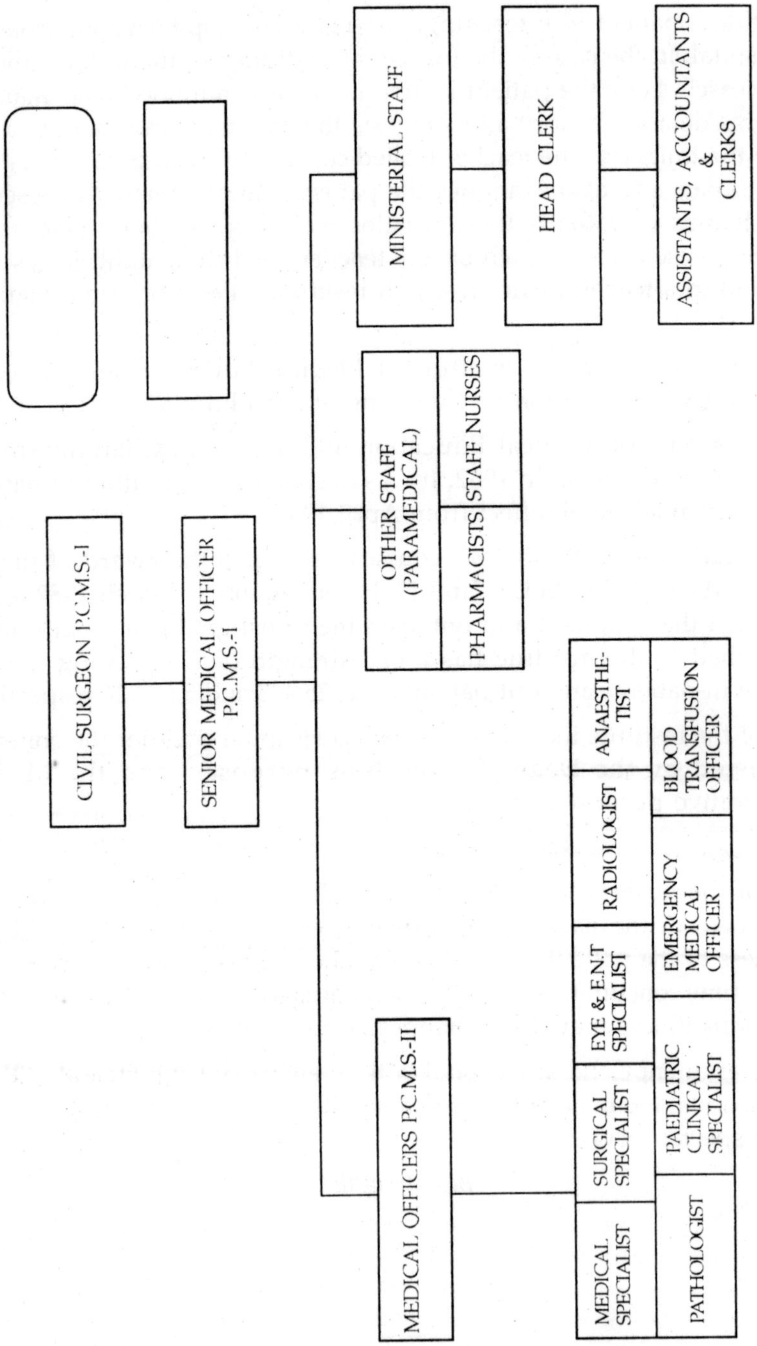

Fig. 2.4

The affairs of the hospital are managed by the Chief Medical Officer (PCMS Class 1); who has under him 12 Doctors, 5 Pharmacists, Radiographer/X-ray Assistant, 4 Laboratory Technicians. I Matron, 2 Nursing sisters, 10 staff nurses. Besides, there are 10 members belonging to ministerial staff, 53 belonging to class IV, one carpenter, one driver, one plumber and one electrician.

We shall explain in the next chapter the working of Primary Health Centres in detail which are like mini-general hospitals.

(iii) *Working of the Special Hospitals*

We shall explain this with the help of Chest Diseases Hospital, Patiala and the Punjab Mental Hospital, Amritsar.

Chest Diseases Hospital at Patiala: The hospital was started with the name, T.B.Clinic, in 1949, with ten beds only. It has been named as Chest Diseases Hospital. It has been serving as Training and Demonstration Centre as well since 1962. The hospital is under the control of Director of Research and Medical Education, Punjab. The day-to-day affairs of the hospital are looked after by the Deputy Medical Superintendent. The details can be seen from the Organisational Chart (Fig.2.5).

Services

The hospital provides patient care—outdoor as well as indoor. It also provides community health services at all levels, i.e., (a) Primary prevention, (b) Secondary prevention, (c) Tertiary prevention.

(a) BCG Vaccination is given to each child immediately after birth.

(b) The hospital has got mobile team, mobile X-ray plant and they move to places where they can detect cases. Such as at fairs where the public is gathered, at factories, industries, camps, schools, etc., through survey and screening of all the population.

(c) For this rehabilitation services are available. Rehabilitation includes everything that is done for the patient.

It also serves as educational centre and provides:

(i) Integration of tuberculosis course. In the general nursing **'A' Grade Diploma Programme.**

(ii) Tuberculosis course for the medical students.

(iii) House job facilities for medical group.

(iv) T.B. health visitors training.

(v) Multipurpose worker's training.

ORGANIZATION OF THE CHEST DISEASE INSTITUTE, PATIALA

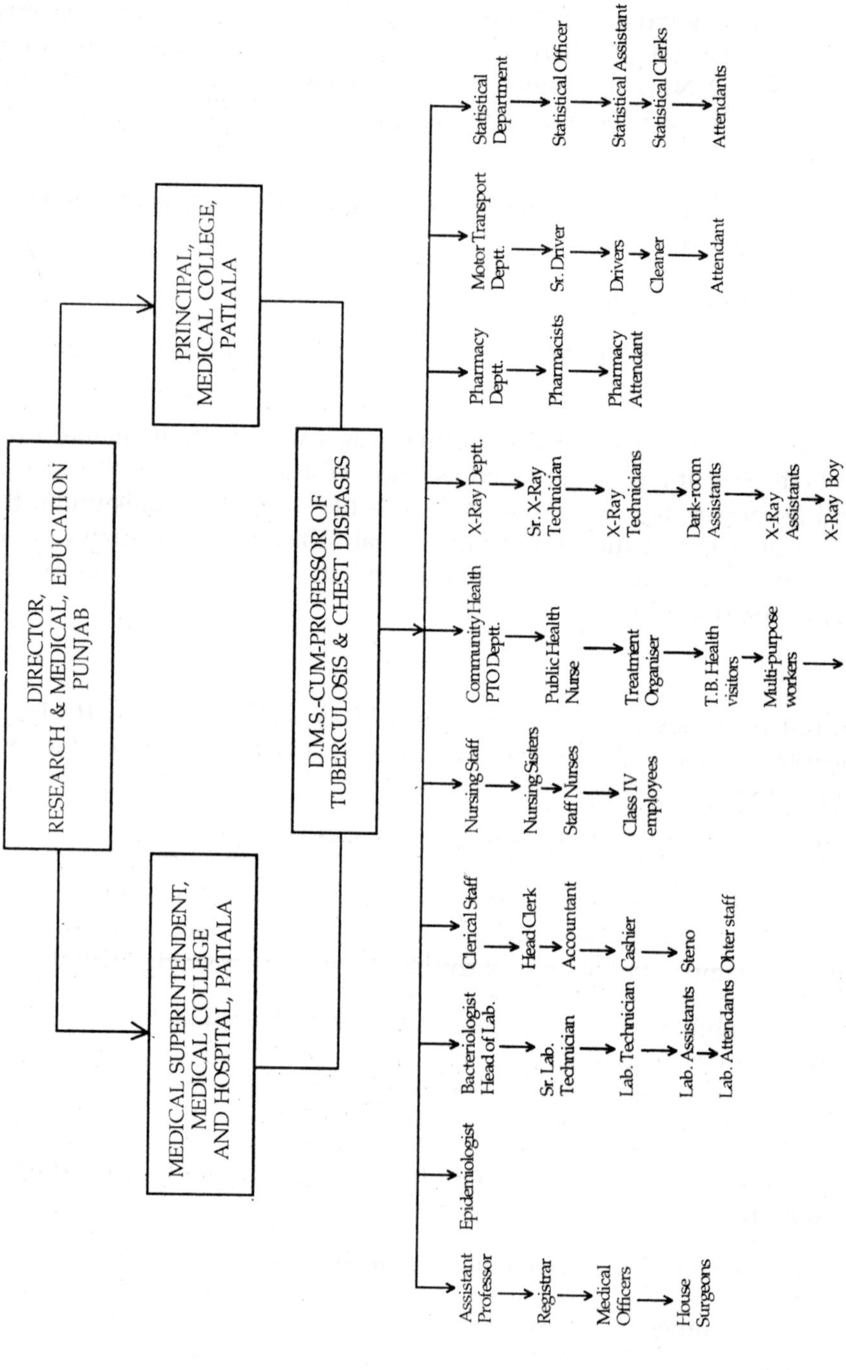

Fig. 2.5

(iv) *Punjab Mental Hospital at Amritsar (2.6)*

The Punjab Mental Hospital, Amritsar, was set up in 1949 with 50 beds. The present strength as 811 (512 male and 299 female). Treatment facilities are available at three levels in this hospital as given below:

(a) *The Indoors*: Certified patients are admitted at the indoors of this hospital from the states of Punjab, Haryana, Himachal Pradesh and the Union Territory of Chandigarh.

(b) *The Out-Patient Department*: Consultation facilities for the patients coming from Punjab, Haryana, Himachal Pradesh, Union Territory of Chandigarh and adjoining areas of Uttar Pradesh and Rajasthan are provided at the out-patient department.

(c) *The Family Care Unit*: This unit consisting of 70 ward-beds and 30 single-seat rooms provides intensive psychiatric treatment to the uncertified patients who need a short duration admission in the hospital. The unit is managed by a team consisting of 1 Medical Officer. 1 Clinical Psychologist and a Psychiatric Trained Nurse.

The hospital administration is looked after by the Medical Superintendent. The hospital staff consists of the following categories of employees.

Categories of Staff	*Sanctioned Posts*
Class I	6
Class II	8
Class III	83
Class IV	141
Warders	232

The hospital besides providing patient care, also serves as a training centre for medical and para-medical personnel in psychiatry, clinical psychology, psychiatric nursing and mental health. Besides, faculty carries out research on various aspects of mental health.

(v) *Working of a Hospital (Homoeopathic System of Medicine)*

Hospital in the traditionals system of medicine are simple as they do not require costly equipments to diagnose the ailments. Let us now describe the working of a teaching-cum-patient care homoeopathic institution located at Chandigarh.

It was set up in 1974 under private management. It has a faculty consisting of 13 staff members—I principal, 9 whole time lecturers and 3 part-time lecturers belonging to the western system of medicine. The intake capacity of the college is 50 students and the course is of 4 years duration.

The college serves as the hospital as well and provides both inpatient and out-patient services. The patient first of all is registered by the registration clerk who maintains the case history (backbone of the system) of the patients. After the registration, the patient is examined by the doctors/faculty members on duty. It takes about half an hour to record the case history of the patient. There is no referral system, since every doctor is competent to deal with all diseases as there is no classification of individual diseases, e.g., Cancer,

STRUCTURE OF PUNJAB MENTAL HOSPITAL AMRITSAR

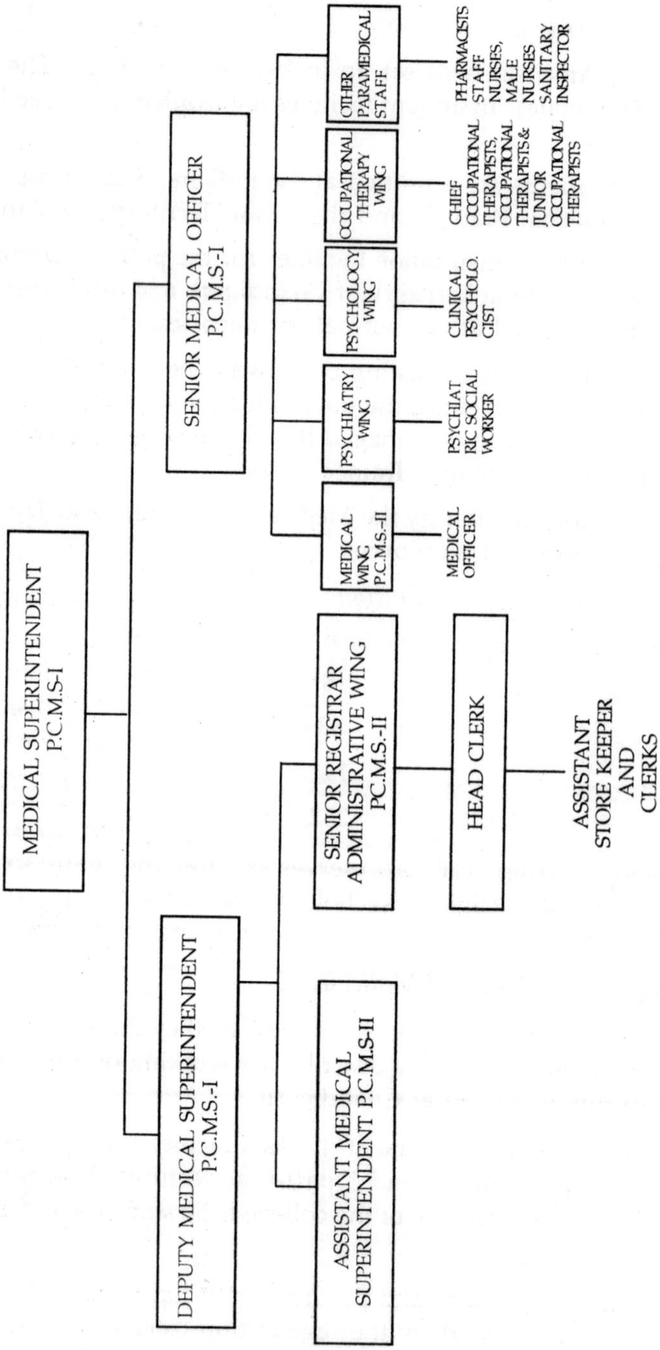

Fig. 2.6

Tuberculosis, etc. The chronic cases are admitted to provide indoor treatment. It has a simple laboratory structure and operation theatre. There is no para-medical staff.

The hospital is visited by about 35 to 80 new patients and 100 to 150 old patients per day. It has 25 beds located in three rooms. The patients are administered medicine through a dispensary. Besides, there is a pharmacy section for the formulation of medicine.

The cost of such a hospital is negligible compared to that of hospitals based on the western system of medicine. The setting up of such hospitals would lower the cost of medical care and would supplement the efforts of allopathic system of medicine.

(vi) *Working of an Ayurvedic Hospital/Dispensary*

The ayurvedic system of medicine is also very simple. After the registration, the patients are examined by the doctor on duty. The patients are treated on the philosophy of *vayu, pitta* and *kapha*. We discuss now the working of an ayurvedic dispensary located in Sector 37, Chandigarh, under the control of the government.

It has 2 doctors—one male and one female. Both are qualified. They have G.A.M.S./ B.A.M.S. degrees. The patients are first of all registered by the Registration clerk and, thereafter, examined by one of the two doctors. It takes about 3-5 minutes to examine the patient. The doctors are taking the help of the stethoscope, manometer, etc. After the examination the medicines are prescribed. The patient gets free available medicines from the dispensary while he has to buy the rest from the market. There is no surgery and referral system. About 60 to 90 new patients and 150 to 200 old patients visit the hospital daily.

The big ayurvedic hospitals have indoor facilities as well, e.g., the hospital at Patiala has 100 beds.

These hospitals are very easy to operate and involve negligible expenditure. The government should encourage such hospitals to reduce the rising cost of medical care.

D. Working of Hospitals

Hospitals are providing medical care only to those who approach them. Hospitals are not serving as the centres of total health care—preventive, curative, promotive and rehabilitative. Hospitals have poor linkages with the community and the family. They are providing expensive medical care and not comprehensive health care. The hospitals has been described by Dorothea Sick as a "Self chosen ghetto of the medical profession" and modern doctors as "Professional Cripples" useless without a hospital. Physicians in developing countries become estranged from their own people in the course of their training. The ablest men and women are not tackling the most acute and difficult problems.[5] Besides, the faith of the people in the efficiency of hospital system is decreasing because of the negligence and indifference on the part of hospital authorities. Lawrence J. Sakarai is very critical of the role of most of the doctors in a hospital. He feels, barring some dedicated doctors, most of them are ruthless and says:

> He (Doctor) exploits the gullible, conspires against the sick and cares little for medicine unless it makes him money...He could murder you through indifference, drugs or just sheer inefficiency all by masquerading under the garb of an ancient Oath rendered superfluous in the business of our times.[6]

Dr. R.V. Rajan, in his article 'Men, Medicine and Misadventure' in *The Tribune* (Nov. 25, 1979), rightly mentioned that,

"It is an unedifying fact, that we have no accurate recorded data on the occurrence and incidence of misadventures in drug administration, diagnostic procedures and surgical operation in hospitals...In a complex hospital, negligence becomes error, scientific detachment and incompetence becomes a lack of specialised equipments...Medicine is still not an exact science in spite of the great advances in bio-chemical sciences. It is imperative for doctors, nurses and para-medical personnel to exhibit utmost precaution, care, judgement and skill in dealing with and treating patients, balancing the relative risk of the disease with the risk involved in the use of drugs, surgery or diagnostic procedures, apart from the cost-benefit consideration."

What can be done to prevent the erosion of the values among the medical professions? What can we do to maintain the confidence of the people in the hospital services? How can we improve the functioning of the hospital system? How can we coordinate the functioning of hospitals? How can we check the rising costs of hospital services? These questions are being raised even in the context of the developed world.The 1968 report of the Secretary's Advisory Committee on hospital effectiveness, US Department of Health, Education and Welfare, Washington, D.C., emphasised the need to improve the internal efficiency of the hospital as a functioning mechanism to provide decent health care to all. We shall discuss in the following pages the answers to these questions. The analysis is based upon the already published documents especially the reports of the Parliamentary Committee and the personal discussion of the author with the health experts, general administrators and the beneficiaries of the hospital services.

Improving Patient-Satisfaction and Harmonious Relationship Between the Patients / Relatives and Hospital Authorities:

Hospitals should try to establish cordial, equitable and, therefore, mutually profitable relations between the hospitals and their beneficiaries. The patients mostly complain of discourteous behaviour of hospital staff especially at the lower level...This irritates the patients and their relatives. The test of the efficiency of a hospital is the satisfaction of the beneficiaries. The sympathetic and courteous behaviour of hospital staff would have a soothing and lasting effect on the patients and their relatives. It is suggested that all hospital personnel must inspire confidence and put the nervous patients and their relatives at ease.

> The hospital today is more than the combination of medical and therapeutic treatment by specialists, greater and refined medical and surgical knowledge and ever better and more effective facilities and equipment. It includes these factors as the core of its efficient operation but an additional dimension—one which is too often ignored or at least minimised—is the human and social element in the structure of the organisation.[7]

The ideal of service must be encouraged among the personnel responsible for health care. It is the responsibility of the hospital authorities to set the pattern for the philosophy of patient care. It was rightly mentioned by Gardern that.

> No society can reach heights of greatness unless in all fields critical to its growth and creativity there is an ample supply of dedicated men and women.[8]

Most of the patients complained of a great distance between the doctors and the patients. This gap between the doctors and the patients must be bridged through personal attention given by the doctors to the patients. According to K.G. Agarwal, "Hospital effectiveness which can be measured in terms of patient satisfaction does not depend on the improvement of hospital service aspect alone but on the medical care aspect. Hospital effectiveness has a positive association with the hospital social system. The hospital social system is almost the measure of its organisational health...some element of democracy must be introduced in the hospitals. This might take care of the alienation of hospital staff that we see all around these."[9] K.K.Kaul, Professor and Head, Smt. Patel Paediatric Centre, Government Medical College. Jabalpur (M.P.) has rightly said,

> To restore their reputation, hospitals need to develop a strong system of public relations and intimate involvement with the community they serve.[10]

Besides these, there are other areas which must be attended to by hospital authorities to build the image of the hospitals. The most irritating factor for the dissatisfaction of the patients is that they have to wait for a long time in the out-patient departments because of the poor planning and management of hospitals. Most of the studies conducted in this regard found the time to be excessive and intolerable, i.e., varying between 2 to 3 hours per patient. The Public Accounts Committee remarked that,

> Although certain delays are inherent in the situation and thus are inevitable, yet to a certain extent these can be overcome by rationalising the existing procedures and strengthening the organisations where necessary.

The patients also complain of the preferential treatment being given to VIPs and influential people. Some of the patients were of the view that these big hospitals are meant only to serve the VIPs. B.L. Agnihotri, in a letter to *The Tribune,* mentioned about the unsatisfactory conditions in hospitals in Himachal Pradesh. He mentioned that,

> After waiting for two hours we were told by some interns that senior doctors were not concerned about the general public and only attended to VIPs and persons with recommendations from the Secretariat. The majority of the doctors agree that conditions in these hospitals are bad but they feel helpless in the matter.[11]

The patients also complained of the lack of coordination between supportive services, and the medical services. Most of the patients complained of the non-availability either of their X-ray report or other laboratory reports. They go on wasting their time in tracing their reports. Besides, many patients complained that preferential treatment is given to friends, and relatives of the hospital staff. Many patients complained of the non-availability of medicines. Besides, patients are referred to other departments which results in great delays for the treatment to be given to them because of unsatisfactory coordination among the various departments of the hospital. In order to improve this relationship, the Public Accounts Committee suggested the following:

(1) To encourage polite and courteous behaviour of the staff towards the patients, orientation and in-serve training opportunities should be provided to the staff.

(2) Out-patients should be properly guided by the doctors issuing prescriptions regarding the procedure to be followed to get their blood, urine, stool, etc., samples tested.

(3) Laboratories may be modernised and out-dated equipment replaced as early as possible to improve the accuracy of the test results because these tests form the basis of the medical treatment which the patients are to be imparted.

Further, it is suggested on the basis of the observations by the author that the patients may be issued the slips on arrival on which may be indicated the probable time of his examination by the doctor.

The following steps could also be taken to improve matters.

(a) Effective coordination should be established between the medical services and the supportive services to ensure promptness and clarity.

(b) Effective coordination and cooperation must be ensured among the various departments of the hospital to help the patients in diagnosing their ailments. It is suggested that a medical board may meet once a week where all the specialities may be represented and the patients needing the attention of more than one speciality may be asked to attend the board.

(c) A receptionist well versed with the functioning of hospital system may be appointed to guide the patients to approach the hospital properly.

(d) There is a need of playcards and signboards to guide the patients and their relatives.

(e) Provision of cheap and quality goods to be used by the patients or their relatives.

(f) Arrangement of stay of the relatives in Dharamsalas specially constructed for the purpose.

(g) Hospital beds may be given to patients according to the severity of the disease rather than other trifle considerations like obliging the VIPs.

In brief, the functioning of the hospital should be organised and re-organised to serve the patients most efficiently. All the personnel engaged in patient care must keep the following definitions of the "patient" in their minds.[12]

The patient is the most important in the Hospital.

The patient is not dependent upon us—we are dependent on him.

The patient is not an interruption of our work—he is the purpose of it.

The patient is not an outsider to our business—he is our business.

The patient is a person and not a statistic. He has feelings, emotions, biases, and wants. It is our business to satisfy him.

The participation of people in the formulation and administration of local and national plans and programmes that affect their well-being is particularly important at a time when developing countries like India are rapidly widening the scope of public services and adopting technological advances for improving their administration. Both developments could make public administration increasingly complex and more difficult for the mass of citizens to understand. Imaginative measures are needed to promote and sustain the interest of citizens in the hospital administration to give them a sense of participation in the decisions of hospitals that immediately affect them and to enable them to contribute to better administration. Citizen participation in hospital administration is also an important safeguard against the abuse of administrative authority. It is a method for tapping human and material resources for development that might otherwise remain inert. It is a means for communicating to people the results of hospital action in fields that are of interest to them. To quote Pt Jawaharlal Nehru, "Administration not only has to be good but also to be felt to be good by the people."

Administration is manned by and meant for human beings. Administration does not exist for itself but for the citizens. Jawaharlal Nehru while delivering the inaugural address at the Indian Institute of Public Administration said, "Administration like most things is, in the final analysis, a human problem to deal with human beings, not with some statistical data...there is the danger that pure administrators at the top (not so much at the bottom, because they come into contact with human beings) may come to regard human beings as mere abstractions... the administrator may think in abstract of the people he deals with, come to conclusions which are justifiable apparently, but which miss human element. After all, whatever department of Government you deal with, it is ultimately a problem of human beings and the moment we forget them, we are driven away from reality."

Thus, Hospital Administration is not to exist in some kind of ivory tower. The true test of Hospital Administration is the welfare of the people visiting the hospitals. The Administrative Reforms Commission has also observed in this very connection that. "If, in the prosperity of the people, lies the strength of a Government, it is in their contentment that lie the security and stability of democracy." In the words of Sir Harold Scot : 'If a wide general knowledge is useful, even more valuable is a knowledge of people. It is very important that the young administrator should not retire into his cell when he leaves his office, but should mix with all kinds and conditions of people. From them, he will learn things that are not in his files.

It, therefore, follows that all the citizens have a right to participate in administration at all levels and they should in the interest of efficient functioning of administration in a democracy exercise this right.

It would be improper to describe this participation as hindrance nuisance, interference or obstacle to efficient administration. Citizen participation, on the other hand is an important part of the unfolding democratic process and not only should it be understood and welcomed but the sooner we all learn to use it, the better it would be for us all.

It the past, the beneficiaries of hospital services were passively receiving hospital services. In modern times, there is a trend wherein the beneficiaries and the community at large wish to participate in the programmes of delivery of hospital and related community services. The hospital authorities must be alive to this emerging change and develop their hospital service plans accordingly.

We must set up the Patient Complaint Enquiry Committee for all hospitals on the pattern of Patient Complaint Enquiry Committee set up in the Directorate-General of Health Services to look into the public complaints regarding the services in government and other hospitals in the Union Territory of Delhi.

Lack of Managerial Training on the Part of the Hospital Administrators

Hospital Administration is a science as well as an art. The hospital administration has become complex and requires administrative capability to solve its managerial problems to provide the optimum care to the patients. It is, therefore, necessary that the persons charged with the efficient running of the hospitals are trained in the managerial techniques and tools which may be applied by them for getting the best out of the resources available. A Diploma in Health and Hospital Administration was started by the PGI in collaboration with the Punjab University (Department of Public Administration). It continued for two years-1975-76 and 1976-77, and was discontinued later on. Similarly, refresher courses are arranged twice a year by the NIHFW. What has been the impact of this training ? Such a training could not make much impact as the trainers were acquainting them with the problems of management without their applicability in the Indian context. It is suggested that,

(a) All the Governments, Union and the States, must ensure that the top officers are appointed in the hospitals after giving them managerial training. What happens is that the persons on promotion become hospital administrators, without any management background.

(b) The trainers in the art of hospital administration must be given intensive training before they start imparting instruction. They should not bewilder the participants with glamorous managerial techniques applicable in advanced countries but should provide them with simple tools, useful and applicable in the Indian context.

(c) A model hospital run on the modern lines may be setup. The participants may be taken to this hospital to let them observe the application of techniques being taught to them.

(d) Training may be restricted only to those who are to shoulder this responsibility at present or in the immediate future.

(e) A regular follow-up of the training programme must be taken up to ensure the utility of training.

The hospital administrators should not be taught merely the art and science of managing formal organisation which would add to the efficiency of hospitals. Rensis Likert, in his article "Motivational Approach to Management Development in *Harvard Business Review* (pp. 37-77, July-August 1959) has mentioned a number of such principles which when taught intensively to the administrators would add to the performance of an organisation. These factors are as follows:

(i) Extent of loyalty to the institution and identification with it and its objectives.

(ii) Extent to which the goals of units and individuals facilitate the achievement of the organisation's objectives.

(iii) Level of motivation among members of the organisation with regard to such variables as:

  (a) Performance including both quality and quantity of work done.

  (b) Concern for elimination of waste and reduction of costs.

  (c) Concern for improving the product.

  (d) Concern for improving processes.

(iv) Degree of confidence and trust among members of the organisation in each other and in the different hierarchical levels.

(v) Amount and quality of the teamwork in units and between units of the organisation.

(vi) Extent to which people feel that delegation is effective.

(vii) Extent to which the members feel that their ideas, information, knowledge of processes, and experiences are being used in the decision-making processes of the organisation.

(viii) Upward, downward, and sideward efficiency and adequacy of the communication process.

(ix) Leadership skills and abilities of supervisors and managers, including their basic philosophies of management and orientation towards leadership processes.

(x) Hospital Services Consultancy Corporation: We may mention here the recent development in India to improve hospital efficiency. The government have set up a company in the public sector under the Ministry of Health and Family Welfare, called "Hospital Services Consultancy Corporation (India) Limited" with an equity investment of Rs. 50 lakhs to provide comprehensive consultancy services both within the country and in developing countries on all aspects of establishment and management of hospital facilities. It is to provide the following services:

  (i) carry out analysis of the requests for hospital services, conduct feasibility studies and prepare initial project reports.

  (ii) undertake preparation of architectural designs for hospitals.

  (iii) undertake hospital construction on turn-key basis.

  (iv) undertake supply of equipments needed for running the hospital services.

  (v) prepare and supply medical as well as para-medical manpower needed for the management of such hospitals.

(vi) undertake administration of the hospital for a period of time on contractual basis.

(vii) provide consultancy services in building up low cost primary health services, family planning services, etc., in developing countries.

Hospitals should make use of this Corporation to improve efficiency.

Medical Audit not a regular Feature in most of the Hospitals

The purpose of Medical Audit is to evaluate impinging on patient care. All the deaths in a hospital where cause of death are not certain are investigated by the Mortality Review Committee. This improved the knowledge of the medical personnel and enchances their capability of handling such cases in future. The Health Survey and Planning Committee (1959-61) recommended the use of medical audit in all hospitals. The Delhi Hospital Review Committee headed any Dr. K.N. Rao (1968) also recommended the appointment of a Medical Audit Committee in each hospital. Such committee will ensure specific checks on the quality of work performed in the hospitals. We have found the following drawbacks in some of the hospitals where such committees are functioning:

(1) Poor recording of a case history.

(2) Sketchy documentation.

(3) Operation notes not properly recorded.

(4) Lack of inter-departmental coordination.

(5) Incomplete case-notes.

(6) Not proper follow-up by the senior faculty members.

Either mortality committees have not been setup in hospitals or function irregularly. The Public Accounts Committee also mentioned that,

> "Although the recommendations of the review committee to carry out hospital mortality review periodically was accepted by the Government in February 1970, it was only after a lapse of six years (May 1976) that the mortality review committee started functioning in Willingdon Hospital (Rammanohar Lohia Hospital)."

The conditions are worse in hospitals under the control of State Governments in this regard. Thus there is a need to setup such committees to ensure efficient and effective medical audit.

Unsatisfactory System of Drugs and Medical Supplies

The efficiency of hospital services depends not only on the competence of medical personnel but also on the availability of drugs in right quantity and quality. We are witnessing a number of problems in regard to the drugs management in hospitals. Some of the important problems are:[13]

(a) Pilferage of drugs.

(b) Purchase of drugs at higher prices from the open market because of lack of advance planning.

(c) Use of adulterated drugs.

(d) Shortage of essential drugs.

(e) Corruption among the authorities in a hospital.

(f) Qualified persons not responsible for drug management.

(g) Absence of regular inspections to check the drug stores.

(h) Use of expired drugs.

The Committee on pilferage of drugs observed,

> "Some government hospital authorities were in league with drug suppliers. By manipulating records and accounts, hospital stores returned part of their stocks to suppliers for a financial consideration, or sold them to chemists at rock bottom prices. Often drugs obtained under the Central Government Health Scheme or the Employees States Insurance Scheme were found to be falsely indented and sold to chemists."[14]

The Public Accounts Committee in its (1977-78) report was very critical of the drug management in three Central Government hospitals in Delhi. The Committee remarked:

> "Certain medicines consumed by patients in the hospitals were sub-standard. . . There have been periodical reports of shortage of certain medicines and it appears that no effective machinery exists to take notice of such shortage in time for remedial action in a coordinated manner."[15]

We give here some suggestions to remove these defects:

(a) Different colours and designs of medicines may be specially manufactured for the distribution through hospitals like the service stamps used in the Government offices.

(b) The machinery to ensure, quality drugs in the States needs to be strengthened.

(c) Advance planning of the requirements of the drugs should be done to ensure regular supply.

(d) Cheap drugs may be manufactured by the Government and all multi-national drug companies may be either wound up or asked to manufacture cheap drugs.

(e) The working of medical depots under the Ministry of Health and Family Welfare needs to be streamlined so that the hospitals may not get the opportunity to purchase drugs from the open market.

(f) *Adhoc* purchases may not be encouraged except under serious circumstances.

(g) The hospital authorities should ensure that only genuine and fully tested medicines are provided to the patients. Time-barred medicines may not be used. Timely action may be taken to ensure that medicines may not become time-barred through the exchange of such medicines from the firms.

(h) Drug stores should be under the control of qualified pharmacists and not semi-skilled compounders.

Less Emphasis on Human side of Medicine

Many people visiting the hospitals constantly turn to doctors without showing any sign of physical disorder. Most of the doctors do not bother to diagnose their problems and administer them sleep inducing drugs which are ultimately harmful. Tranquillizers and barbiturates are being dispensed on a large scale. "It is because medicine has become so accustomed to searching for technical answers to its dilemmas that quests for answers on the behavioural side continue to be deferred."

What can be done to make the doctors understand all this ? The situation can be improved by providing courses in anthropology, sociology, and psychology to the doctors. According to Maureen A. Bailey,

> "In the face of a virtual epidemic of behavioural disorders, modern health care must place a new emphasis on solving the human side of medicine."[16]

Absence of Cost Consciousness among Hospital Authorities and Staff

The budgets of hospitals are increasing beyond proportions over the years which is beyond the capacity of poor countries like India. The whole of the health budget is spent in maintaining few hospitals neglecting the vast population needing health and medical care. According to H.A. Goddard,

> "In the management or administration of any enterprise, the quality, quantity, timing, and cost of the work necessary to reach the objectives of the enterprise are inter-related factors which must be given constant attention. If the resources for health work, in trained persons and in finances, were unlimited the need for constant attention to these factors would not be so great. But the limitation in the number of trained personnel and the lack of adequate financial resources are major obstacles to greatly improved health in the world today. We must, therefore, husband our resources carefully to accomplish as much as possible with what we have available."[17]

A serious problem in health care administration is the absence of cost-consciousness among the staff of public health administrations. All over the world, health service staff—even of the highest professional cadre—are taught little about the economics of health services and know little about the costs of the equipment and supplies they use. Doctors tend to employ what is new without regard to cost. It is a fashion to prescribe costly drugs. They are also subjected to considerable sales pressure from manufacturing firms. A cheaper drug or cheaper equipment may give just as good a result for the vast majority of patients. Cost consciousness is not just a matter for central administrators or planners but should be inculcated in all those working in health care. More people can be provided with services if no services cost more than what is a must to provide the necessary level of care. The price paid for high-cost technology for a few is no technology at all for the many.

Another aspect of this problem is the use of hospital non-judiciously. In the more developed countries, the majority of secondary care is generally given in hospitals, and increasingly the hospitals in which it is provided tend to be large, i.e., 500 beds or more. The larger hospital offers the opportunity for a high degree or specialisation and for achieving the fullest use of expensive specialised equipment. The larger the hospital and the more specialised its work, the larger catchment area it needs to serve. The higher average transport costs for staff and patients may be justified by the quality of service that a large hospital should be able to provide.

In the developing countries like India where the bulk of the population live in rural areas with limited public or private facilities for long distance travel, such transport is costly, except for the few patients who can be transported to hospital in vehicles travelling for other purposes. Moreover, in-patient care must be provided much more selectively if it is not to absorb an excessive share of the health budget. It must be confined to those with a high probability of deriving clear and lasting benefit from it. The emphasis should be on ambulatory services.

For these reasons, hospitals should on average be smaller in developing countries than in more developed countries and they should not be used to provide the most sophisticated technology. Costs can be saved if limited number of relatives accompany the patient and take responsibility for preparing food and providing basic patient care. But many developing countries have followed the example of more developed countries and concentrated on a high proportion of their health service expenditure on large urban hospitals, many of them teaching hospitals, equipped to provide tertiary care with high technology. These hospitals have been set up before smaller district hospitals have been developed and as transport is not normally developed they tend to be used to provide secondary care to the urban population. Moreover, they are mainly used for patients who do not need their special facilities, e.g., the chronically disabled, children suffering from malnutrition, and patients with minor illness who could be treated in a much simpler hospital or at home. In some countries, the out-patient department of a regional hospital is even used to provide primary care as there is no referral system and time of super-specialists is wasted on minor problems which could be dealt elsewhere. It is suggested that the referral system must be made statutory to screen the patients.

Absence of Proper Space Planning

A large number of hospitals in the country have come to be established and housed in buildings which were not originally designed for the present needs and technology. The new hospitals have also to undergo changes as new facilities are provided to the community. The planning of hospital facilities in such a changing situation within the constraints of the existing space availability is one of the biggest problems that any hospital faces.

> "Moreover, hospital development is often designed in an *ad hoc* way or based on `type plans', with the result defects are repeated in new hospital construction and remains unremedied in the existing ones."[18]

There is also lack of coordination between the hospital authorities and transport authorities resulting in the poor transport facilities available to the patients. The buildings and equipment are not maintained properly. It is suggested that:

(a) Hospital Engineering section must be setup in all big hospitals to take care of the building and equipment.

(b) Hospitals may be located at places wherefrom transport facilities are easily available so that the patients can reach back home the same day.

(c) Proper maintenance of hospital equipment should be ensured otherwise these would tell upon the efficiency of the hospitals.

(d) Hospital planning and administration should receive greater attention.

(e) Operational studies on such aspects as the utilisation of hospitals, over-crowding and referral system would help to define requirements realistically and bring improvements and economy in hospital design.

Poor Management of Dietary Services

The dietary unit stands as the second major department of a hospital from the point of view of expenditure. It needs careful analysis and control. Most of the patients always complain of poor and costly diets served in the hospitals. There is a problem of excess diets issued as compared to the number of patients resulting in huge expenditure. Besides, many of the patients do not consume all that is served to them. Patients generally prefer food from their houses as they do not like hospital food. The Public Accounts Committee (1977-78) has mentioned in this connection:

> "The Committee are constrained to note that whereas economy on expenditure on diet is being thought of by reducing quantum of diet, other measures to effect economy without diminishing the quality and quantity of diet such as plugging leakages of diet, have not been given the attention they deserve. In the opinion of the committee the leakage of diets may be possibly one of the reasons for issue of excess diets over the census figure. Therefore, it is necessary that institutional arrangements are made to watch that leakages of diet and dietary materials do not take place."

It is suggested that the efficient management of dietary services may be done to achieve economy and quality. The hospital authorities must compare the cost of dietary services with other hospital dietary services and thus try to locate the defects and remedy them.

Non-Availability and Non-Judicious Utilisation of Blood

There is a lot of resentment among the patients and their relatives regarding the availability of blood required for certain ailments. Most of the patients complain about the prevalence of corruption in the supply of blood to patients. Besides, it is mentioned that only high ups in the Government can get the required supply of blood while the poor people are denied this right. It is suggested that the supply of blood must be made according to the needs of the patients rather than on the basis of their status. This would motivate the general public to donate blood for saving the lives of the people—a noble cause. The present author was entrusted with the task of arranging a camp to donate blood. The people when approached were very critical about the use of blood taken from voluntary workers. This feeling prevents most of the potential donors of blood to contribute to this noble cause. It is necessary to manage the blood banks in the hospitals judiciously to inspire confidence among the people in general-donors as well as consumers of the service.

Absence of Effective Personnel and Materials Planning

In most of the hospitals, there is no personnel planning, resulting in the under-utilisation of resources. Expenditure on personnel is mounting high and care must be taken to ensure optimum utilisation of resources. After the personnel, materials constitute about 50 per cent of the total expenditure of an organisation. Optimum utilisation of these resources must be ensured to achieve high productivity. There have been many cases where articles lying in bulk quantities in one department were purchased by the other and sometimes in emergency at exorbitant prices. The situation can be improved by designing a proper system of purchase, storage and utilisation. The hospital authorities must ensure whether the existing staff in the various departments has been deployed consistent with the work-load and are accordingly to prescribed norms. Besides, they are to ensure economy by avoiding wastage, duplication through inventory control. A study may be carried out in every hospital after three years in the following areas to ensure optimum utilisation:

1. Corporate Planning.
2. Manpower Utilisation.
3. Materials Management Drugs Control.
4. Management Information System.
5. Organisational Planning and Development.

Thus, periodic studies of the functioning of hospitals are needed to enable the administrators to manage them efficiently.

Absence of Planned Regionalisation to ensure Graded Patient Care

At present, all hospitals whether at the state, district or local levels are working in isolation and their services are not provided in a coordinated manner. Most of the patients visit all these hospitals and are examined afresh by all of them resulting in wastage of efforts and resources. The medical staff prescribe medicines to patients without having a proper awareness of his previous treatment.

Recently Mrs Indira Gandhi, Prime Minister of India, while presiding over a function at Lady Hardinge Medical College at Delhi, rightly mentioned (quoted by Dr P.N. Chhuttani, Ex-Director, PGI, in his article "Decentralisation Needed" published in *Medical View Point* column of *The Tribune*, dated 4-5-1980) that "The referral system has entirely failed in almost all our larger towns and cities. Consequently, there is growing overcrowding at our major hospitals whose services stand diluted. In the larger cities there is the multiplicity of the controlling authorities—The Government, the Municipal Corporation, the Municipal Committee, Voluntary Organisations. Private Hospitals etc." She further stated that "there is no common meeting ground and hospital services have become almost totally unregulated. Consequently, the conditions in our capital city are chaotic. The poor and the needy flock towards the larger, better known hospitals in the hope of better treatment and care only to find that they have to wait for days to be examined, much less to find a place to stay. Patients wander from hospital to hospital. Besides facing considerable inconvenience, their efforts to seek relief cause duplication of work and expenditure. It is thus necessary that every big city must have an apex body, perhaps called the hospital board, to establish referral hospitals for every zone."

REFERRAL SYSTEM

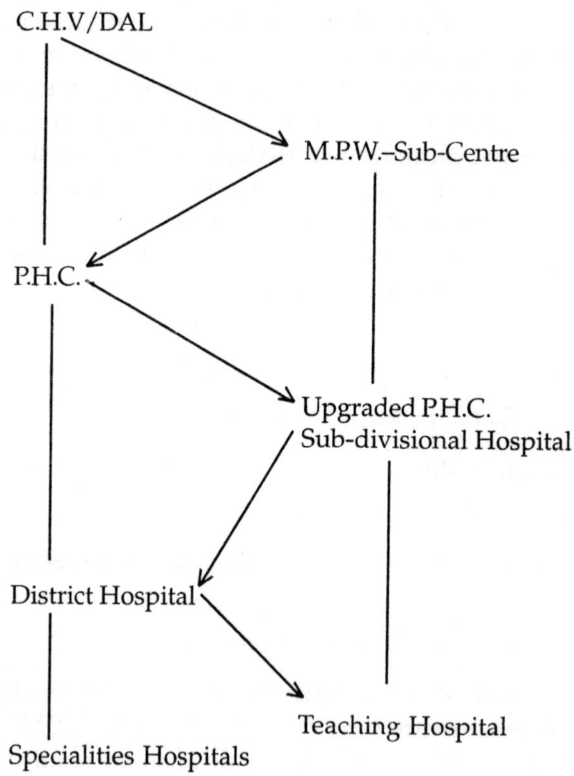

Fig.: 2

How can we get out of this chaos to design a system of patient Care ? The answer is— introduction of Regionalisation. Regionalisation connotes the development of graded patient care within a defined geographical or functional area from lower to higher levels adapting the health services to the characteristics and needs of the area and, thus, ensure the optimum utilisation of resources. The essential characteristics of regionalisation are:[19]

(a) Two-way flow of patients
(b) Two-way flow of records
(c) Two-way flow of services
(d) Two-way flow of personnel
(e) Mobile units
(f) Centralised administration and decentralised execution
(g) Coordinating education programme for the region
(h) Communication and transport between components
(i) Coordination with other community health services.

Thus regionalisation would ensure the best utilisation of time of the specialists and provision of comprehensive health care to the patients nearer their homes with all the benefits of specialities. The regional area should neither be too large nor too small but should be such as to ensure adequate span of attention. It would also automatically develop referral system scientifically.

The referral system presents the following five aspects:[20]

(a) It has to be built into the organisational structure of the medical services of a country. The rule should be that only when one unit cannot provide what a patient needs should the patient be referred to the next higher unit in the chain.

(b) The referral system has to be organised both internally and externally. 'Internally' means that patients in the hospital have to be referred from the in-patients to the out-patients department just as soon as their health situation permits. The 'externally' referred system exists among the several institutions on different levels of the hierarchy.

(c) The referral system, must be established for the purpose of diagnosis and treatment and used for both in-patients and out-patients.

(d) It is a two-way system. Patients should be referred to higher level institutions for diagnosis and treatment when necessary, but they should also be referred back to the referring institution as soon as possible.

(e) The referral system concerns not only patients and diagnostic facilities but also the personnel of the medical services. This is also a two-way system, so that human knowledge and skills are utilised fully and are continually developed through consultations and the interchange of ideas and experience.

The specialists from the regional hospital must come to the District hospital and the specialist from the District hospital to the health centre on a regular basis as consultants, to hold specialist clinics and give guidance; the medical and para-medical personnel should go to the higher level institution regularly for in-service training.

Absence of any Legislation for the Organisation and Functioning of Hospitals

At present there is no comprehensive legislation to guide the organisation and management of hospitals. There is need of a hospital legislation to ensure maintenance of standards, to define rights and duties of the hospital staff and to ensure the efficient functioning of hospitals. It is suggested that the Government of India may set up a body Development Council for Hospitals with its branches in the States like the Medical Council of India, to lay down policies to ensure that the hospitals have requisite facilities and provide efficient services to the patients. It has become a common practice to set up nursing homes in the private sector. These so-called 'nursing homes' are often huge money-making projects devised by the specialists in league with one another. All these nursing homes must be under the control of the proposed council. It should be the duty of the council to see that the specialities like the private industry do not fleece the people and provide medical care of right quality and at a reasonable price. Besides,the proposed council may attend to the complaints of the patients to ensure smooth relations between the hospital authorities and

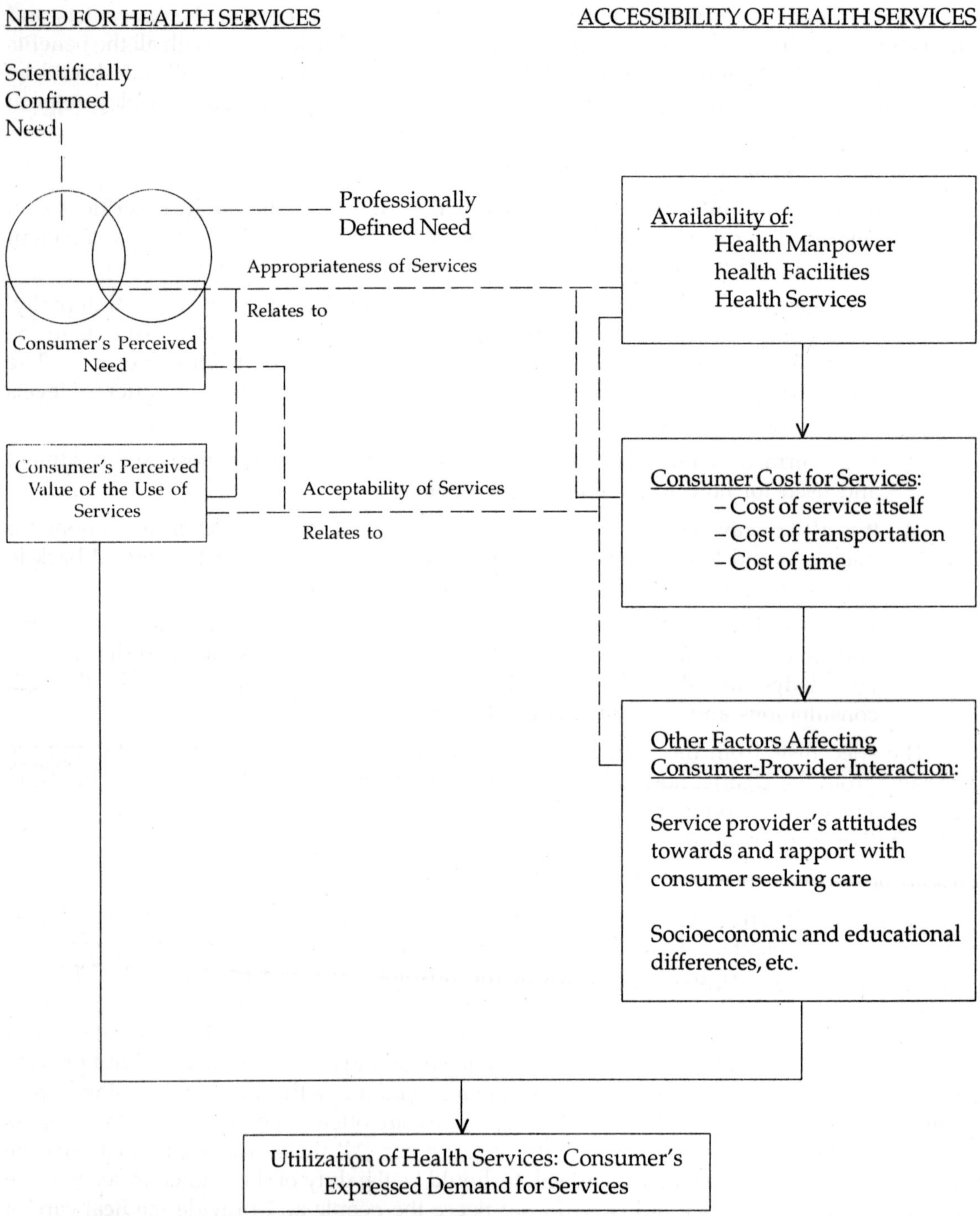

the beneficiaries and thus help in the building of a Welfare State, a cherished ideal in the constitutions of most of the states in the world.

We must attend to all these problems to ensure efficiency of the hospitals. These problems also emanate from a number of constraints on hospital authorities, e.g., shortage of staff at all levels, absence of proper accommodation to provide space to the ever increasing number of patients, shortages of funds, shortages of medicine, shortage of equipment, political and administrative inference, etc., which need to be attended to by the governments at the Union and State level to provide satisfactory hospital services. Besides, the patients and their relatives must cooperate with the hospital authorities to make the best use of the available resources. Thus, we shall have to have a three-pronged attack-increasing internal efficiency, mobilising government support and enlisting people's cooperation to ensure the reputation, prestige, credibility and viability of the hospital services.

References

1. WHO, *Technical Report Series*, 1968, 395, p. 6.
2. WHO, *Technical Report Series*, 1957, 122, p. 4.
3. Pubjab Govt. Memo. No. 11875-4 BI-66/30459 dated 25.10.1977 (from the Secretary to Govt., Punjab, Medical and Health Department to the Director Health Services, Punjab).
4. Tiny M. Calender, *Unit Administration*, W.B. Saunders Co., London, 1962, p. 66.
5. V. Ramalingaswami, "Medicine Health and Human Development" in *Health and Basic Services; Key to Development by UNICEF*, New Delhi, p. 10.
6. Lawrence J. Sakarai, "The Hippocratic Oath; License to Kill" in *Sunday Standard*, Chandigarh, 12, August 1979 (Sunday Magazine, p. 1).
7. Mary D. Shanks and Dorothy A. Kennedy, *The Theory and Practice of Nursing Service Administration*, McGraw-Hill, London, 1965, p. 95.
8. John W. Gardner, *Excellence*, New York, 1961, Harper and Brothers, p. 154.
9. K.G. Agarwal, "Managing Patient Satisfaction in Hospitals" in the *Indian Journal of Public Administration*, Vol. XXII, No. 2. April-June, 1976), p. 277.
10. K.K. Kaul, "Hospitalisation of Children" *Health and Population Perspective and Issues* 2(1); 49-53, 1979.
11. *The Tribune*, Chandigarh, November 1, 1979.
12. Edythe Alexander *et al.*, *Nursing Service Administration* (ed.), New York C.V. Mosby Co., 1962, p. 63.
13. Based upon personal discussion with hospital staff at Chandigarh.
14. *Indian Journal of Hospital Pharmacy*, Vol. VII, No. 3-4/70.
15. Lok Sabha Secretariat, Public Accounts Committee, *Forty-ninth Report*, Sixth Lok Sabha, December, 1977, p. 142.
16. Maureen A. Bailey, "The Human Side" in *World Health*, December, 1975, p. 4.
17. H.A. Goddard, *Principles of Administration applied to Nursing Service*, World Health Organisation, Geneva, 1958, p. 84.
18. WHO, SEA/RC/21/2, p. VIII.
19. Timmappaya *Regionalisation of Health Care* (Mimeographed).
20. WHO, SEARO; SEA/RC 23/1, pp. 39-40.

3

Administration, Finance and Implementation

In this Chapter, we shall discuss some of the issues relating to the creation of the alternative model of health care services which have not been discussed earlier.

Administration

Redefinition of Roles at the Central, State and Local Levels

In the existing health services, the pyramid of power is inverted, most of the power is vested at the top while the people become the dependent and neglected 'periphery'. The alternative model of health care services is based on an opposite assumption. The people are not the periphery but the nation; they should be, not dependent, but self-reliant; they should have the authority to decide the health care services they need and also to provide them; and the health needs of the people should not be neglected and, in fact, the larger part of the health care expenditure should be incurred in the community. Quite obviously, this radical change has far-reaching implications for the administration. Among these, mention has been made of the need for a total redefinition of the roles, responsibilities and functions of the health services at the Central, State and local (district and below) levels. In so far as the roles, responsibilities and functions of the health care services at the village, sub-centre, community and district levels are concerned, these have already been discussed in detail in Chapter VII and need not be repeated here. Some explanation is, however, needed regarding the consequential changes at the national and State levels.

At the national level, the continuing concern will be with the overall planning of health services and the integration of these plans with those of overall development. It is the responsibility of the Government of India to provide stimulating leadership and the bulk of the financial support. The proposed Medical and Health Education Commission will be an important instrument for this purpose. The Centre will also ensure that the less advanced States are properly guided and assisted and that a minimum of health care services becomes available to the citizens, and especially to the poor and underprivileged groups, in all parts of the country. The Centre will also have large responsibilities for research, for coordination and maintenance of standards in teaching institutions, for control of communicable diseases, for the maintenance of national institutions of excellence, for the proper development of an information system and for periodical evaluation. The central health administration will have to be reorganised to carry out these responsibilities effectively.

At the State level, the main change will be that the State Governments will be relieved of the taxing responsibility of providing day-to-day health services to the community. This is an immense advantage because they will now have adequate time to deal with the more important and broader questions of policy which can be dealt with at the state level alone and which tended to be neglected in the past. The concentration will now be on planning; ensuring equity of development in different districts; constant vigilance to see that the poor and the deprived do get adequate access to the health services and that the vested interests in the community which prevent this are curbed; management of state health cadres and state-level health institutions; providing guidance and expertise to local bodies or district-level authorities and to the community-based health services; adequate provision of financial support; and periodical evaluation.

Following this change in the role and responsibilities of the State Governments, the character of the state-level administration of health services will also undergo a radical change. Their main responsibility now will be to assist the State Governments to discharge their onerous responsibilities in planning and financing of the health care services and in their evaluation and supervision. They will no longer be responsible for the day-to-day administration of health care and their main responsibility in this regard will be to provide technical guidance to the health services at the local levels. They will also have to deal with democratic bodies at these levels. The changes offer more exciting and more challenging opportunities to serve the people than the earlier centralized and bureaucratic set up. We hope that the state level health services will welcome these changes and rise to the immense new challenges they imply.

Voluntary Agencies

Voluntary agencies have a long tradition of providing valuable health services and are doing pioneer work in the health field; and as the philanthropic tradition is deeply rooted in the culture of the people, voluntary effort will always continue to be a valuable asset to society. We, therefore, recommend that the State should preserve and promote this tradition through appropriate policies in view, not of its size, but of its quality and significance. Voluntary agencies should, however, be required to work within the overall plans and policies of Government; and special assistance should be available to those agencies which are fighting at the frontiers and doing pioneer work of significance.

Readjustment Within the Health Services

The alternative model of health services will need a redefinition, not only in the roles of Centre, State and local governments, but also of the roles, responsibilities and functions of the different cadres of health services and their mutual relationships. For instance, the health services will have to deal with the very large army of Community Health Volunteers (about two million) and about ten times that number of voluntary health leaders, who will be trained to participate in and assist the development of promotive and preventive health care services at the local level. The vast problems of their training, organisation and guidance will present unprecedented and stimulating challenges to the regular health services. Similarly, there will be a tremendous increase in the middle-level personnel of all categories; a massive improvement in the production and status of nurses is critical; a new and large integrated cadre of male and female Multipurpose Workers is emerging; and the roles and numbers of other paramedical personnel will also undergo radical changes. In fact, the ratio between the middle-level personnel and the top leadership which is now almost 1:1 may increase to 10:1 or so. At the top level, the doctors, specialists and superspecialists will still have a very important role. But they will not dominate the situation totally as they did in the past, and will have to share the leadership with other health functionaries at this level. The new policy has also created a great shortage of functionaries in several fields which were neglected in the past (e.g. epidemiologists, public health engineers and other public health specialists) and these will have to be made up very soon. It will thus be seen that the transition to the new model will pose three main challenges. Firstly, it throws the entire policy regarding manpower and training into flux and necessitates a continuous review of the changing position and prompt action. This should be a major responsibility of the Medical and Health Education Commission we have recommended elsewhere. Secondly, it poses vast problems of recruitment and training which will have to be dealt with carefully and competently. Our recommendations on the subject have been given earlier in Chapters VII and X. Finally, the emerging tensions between the different cadres will have to be resolved and their mutual relations placed on a proper footing to enable them to function as a team. This is essentially a task of leadership and will be the main responsibility at the State level. We also trust that the services themselves will see the challenges and opportunities involved and adjust themselves to the new roles expected of them and function as a well-knit, homogenous and efficient team.

There are three aspects of the existing system of health care which will become far more significant in the alternative model, and especially because our total investments in health care will increase substantially. viz, referral services, information system and coordination. These deserve special attention.

Referral Services

The organisation of referral services will have to be streamlined and strengthened in the alternative model much more than at present. To begin with, the rural people in general and the poor and deprived social groups everywhere will have to be convinced, through personal or readily 'visible'concrete evidence, that they have a much better and more equitable access to the referral services in the alternative model than in the existing system. This will give them greater confidence in the new system and enhance its credibility. At present, many people by-pass the peripheral services and make direct approaches to the hospital which is thus converted into a sophisticated Primary Health Centre for the people in the neighbourhood. This trend should be discouraged and as has been stated earlier, a sub-centre meant for the people in the neighbourhood, should be attached to each large hospital. When this step will begin to yield results, the large hospitals can be better and more enonomically utilized for the more difficult referral cases for which they are essentially designed. The overall quality of the health services will also improve because hospitals will then begin to perform their proper function, viz. to support community-based comprehensive care. In the present pattern, hospitals are the central focus of health activity and primary care services serve mainly to provide them with patients. The alternative model will help us to get away from this unhappy situation.

Information System

The main problems in the existing information system are: (i) there are so many useless forms and reports clogging the system that relevant information hardly reaches the point where it can be meaningfully used: (ii) the time lags in data collection and analysis are very large; and (iii) the relationship between the data collected and policy formulation, implementation and evaluation is very tenuous. All this will have to be changed. A selective process of abolishing most of the present forms and reports is the obvious way to start. No part of datagathering should be retained or included unless there is clear evidence that it helps to improve the services. A streamlined national information system should then be set up and the local community should be involved in data collection. The data should be simple, reliable and honestly filled out. They should be collated and analysed for all the five levels of administration (village or sub-centre, community, district, State and nation) in formats appropriate for evaluation, policy formulation and action at each level. Such feedback at lower levels will cease to be statistics; they get readily converted into people whom one knows and the delivery of health services becomes more prompt and effective. At higher levels, the data activate the "information-evaluation-better planning (or action)" loop and result in improved services or greater economies.

Coordination

Health is not a responsibility of the Health Ministry (or Departments) alone; it is a total societal responsibility of the Government and the people. Moreover, the action for health is more often needed in the non-health sectors (e.g. nutrition or improvement of sanitation). Coordination of the health-supportive activities of all concerned official and non-official agencies is thus a very important need as well as instrument of raising health status. The Ministry of Health (or the State Health Departments) have not been known for their political weight or administrative stature and have not been able to discharge their responsibilities for coordination adequately in the past. In view of the great significance of health for human and national development, however, it is essential to make adequate arrangements for this coordinating role at all the important levels-national, State, district and community. No one method can or need be prescribed and each State can devise its own appropriate procedures for the purpose.

Finance

It is a pity that problems of the economics of health and financing of health care services have received little attention in this country. Very little meaningful data is available on the subject. There is hardly any analysis of issues like the different sources and objectives of the total expenditure on health, costeffectiveness of different programmes, efficiency and waste in the system, and so on. A fairly large-scale and intensive programme of research on the subject needs to be developed on a priority basis. Perhaps, it would be desirable to set up special units for the study of this problem in two or three strong centres of economics research.

The main features of the existing situation regarding the financing of health services in India may be briefly stated. Social services, as a rule, receive stepmotherly treatment in our system. Even among them, health has a far lower priority and the total public expenditure on health services of all types is even less than half that on education. The present total expenditure on health (private and public) is about two per cent of the GNP only. Within health, the large bulk of our expenditure is incurred on curative services, or within urban areas, and the largest beneficiaries of it are the top 20 or 30 per cent of society. The waste and inefficiency of the system is colossal and almost criminal in a poor country so directly in need of good health services. The alternative model moves in the opposite direction and tries to alter this sad state of affairs radically. It assumes that the priority given to health in our system would be very high—equal to that of education—and that each of these social services should ultimately get about 6 per cent of the GNP. This will mean that the total expenditure on health will rise be A.D. 2000 to about six times that at present (at constant prices) on the assumption that the GNP per head would also be doubled by then. The bulk of this expenditure would be in the public sector and on promotive and preventive aspects, in rural areas or within the community, and its benefits will go directly to the people, and particularly to the poor and underprivileged. It also proposes to make the system more economic and efficient. It is therefore obvious that the financial basis of the health care services will have to be radically restructured to suit the needs of the alternative model. The main changes needed will include:

- a substantial increase in the total public expenditure on health at about 8 or 9 per cent per year (at constant prices) over the next 20 years;
- investment of the vast bulk of available additional funds in promotive and preventive aspects and holding down the expenditure on curative aspects to the genuine real needs so that, over time, the bulk of the health expenditure is devoted to promotive and preventive aspects;
- increasing the expenditure on health services within the community very substantially and keeping down that on urban hospitals and specialities and superspecialities, so that, over time, the people who now occupy a peripheral position, will get the bulk of the expenditure on health care services;
- increasing the expenditure in rural areas and in programmes whose benefits go directly to the poor and underprivileged groups; and
- improving the efficiency of the system by moving away from the existing borrowed model and creating another model more suited to the life and needs of the people, by vesting control in the beneficiaries of the system, and by continuous monitoring and evaluation.

When any radical changes of these types are to be brought about, both positive and negative decisions are needed. It is the general experience, particularly in 'soft' politics, that the positive decisions are more readily taken because they express a desire to do something good and have no connotation of harming any vested interests. If somebody is going to benefit without harming any one else, who will object and why? On the other hand, a negative decision is rarely taken because this needs great political courage and strength.

When taken, its form shows that it definitely harms some vested interest without indicating specifically who will benefit therefrom. The interests adversely affected raise a howl against the proposal which no one is particularly interested in defending and it soon gets thrown out. What is not realised, however is that the positive decision remains unimplemented on paper unless it is accompanied by a corresponding negative decision which destroys an evil and makes it possible for a good thing to grow. If one desires to grow a good harvest, for instance, it is not enough to sow seeds; it is even more important to decide that all weeds shall be rooted out.

This is very relevant to the discussion under issue, viz a radical change in the existing pattern of expenditure on health care services and its priorities. If this change is to be brought about, both positive and negative decisions are needed and they will have to go together. For instance,

(1) A decision to give a promotive and preventive orientation to the health care services is not possible unless, from a financial angle, the easy positive decision to invest more funds in these services is taken simultaneously with the hard negative decision that the expenditure on large urban hospitals and on the specialities and superspecialities should not be increased without a very close scrutiny of its essentiality and priority.

(2) A decision to give a promotive and preventive orientation to the health care services is also not possible, from the personal angle unless the easy positive decision of creating the cadres of CHVs or MPWs or other needed public health functionaries is taken side-by-side with the hard negative decisions to redefine the role of the doctor, change his training, and above all, stop all over-production by refusing to establish new medical colleges or increasing the capacity of existing colleges or creating a new cadre of 'quick' doctors.

(3) A change in the existing pattern of drug production in the country to suit the disease pattern and particularly, to meet the needs of the poor and underprivileged groups, is not possible unless the easy positive decision to produce the basic drugs is taken side-by-side with the hard negative decision to restrict overall drug production and even to ban the production of profit-making, costly but useless or even harmful drugs.

It is easy, but not necessary, to multiply such instances. What we desire to highlight is the need to take and implement hard, unpopular, negative decisions if our objective of implementing the positive decisions is to be realized in practice.

In the present system, resources, authority and responsibility are all concentrated at the top. A common experience in implementing plans based on decentralization in such a situation is that responsibilities are decentralized to lower levels with alacrity while there is a great hesitation to make a corresponding devolution of resources and authority. Consequently, there is a mismatch between responsibility, authority and resources at every level and this is generally the largest at the lowest level where one finds the heaviest responsibility matched with little authority and even less resources. This error will have to be avoided and care will have to be taken to see that adequate resources are transferred to *every* level and that each level has adequate resources and authority to enable it to discharge its responsibilities.

The total expenditure needed for health services is very large and the vast bulk of it will have to come from Central and State taxes. It would, however, be desirable to levy a local health cess and make the community pay a share of the total cost, however small. As suggested earlier in Chapter II, we could move in the direction of a system where a patient ordinarily pays for the cost of drugs, except for a rather small percentage of patients who are defined by local community representatives as being so poor that they deserve free medicines also.

A National Health Service

The alternative model proposed here is a very major step in the eventual creation of a national health service. It tries to ensure that by A.D. 2000, morbidity will be considerably reduced through better nutrition, improvement of environment and health education and that all citizens shall receive adequate primary health care and equitable access to a prompt and efficient system of referral services. In particular, the model provides that special attention will be given to the needs of the poor and underprivileged groups. What is even more important, it refuses to create dependency among the people and strives to build their capability to understand and solve their own health problems. All the same, it is necessary to point out that the alternative model is not a programme of national health service. We do not think that the time is ripe for such a measure. If introduced in haste, without adequate preparation, and in the absence of the social ethos necessary for its success, it is likely to do more harm than good. We do not also think that one can abolish the private sector in health alone. It will involve the abolition of the private sector in all important walks of life, including the abolition of the mixed economy. Our proposals, therefore, have a limited approach: they aim to provide good and adequate health services to the poor and the underprivileged sectors of the population who get little benefit from the existing services, either free of charge, or for payment of the cost of drugs (which is, anyway, a very small portion of the total cost). Our aim also is to improve the quality of these services so that there will be less and less need for citizens to go to the private practitioner. If this process is carried on far enough, the domain of private practice will get considerably reduced. The problem of creating a national health service and abolishing private practice altogether may be reviewed then, say about ten years from now.

We also believe that there will have to be some restriction on private practice. No private practice should be permitted to employees of the public health services. There should be adequate control on private practitioners also to see that they do not indulge in malpractices.

Conditions Essential for Success

What are the conditions essential for the success of the alternative model? Since good health and good societies go together, health is a function of social, economic, cultural and political factors and action to raise the health status of the people will have to be taken on several fronts, both within and without the health sector.

Action Outside the Health Sector

The intensive efforts of the State and the people should be directed at bringing about the socio-economic-political transformation visualised in the Constitution. The development of good health care services will succeed in proportion to the extent to which these basic attempts to eradicate poverty, inequality and ignorance make headway.

The basic objective of this proposal is to improve the health status of women and children and of the poor and under-privileged social groups like Scheduled Castes, Scheduled Tribes, landless agricultural labourers in rural areas and the lumpen proletariat of the urban slums. This cannot be done unless their overall status is improved. This is basically a political issue and implies the need to take them out of the present marginalised existence and vest them with effective political power. This can only be done through organisation and political education. The health programme (like programmes in other fields) can be a great instrument for this just as the political awakening and organisation of the poor and the underprivileged can be a sure path to an improvement in their social and health status. This is what the country has failed to do in the last 30 years, and this is what its young men and women will have to concentrate on during the next two decades. This alone will create the foundation on which a good and equitable programme of health services can be built.

Action Within the Health Sector

This action outside the health sector is necessary but not sufficient. The socialist countries have taken these measures and that explains the great and rapid advance of their health care systems. But even these countries are paying a heavy price because of the continuance of the consumer-oriented over-professionalized and dependency creating model of health care services and because of a false value system regarding pain, ageing and death. It is therefore necessary for us to abandon the Western model of health care services which was initially imposed on us, but which we have continued uncritically to retain and expand and it will have to be replaced by the alternative model of community-based health services we have proposed. This programme will need financial investments no doubt. But money alone will achieve very little. The programme will succeed only if better human inputs are made, among which the following three may be highlighted:

(1) The alternative model is *not* to be imposed upon the people. Such a step will not be justified even on the grounds that it is in the interest of the people. What is necessary is that the people are educated to realise the weaknesses of the existing model and are convinced, as a result of rational discussion, that the alternative model will give them better health services at lesser cost. It is only this realisation and conviction that will secure the full co-operation of the people without which its effective implementation is not possible. It is, therefore, necessary to publish this report in all the Indian languages and take the discussion of the basic issues it raises to all the people. The mass media, the press, and official and non-official agencies should play a major role in this essentially educational campaign and create the necessary intellectual and social climate for the acceptance and implementation of the Report.

(2) The present model of health services is centralized and bureaucratic. This creates a certain set of attitudes, both in the services and in the people. For instance, the services

develop an authoritarian and paternalistic attitude towards the people who, in their turn,become dependent. The alternative model which is decentralized and participatory will require a very different set of attitudes. The bureaucrats and the professionals will have to cultivate respect for the people and a faith in their ability to identify and find solutions to their problems. This alone will give them the courage to allow the community 'the right to sin'. They have also to realise that their responsibility is not to provide the services, but to build a capability among the people to provide the services to themselves; and that the measure of their true success is not to do things for the people, but to enable the people to look after themselves. On their part, the people will have to develop self-confidence and abandon the *ma-bap* attitude towards the services. They will also have learn to organise themselves, not on the basis of the law of the jungle where everyone tries to get away with whatever he can and exploitation and competition reign supreme, but on the basis of a community based on principles of mutual respect, tolerance and goodwill, cooperation and sympathy for the underdog. It must be realised that these changes in attitudes and value will be the result of the successful operation of the alternative model, just as it is the deliberate cultivation of these attitudes and values that will itself make a major contribution to the success of the model.

(3) Finally, the success of the alternative model will depend largely upon the quality of the health services. This will, of course, include the usual problems of proper selection, training, creation of proper conditions of work and service, adequate supervision and guidance and good administration which will ensure justice and fair play and relate rewards visibly to quality and punishment to failure. But this is not sufficient. Health care differs from other societal activities in the greater expectations of the public that in addition to technical competence, personnel should have an abiding spirit of social services and should bring concern and humanity to bear on their activities. Unfortunately, the current trends in this regard are far from happy. The impersonal callousness which is bred in large hospitals is spreading and the system is getting dehumanised and even mercenary and corrupt. The public dissatisfaction against these trends is manifest and growing. But only a few citizens can resort to private practice; and the only way out is to reverse these trends and reinfect the health services with a spirit of service. This is partly a responsibility of the training process. Moreover, the doctor as the leader of the team can play an important role and influence the values and quality of caring among the whole staff if he shows these concerns himself. Ways should be found to discover and reward such leadership. This also highlights the need to vest the control of its health services in the community itself. Just as doctors in private practice have to behave courteously and show concern in order to satisfy their patients, the quality of care will be improved by making personnel responsible to local users of each facility.

4

Issues Related to Health and Hospital

We are optimistic about the possibilities of bringing better health to the people of India. A new partnership between the health system and the people can release their tremendous capacity to solve their own problems. The remarkable scientific advances of recent years can be adapted specifically to meet the needs of the poor and deprived rather than being focussed mainly on sophisticated care for the elite. Abundant demonstrations have shown what needs to be done to produce dramatic changes in the health and welfare of those in greatest need, especially women and children. We are, therefore, convinced that the goal of health for all by A.D. 2000 is realistic and practicable. The plan we have presented here is expected to help the country to achieve this goal through vigorous and sustained action. Its principal message is that this goal cannot be achieved by a linear expansion of the existing system and even by tinkering with it through minor reforms. Nothing short of a radical change is called for; and for this it is necessary to develop a comprehensive national policy on health and to create an alternative model of health care services.

The basic challenges presented in this plan are to initiate an integrated plan of health, development and family planning, based on a hopeful vision of what can be achieved by the year 2000. It necessarily implies the adoption of several alternative policies which have been broadly outlined in this Report. No twenty-year perspective should try to provide detailed prescriptions for implementation. Tjat is essentially a task for the five year and annual plans, and in a vast and plural country like India, for each State Government and district authority to decide in the light of the national policies laid down by the Government of India. What this plan provides—and that is all what a plan of this type can ever hope to provide—is a frank analysis of the existing health situation, highlighting the gap between even minimal aspirations and the actuality, a comprehensive conceptualisation of where the country might be at the end of this century if this challenge is taken seriously, critical analysis of constraints and major policy options, a discussion of interlinkages and priorities, and an indication of the best strategy available to realise our objectives, with some idea of its administrative and financial implications. These are presented here in a format designed to be used by all those who will be most concerned with these issues, including leaders of public opinion. The various Chapters of this Report present the rationale and justification for the new directions proposed in the different health sectors and a fairly detailed indication of the changes needed in programmes and strategies. In this concluding Chapter, we shall bring together our major conclusions and recommendations to facilitate the consideration of this document and to expedite action thereon.

Health for all by A.D. 2000

Targets

What does this goal of health for all by A.D. 2000 mean in precise terms? We have suggested that his should mean the provision of good and adequate health care for all citizens —and especially for the poor and underprivileged groups. In our opinion, this will imply a tremendous reduction in morbidity and mortality resulting in a fall of the total death rate from 15 to 9 and in the birth rate from 33 to 21. This will also imply that the net reproduction rate (which is now 1.67) will be reduced to one, that infant mortality would be reduced from 120 to 60, that the average family size from 4.3 children to 2.3 children, and that the total population of India may stabilise at about 1,200 million by about 2050. This would indeed be a great breakthrough, not only in health, but also in development and family planning. We consider these targets as realistic and practicable.

If this goal is to be realised, a major programme for the development of health care services is of course *necessary*, but it is not *sufficient*. Health is a function, not only of medical care but of the overall integrated development of society— cultural, economic, educational, social and political. In fact, as we said earlier, good health and good societies go together. Health also depends on a number of supportive services—nutrition, improvement in the environment and education; and the influence of these services on health status is far greater than that of medical care. The major programmes which will improve health are thus outside the realm of health care proper. These were comparatively neglected in the last 30 years and that is one of the major reasons why the country has obtained such meagre results for its large investments in health. This error should not be repeated, and during the next two decades, the three programmes of (1) integrated overall development, (2) improvement in nutrition, environment and health education, and (3) the provision of adequate health care services for all and especially for the poor and underprivileged, will have to be pursued side-by-side.

Integrated Development

Poverty, inequality and ignorance are the greatest illnesses of the Indian society. The status of its women and children is low: they are both cheap and expendable. Health for all is an essentially egalitarian goal and it cannot be achieved in a society of this type. The integrated programme of development of be pursed over the next 20 years should therefore be basically aimed at reducing poverty and inequality, spreading education, and improving the status of women and children as well as of the poor and deprived social groups. This will include the following:

1. Rapid economic growth with the object of doubling the national income per capita (at constant prices) by A.D. 2000.

2. Full-scale employment, including a guarantee of work on reasonable wages to every adult who offers to work for 8 hours a day . Creation of adequate opportunities of gainful employment to women, with an emphasis on equity of remuneration and reservations to make up for past neglect, so that women become 'visible' assets to their families.

3. Improvement in the status of women a determination to check the adverse sex-ratio and to make it rise substantially upwards, say to 972, the level it was in 1901

4. Adult education with emphasis on health education and vocational skills, the targets being to cover the entire illiterate population in the age-group 15-35 by 1991 and liquidation of illiteracy by A.D. 2000.

5. Universal elementary education for all children (age-group 6-14) to be provided by 1991.

6. Welfare of Scheduled Castes and Scheduled Tribes.

7. Development of an intensive and integrated programme of family planning.

8. Creation of a democratic, decentralised and participating form of government.

9. Rural electrification and

10. Improvement in housing, with emphasis on the provision of houses for the landless and slum clearance.

We have recommended that the details of these programmes should be worked out and that they be implemented fully over the next 20 years.

Family Planning

Family Planning should become a people's movement. This process would be facilitated by the efforts at integrated development and the education and organisation of the poor and underprivileged groups. It is desirable that there should be a National Population Commission set-up by an Act of Parliament to formulate and implement an overall population policy. The objective should be to reduce the net reproduction rate from 1.67 to 1.00 and the birth rate from 33 to 21. This will imply effective protection of 60 per cent of eligible couples (against 22 per cent at present). While the emphasis on terminal methods should continue, there should be far greater use of other methods as well. The accent should be on education and motivation, especially through inter-personal communication and group action. Incentives, especially those of a compensatory character, should be used. There should be concentrated effort to work with women as well as men. While the health care services have a role to play in motivation also, their main responsibility is to supply the needed services, and to undertake follow-up care. The alternative model of health care services has been designed to meet these challenges fully and squarely.

Nutrition

Among other supportive programmes, nutrition deserves priority because it is a major foundation of health. For this purpose, it is necessary to grow adequate food, to reduce post-harvest losses, to create an adequate system of storage and distribution, and to increase the purchasing power of the people by creating employment for men, and especially for women. It will also be necessary to give special attention to improving the nutritional status of women and children. Breast feeding should be encouraged and women trained and assisted to take better care of children through weaning at the right time and through a more efficient management of the child's diet in the immediate post-weaning period. Pregnant and lactating mothers should be given the special protection they need. Special programmes should be developed for specific nutritional disorders like iron-deficiency anemia, or Vitamin A and iodine deficiencies. In addition, supplementary feeding programmes may have to be organised for carefully identified target groups at risk.

Improvement of the Environment

The second supportive service is improvement of the environment. It will reduce infection and make programmes of nutrition itself more effective. Several programmes will have to be developed from this point of view. Safe drinking water supply should be provided to all urban and rural areas at an average annual estimated cost of Rs. 7,500 million. In urban areas, the sewage disposal system will have to be improved by eliminating the basket service system in ten years, providing water-seal latrines to all households who have no facilities at present, during the same period, and ultimately, installing good sewage disposal systems with essential purification works in all urban areas by A.D. 2000. The estimated costs of this programme will work out to Rs. 1,125 million per year. A massive programme of proper collection and disposal of solid wastes and their conversion into compost will have to be developed in all areas, the estimated cost being Rs. 4,000 million a year on an average. In rural areas, an intensive programme of improving sanitation, with special emphasis on proper disposal of night soil, will have to be developed at an estimated cost of Rs. 5,000 million a year. Greater attention will have to be paid to town and village planning (with special emphasis on removing the segregation of the Scheduled Castes), and large-scale programmes of housing for the rural poor and clearance of urban slums will have to be undertaken, with emphasis on the development of a low-cost building technology. Urgent steps have to be taken to prevent water and air pollution, to control the ill-effects of industrialization and to provide better work-place environment.

Health Education

The third supportive service is health education. It gives information, teaches skills and cultivates attitudes and values which help an individual to be healthy. Health education is not also a one-short affair: an individual will need it throughout his life. The best way to universalize health education therefore is to make it an integral part of general education which, in its turn, will have to be life-long. In early childhood (0-5 years), it is primarily the responsibility of the mother to give it to her child and she must be trained to do so. For older children (6-14 years), health education should be an integral part of general elementary education which should be universal. Health education suited to adolescents and youths should be an integral part of secondary and university education also. What is extremely important, health education should be an integral part of adult education.

The health personnel have three major responsibilities for health education. They should assist the general education system to provide health education by devising suitable programmes, training of teachers, production of materials and conduct of experiments. They have also an educational role with regard to every patient because all proper medical treatment often includes an element of health education. Finally, they have a very important role in which they try to give health education to the poor and underprivileged groups who need it most. The Central and State Health Bureaux should be reorganised and strengthened to help the health personnel to discharge these responsibilities. The mass medcial should be harnessed fully for purposes of health education.

The Alternative Model of Health Services

This brings us finally to the central problem of the action required within the health field itself to reach the goal of health for all by A.D. 2000. As stated earlier, no meaningful results can be obtained by a linear expansion of the existing health services or by tinkering with them through minor reforms. We have, therefore, proposed that this model should be totally abandoned and a new alternative model should be created in its place. This is described in detail in Chapter VII.

This new model differs from the existing model in several important respects. It abandons the top-down and elite oriented approach of the existing services and is based or rooted in the community (which means a population of 1,00,000 which will have a Community Health Centre, a sub-centre for every 5,000 population and a village/neighbourhood centre for every 1,000 population) and then rises to specialised referral services at the district and regional levels. It gives up the over-emphasis which the present system places on large, urban hospitals and creates a small community hospital of about 30 beds in each community to meet the vast bulk of its referral needs. It moves away from the predominantly curative orientation of the existing services and integrates promotive, preventive and curative aspects at all levels. It redefines the role of drugs and doctors so that they remain the best agents of health care and do not develop a vested interest in ill-health. It gives up the centralized and bureaucratic character of the present system and adopts a decentralized, democratic and participatory approach which will involve the community intimately in planning, providing and maintaining the health services it needs. It strives to integrate the valuable elements in our culture and tradition (e.g. the *ashrama* concept of stages in life —non-consumerist attitudes, sense of individual and community responsibility, yoga and simplicity and self-discipline as the core of a life-style). It also strives to create a national system of medicine by giving support to and synthesizing the indigenous systems. Finally, it abandons the over-expensive model of the health care systems in the developed countries and creates an economic model which will provide a better quality of health service at a much smaller cost which will be within the reach of the country. It is our considered view that health should have the same priority as education and that both should receive about 6 per cent of the national income by A.D. 2000. This would provide all the funds needed to implement this model and to develop its essential support services. It is our recommendation that this model should be fully created, in a phased and planned manner, by A.D. 2000.

MCH Services

In this new model, special efforts will have to be made to expand and improve MCH services which are now patchy and rudimentary. There should be an attempt to cover all women and children with basic services with special attention to those at risk The *dais* should be trained and fully utilized, along with CHVs, at the village centre level with strong referral support from the MPWs. These services will be largely domiciliary. A detailed programme should be drawn up of the different services that will be provided at the village, sub-centre and community levels, and priorities in MCH activities should be clearly laid down. The MCH staff at each level should be adequate and should receive job specific training. Health education of the mothers should be an important component of MCH services and care should be taken to see that these services retain their essential character as services for women and children even while laying adequate emphasis on family planning.

Communicable Diseases

The communicable diseases still form the largest cause of morbidity and mortality and the fight against them will have to be continued with still greater vigour in the years ahead. The existing programmes against malaria, tuberculosis, leprosy, filariasis , poliomyelitis and Japanese encephalitis will have to be strengthened, broadly on the lines indicated. Diarrhoeal diseases, especially those of children, need special emphasis. To develop these programmes on proper lines, it is necessary to develop a good surveillance system and a coordinated effort of all research institutes and the administration. By A.D. 2000, our object should be to eradicate (or at least effectively control) diarrhoeal diseases, tetanus, diphtheria, hydrophobia, poliomyelitis, tuber-culosis, guineaworm, malaria, filariasis and leprosy.

Rehabilitation Services

There are an estimated 60 million physically handicapped in the country. Every year, 5 million more are added. Despite this the rehabilitation services are poor and inadequate. Rehabilitation services should be integrated with other community health services. Rehabilitation workers should also be drawn from the community and health education will include rehabilitation education. New technologies suited to our life should be evolved, using local materials and artisans.

Personnel and Training

Under the new alternative model, the organisation of the health services will be radically different from that in the existing system. A new personnel and training policy will, therefore, have to be adopted on the broad lines indicated. A new category of personnel, the CHVs, will be introduced and will be the main bridge between the community and the services. The middle level personnel will increase very substantially. This will include health assistants, MPWs, nursing personnel whose numbers will be much larger and whose status will need considerable improvement, and paramedicals. Very important questions about doctors will have to be sorted out: these relate to their numbers, training, remuneration and social conditions, value system and proper development of postgraduate courses. The training and utilization of specialists and superspecialists will have to be reorganised from the point of view of effective utilization. Facilities for training in public health should be increased. There should be adequate arrangements for the continuous in-service education of all categories of health personnel. The Government of India should establish, under an Act of Parliament, a Medical and Health Education Commission, with comprehensive terms of reference. A continuing study of personnel and training and taking effective action thereon should be a major responsibility of this Commission.

Drugs and Pharmaceuticals

There is need for a clear-cut drug policy and a National Drug Agency to implement it properly. The pattern of drug production in the country should be modified to suit the disease pattern. The drugs required by the poor people should be produced in adequate quantities and made available at the cheapest prices possible. This applies specially to the few simple drugs required at the community level. It is also necessary to compile a list of other essential drugs. The quantities needed of all essential drugs should be calculated and steps taken to see that they are produced. The production of high price and useless drugs needs to be controlled, the tendency of the profession to over-prescribe should be curbed. The production of basic drugs has to be made more self-sufficient and in this, the small-scale sector needs to be encouraged subject to strict quality control. The dominance of the foreign sector should be reduced still further. Price control should be more effective; the cost on packaging and overheads should be reduced; the introduction of new drugs should be strictly controlled and proliferation of drugs by minor variations should not be allowed; the prices of essential drugs should be kept to the minimum, a higher mark-up being allowed, if necessary, in other drugs; and all essential drugs should be sold only under generic names. There should be adequate arrangements for quality control of all drugs, including indigenous medicines and R&D in drugs needs to be greatly encouraged. There is considerable imbalance in the consumption of drugs in urban and rural sectors of the health system which needs to be corrected and it may be desirable to move towards a system when the patient pays for the cost of drugs.

Research

The main problems in research are selection of priority areas, quality and utilization of research, improvement in research capability, and attainment of indigenous self-reliance. The priority areas obviously are: primary health care, epidemiology, communicable diseases (with special emphasis on diarrhoea), environmental research, and research on drugs and problems of rural water supply and sanitation. It is also necessary to promote research on social aspects of medicine jointly under the ICMR and ICSSR, especially on the economics of health and financing of health services. Other important areas are indigenous medicine, health implications of industrial development, and family planning. Considerable attention has to be given to the development of appropriate technology. Side-by-side, there should be an emphasis on the development of clinical and basic research, particularly in the field of biology, and a determined bid to build up high level indigenous research capability with a view to attaining self-reliance.

Administration, Finance and Implementation

The introduction of the alternative model has large administrative and financial implications. From the administrative point of view, it is necessary to redefine the roles of the Central and State Governments in view of the large powers delegated to the local bodies at the district level and below. Voluntary agencies will have to function within the overall policy laid down by the State. But they should receive encouragement and aid, especially when fighting at the frontiers and doing pioneer work. There will be considerable tensions within the new health care services and need for redefinition of roles and mutual adjustment. This is the responsibility of the administration to secure through good leadership and proper training. The referral services should be strengthened and streamlined; a new and efficient national information system should be created; and adequate arrangements made for more effective coordination at all levels.

On the financial front, the total investment in health services will have to be substantially stepped up and the health expenditure will have to rise by about 8 to 9 per cent per year (at constant prices). The existing priorities will have to be radically altered and the bulk of the additional resources will have to go into promotive and preventive activities, in rural areas in the development of supportive services like nutrition, sanitation, water supply and education, and for providing health care services to women and children and the poor and underprivileged groups. This will need taking of both positive and negative decisions. There should be adequate grants to local bodies and communities to enable them to discharge their responsibilities; and while the basic responsibility of financing health will continue to rest with the Centre and State, an effort should be made to tap local taxes and individual payments to cover drug costs.

The alternative model proposed here is a large step in the creation of a national health service, but it does not create it. In our opinion, the time is not ripe for the purpose and the issue may be examined in due course, say, ten years from now. There is, however, need to control private practice and it should not be allowed to employees in the public health care system.

Conditions Essential for Success

This, in brief is the plan we have proposed, for realising the goal of health for all by A.D. 2000. There can be no two opinions about its desirability, and what we have outlined is enough to show that the goal is realistic and feasible.

As we said at the opening of our Report, the country dedicated itself, when it adopted the Constitution in 1950, to create a new social order based on equality, freedom, justice and dignity of the individual and to eliminate poverty, ignorance and ill-health. This 'mid-term' review after three decades shows that, in so far as health is concerned, the country is still far short of its objective in spite of major advances in several areas. It also shows than an attempt to eradicate ill-health will not succeed in isolation and that it can be pursued side-by-side with the other two interdependent and mutually supportive objectives of eliminating poverty, inequality and ignorance, and against the back-drop of a socio-economic transformation which will give effective political power to the poor and deprived social groups. It is, therefore, necessary that the country rededicates itself to this task and strives to achieve its goals by A.D. 2000. Succeeding generations will never forgive us if we fail to do so.

The attainment of this goal depends, above all, on three things: (1) the extent to which it is possible to reduce poverty and inequality and to spread education; (2) the extent to which it will be possible to organise the poor and underprivileged groups so that they are able to fight for their basic rights; and (3) the extent to which we are able to move away from the counter-productive, consumerist Western model of health care and to replace it by the alternative model based in the community which is proposed here. These are our tasks and it needs millions of young men and women, both within and without the health sector, to work for them. If a mass movement for this purpose can be organised and the people rededicate themselves to the realisation of their national goals, the country will be able to keep its tryst with destiny at least by A.D. 2000, if not earlier.

5

X-Ray Department

General During the course of their training most doctors acquire a useful degree of skill in the interpretation of radiographs, without at the same time acquiring any knowledge of the way they are taken. Because this knowledge is very useful in a rural hospital, this chapter makes some attempt to supply it. These few pages will, it is hoped, give the doctor enough insight into the work of a small X-ray department to enable him to supervise it satisfactorily, and to use it to the best advantage. It will also give him some ideas on the type of plant available and its installation.

Theory. At its simplest an X-ray tube is an evacuated glass vessel containing two electrical conductors or electrodes, a negative electrode or cathode, and a positive electrode or anode (Figure 5.1). The anode is usually a dise of tungsten set in a block of copper; the cathode is a thin wire filament heated by current of about 12 volts. When a potential difference of upwards of about 40 thousand volts-40 Kilovolts or 40 kV—is applied between these electrodes, a stream of electrons leave the hot filament (the cathode) and flow across the vacuum to hit the anode. In striking the anode these electrons produce X-rays, which are given off in all directions. Of this radiation, a small part is allowed to pass through a window in the X-ray tube and the shielding around it, and so through the patient and on to the X-ray film.

The *quality* or penetrating power of the X-rays is determined by the kV across the electrodes, the *quantity* of X-rays produced is determined by the current in milliamps—'the mA'—flowing through the filament, and the time for which it flows.

Circuits. Electricity at two quite different potentials is needed to produce X-ray. It is required at a high potential of many kV across the two electrodes, and also at a low potential of a few volts to heat the filament of the cathode. These two types of current have both to be produced from the normal AC mains. A step-up transformer is thus required to produce the kV, and a step-down transformer to produce the low voltage for the cathode filament.

The simplest type of transformer has two coils, one wound over the other—the primary coil for the electricity going into the transformer, and the secondary coil for the electricity coming out of it. The greater the number of turns in the secondary coil as compared with the primary, the higher the voltage of its output and vice versa. Thus, by altering the ratio of the number of turns used in the primary and secondary coils, the output voltage of a transformer can be varied within wide limits.

X-RAY APPARATUS

A. THE X-RAY TUBE

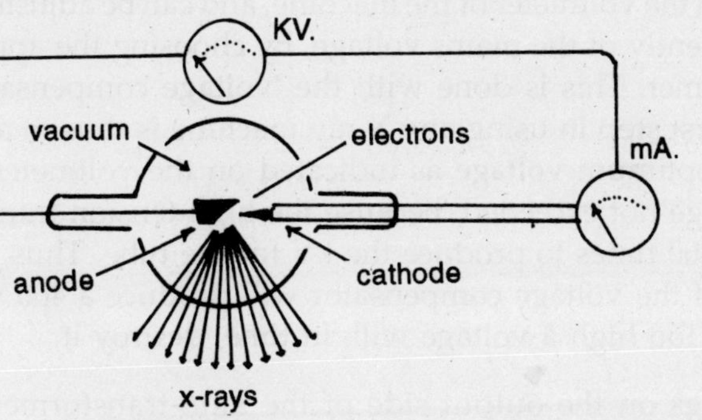

B. SIMPLE CIRCUIT DIAGRAM

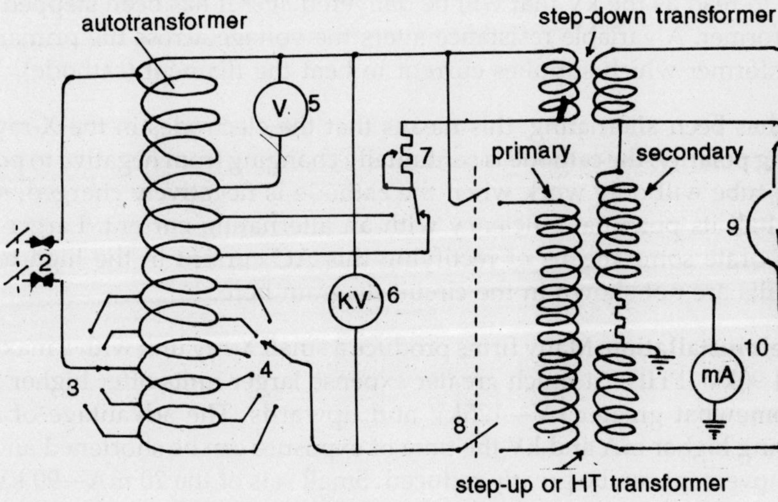

1. Double pole mains switch	6. kV meter (pre-reading).
2. Fuses	7. mA control
3. Voltage compensator	8. Exposure contactor
4. kV selector	9. X-ray tube
5. Voltmeter	10. Milleammeter

The coils need not be separate and can be combined together as an 'auto-transformer'. The first transformer of an X-ray set is usually of this kind and serves several functions, one of which is to compensate for variations in mains voltage. The mains are led into such an auto-transformer through a number of alternative tappings controlled by a knob on the panel of the set—the 'voltage compensator'. The voltage actually developed by the auto-transformer is measured with the voltmeter of the machine, and can be adjusted to an optimum value more or less independently of the mains voltage, by choosing the appropriate tapping on the input of the transformer. This is done with the 'voltage compensator' knob on the panel of the machine. The first step in using any X-ray machine is thus to adjust the voltage compensator to secure the optimum voltage as indicated on the voltmeter. This should be done carefully and the voltage not exceeded, because the high tension transformer steps up this voltage approximately 400 times to produce the kV for the tube. Thus, the difference of a single volt in the setting of the voltage compensator will produce a 400 volt difference in the KV applied to the tube. Too high a voltage will, in time, destroy it.

A further set of tappings on the output side of the auto-transformer determines the voltage led into the primary coils of the high tension transformer. These tappings enable any desired kV to be chosen in advance, the knob which controls them being called the 'kV selector'— the greater the number of turns of the secondary coil included in the circuit, the greater the kV. The voltage across this part of the auto-transformer is read by another voltmeter— 'the prereading kV meter'. Because it is not easy to measure the kV directly, this voltmeter is calibrated to read as the kV that will be delivered *after* it has been stepped up in the high tension transformer. A variable resistance alters the voltage across the primary coil of the step-down transformer which supplies current to heat the filament (cathode).

So far all current has been alternating, this means that the electrodes in the X-ray tube are continually changing polarity; the cathode is continually changing from negative to positive and vice versa. As the tube will only work when the cathode is negatively charged, such a tube only operates at half its potential efficiency with an alternating current. Larger X-ray plants therefore incorporate some means of rectifying this AC current in the high tension circuit - such refinements are not shown in the circuit diagram here.

Machines and their installation. Many firms produce a small X-ray unit with a maximum capacity of 20 mA and 90kV (PHI). At much greater expense larger units offer higher mA—500 and more, and somewhat greater kV—125kV and upwards. The advantage of larger machines is, that by using higher mA and kV the time of exposure can be shortened and thus the disadvantages of movement can be greatly reduced. Small sets of the 20 mA—90 kV type enable limbs to be X-rayed and fairly satisfactory straight chest films to be taken. Views of the skull, the spine, the pregnant uterus, etc. are normally taken using a stationary grid (see below), and require such long exposures with these machines that they are usually unsuitable for these purposes, except on very co-operative patients.

All X-ray plant requires alternating current, the smallest sets requiring 18 amps at 220 volts (4 KVA). However, because this current is required for such a short time only, such sets can be operated with safety from a 13 amp mains socket.

The short heavy load drawn by an X-ray plant imposes severe demands on a small generator on which it acts as a sudden break. Unless the generator has been specially designed for X-ray plants, and equipped with a very heavy flywheel to enable it to cope with this sudden load, the output of the generator should be at least twice that demanded by the X-ray plant. A special petrol generator delivering 5.5 kVA is available (PHI) which will run small X-ray plants requiring 4kVA, as well as supplying electricity for such purposes as dark room illumination.

Altitude should also be considered in specifying the output required for the generator of an X-ray plant, for the output of an internal combustion engine falls 5 per cent, with each increasing 1,000 feet (300 metres) of altitude above sea level.

The generator should be near the X-ray department, for they have to be joined by a heavy copper cable the size of this cable being determined, not by its current carrying capacity, for which a much smaller cable would do, but by the necessity for it to have a very low resistance.

The X-Ray exposure. Besides the X-ray machine and the film, it is usual to use two other pieces of apparatus each time an exposure is made. One is an intensifying screen and the other is a grid. An intensifying screen is a thin piece of cardboard that is normally coated with calcium tungstate and is placed inside the cassette close against the film itself. A screen of this kind converts some of the X-rays reaching it into light to which the emulsion is more sensitive than it is to X-rays. An intensifying screen therefore makes possible a considerable reduction in the exposure required.

When X-rays strike tissue some of them are scattered and impair the quality of the radiograph. It is therefore, usual to cut down these scattered rays by interposing a grid between the part to be X-rayed and the plate. A stationary grid is composed of fine alternating strips of opaque and translucent material, but though it improves the definition of the film, it covers it with a series of fine lines. The only way to remove these lines is to cause the grid to move slightly during the course of the exposure—such a moving grid is called a Bucky diaphragm, or more simply, a 'Bucky', and is an invariable fitting on bigger machines. An equally important method of ensuring radiographs of the best possible quality is to restrict the area irradiated to the minimum practicable, by the use of a series of interchangeable metal cones attached to the X-ray type.

An intensifying screen decreases the exposure required and a grid increases it, but these are only two of many factors which influence the quality of a radiograph.

When films are processed in a standard manner the quality of a radiograph depends on the following variables:

1) The time of exposure—long exposures tend to be associated with poor definition due to movement of the patient and/or the X-ray tube.

2) The kV used—the higher the kV, the greater the penetrating power of the X-rays but also the poorer the soft tissue contrast.

3) The mA—the greater the mA the larger the quantity of X-rays produced and in consequence the shorter the time needed for an exposure. Thus, if the mA are doubled the time can be halved.
4) The focus film distance—the greater the distance the sharper the detail, but a longer exposure is required. The distance factor is a powerful one, for the intensity of the radiation falling on the film decreases with the square of the focus-film distance.
5) The sensitivity of the film; 'slow' 'medium' and 'fast' films are made. Fast films mean a loss in detail and poorer keeping qualities, but they make shorter exposures possible.
6) The intensifying factor of the intensifying screen, 'slow' 'medium' and 'fast' screens are available—again fast screens mean poorer detail.
7) The 'grid factor'—this is a measure of the radiological opacity of the grid or Bucky.
8) The thickness and density of the part being X-rayed.
9) A factor dependent on the efficiency of the machine itself.

All these nine variables must be considered when taking any radiograph. How are they all to be balanced against one another? No neat formulae are available and radiography is something of an art—experience is the only answer. However, it is usual to use medium speed intensifying screens, except for thin parts like the hand, for which paper wrapped film can be used without grids or intensifying screens. This leaves only the following variables, time mA, kV, focus-film distance and the part to be X-rayed. Tables are supplied with most machines to relate these variables: these give suggested exposure times for every part at given values for mA, kV and focus-film distance. Experience of local conditions may show however that some modifications need to be made to these average figures.

Low mA can be compensated for by increased time and vice versa. It is therefore usual to consider these together as milliamp-seconds or mAS. It is a useful rule that if the kV increases by ten in the range 40-90 kV, the mAS can be halved.

Radiographic assistants soon get to know the standard exposures for their machine, but when posted to a new plant they are advised to take a postero-anterior chest film of an average man at the standard 2 metres (6ft) at 6 mAS and 72 kV. This film when developed under standard conditions will give them some idea of the efficiency of their plant and they can adjust their other exposures accordingly.

When money is scarce screening may appear to offer a substantial economy in the use of X-ray film. However, a special screening plant is needed before patients can be safely screened and the usefulness of a low powered plant for barium studies of the stomach and colon is very limited. No radiographic assistant is competent to screen—this must be done by a doctor wearing lead gloves and a lead apron.

When a radiographic assistant has been properly trained he should take the correct precautions against exposure to radiation as a matter of course. Many radiographic assistants have not been so trained and even trained ones sometimes become slipshod in this matter. They must stand behind the X-ray machine when an exposure is taken and wherever possible behind a lead screen, should one be available. An X-ray tube should always be pointed away from other people, that is at the floor, or a wall.

6

The Outpatient Department

The work of the outpatient department. When the pattern of illness in a community is looked at as a whole, it will be seen that comparatively few diseases are severe enough to confine the sufferer to his bed. Most of them permit him to walk about, and if given the choice, many patients prefer to be up and around. In addition to this bed rest is now coming to be considered of less value in some diseases than was formerly the case. Because of the great volume of ambulant disease in most communities, an efficient outpatient department is clearly of critical importance. This is increased by the cheapness of outpatient as compared with inpatient care. But besides treating outpatients of the traditional type, this department also serves another useful purpose; it is the place where 'self-care' patients are often best given their daily treatment.

An outpatient department is usually thought of as being part of hospital, but general outpatients are also seen by health centres. Their are thus many aspects of outpatient care which apply equally to has institutions. But one important difference between them is the differing scale of their activities; so many more outpatients are apt to seek attention from a hospital. It is this problem of scale, the vast numbers of patients to be seen, that is the critical determinant of outpatient practice. But before considering this in more detail, it should be mentioned the a health centre has been defined as a unit which supplies all the medical needs of a family other than those which can only be supplied by a hospital. Health centres should therefore provide all the ordinary on patient services, and be so sited that they can relieve hospital outpatient departments of all but their most specialized functions. Ideally therefore outpatient departments should only see patients referred to them by health centres; but in practice the ideal seldom happens, and most outpatient departments have to see anyone who comes to them. Health centre outpatient practice has already been considered in detail in Chapter Three and will not therefore be considered any further here.

The numbers of people seeking outpatient care would not matter so much if there were staff and facilities in proportion to the demand. Usually, there are not, and doctors in particular are almost always critically scarce. Not only this, but the services that outpatients require are both complex and varied. There are 'general outpatients' with a multitude of different conditions, there are children as well as antenatal and postnatal mothers. There are also cases with diseases of particular frequency and importance, such as tuberculosis and malnutrition. Several special clinics may therefore be required which have often to be organized in buildings of poor design.

The key to making the best of the facilities available is a proper appreciation of the role of the doctor and the auxiliary. Nowhere is *the doctor's role as organizer, teacher and consultant to a team of auxiliaries* more important than it is in the outpatient department. The only way in which huge numbers of patients can be seen is for medical assistants, and even dressers, to see most of them. Some means must be found whereby the common mild and easily recognizable complaints can be dealt with by these auxiliaries, without their wasting the scarce time of a doctor.

There are medical services which require that all patients be seen by a doctor no matter for how short a time. Pressure must be exerted to try to set such regulations altered and a sorting system instituted. This should make it possible for a doctor to spend not less than a minimum of say, ten minutes on each previously screened or sorted case. Depending on his experience he will of course be able to see cases much more rapidly, but this should not generally be his job.

Before considering sorting systems in more detail there are two things to be stressed. The first is the value of separating children from adults and organizing an under-fives clinic after the manner described in next chapter. This incidentally serves as a fine example of the general principles of organizing outpatient services. The right use of auxiliaries, the principle of sorting and the value of simple standardized regimes of deatment are all well demonstrated as too is the importance of carefully designed records.

The second is to are if it is possible to reduce the load on the outpatient department. Thus there is a general impression that those living near a hospital are see there other more frequently than perhaps they should be. There it will be seen that at zero distance from the hospital the average outpatient attends about six times yearly, or about once in two months. Quite apart from the question as to whether or not this is excessive, it is certainly fairer to discourage those living in the vicinity by first attending to those who come from a distance. Where record clerks ask for the patients' address, this is easily arranged.

In some hospitals the same excessive attendance is also true of policemen, prison officers and other government employees as well as schoolboys, all of whom frequently attend with only minor complaints. Many want light duty of time off work, and there are departments where they form as much as a third or even half of the entire outpatient load. Their employers and teachers complain about the hours spent at the hospital, and doctors about their wasted time. This unnecessary work can be reduced by restricting routine cases in these categories to special clinics that are held only once a week, say government employees on Wednesdays between 2 and 3 p.m. and schoolboys from 3 p.m. onwards. Urgent cases have to be seen at any time, but if they turn out not to be quite so urgent, they can be referred to this clinic (3).

Sorting systems. There are several ways in which patients can be sorted or screened and the particular method adopted will have to depend upon the staff available and the way in which the building is designed.

A THREE STAGE SORTING SYSTEM

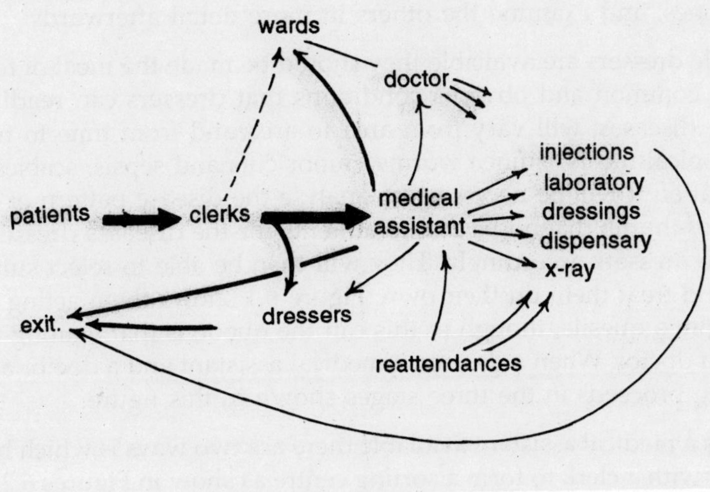

Fig. 6.1

THE SORTING CENTRE

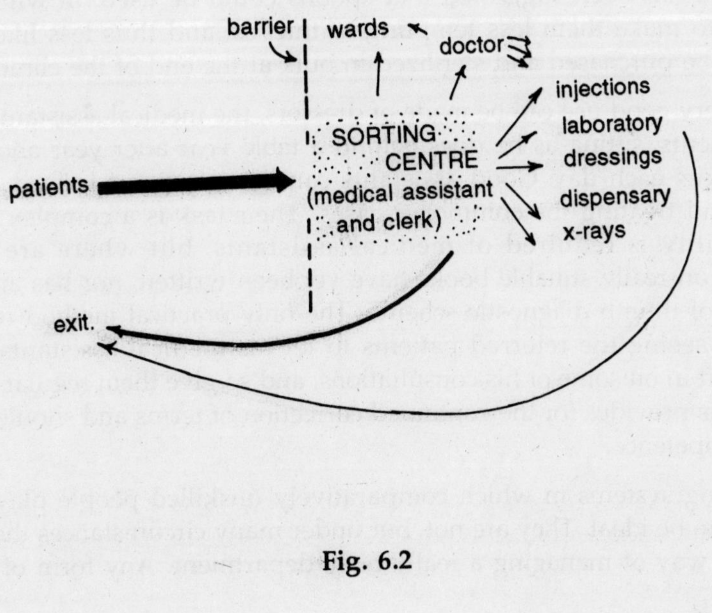

Fig. 6.2

The simplest situation is that where no suitable auxiliary staff are available whatever. Under these conditions the best thing a doctor can do is to stand his patients in a queue, and quickly screen or sort them himself. He can then rapidly prescribe treatment for the straightforward ones, and examine the others in more detail afterwards.

When suitable dressers are available they should be made the most of for many patients attend with such common and obvious conditions that dressers can readily diagnose and treat them. These diseases, will vary from area to area and from time to time and include such things as tropical ulcers, guinea worms, minor cuts and sepsis, scabies etc. Because of this regional variation it will be necessary to analyse the disease pattern of the department, to work out rule-of-thumb diagnoses and treatments for the diseases dressers can deal with and to teach these dressers accordingly. They will then be able to select suitable cases from waiting queues and treat them on their own. Figure 6.1 shows them acting in this way and diverting cases from a quesile, though in this can the queue is that waiting to see a medical assistant and not a doctor. When a dresser, a medical assistant and a doctor all work together in this way sorting proceeds in the three stages shown in this figure.

When there is a medical assistant available there are two ways is which he can work.One is for him to work with a clerk to form a sorting centre as show in Figures 6.2 and 6.3. He can also work on his own in an office like the doctor. This has been shown diagrammatically in Figure 6.1. No firm answer can be given about which is the best arrangement; but the closer a medical assistant approaches a doctor in skill the more use will he make of the facilities of an examination couch, and the more he will need a room on his own. The average medical assistant is probably better employed in a sorting centre. At his desk he will require a stethoscope, an auriscope, a magnetic headed Heaf gun , records on which to enter notifiable diseases, the common drugs in prepacked envelopes and some prescription forms which patients cantake to the dispensary for the less common drugs. Tongue depressors are a problem, and it has been suggested that spoons could be used, in which holes had been drilled, so as to make them less tempting to thieves, and thus less likely to be stolen. A number could be purchased and sterilized in bulk at the end of the clinic.

Though very good use can be made of dressers, the medical assistant is the backbone of many departments, sitting as he does behind a table year after year and seeing up to two hundred patients each day. Good assistants can be very good indeed at picking out the gravely sick and treating the commoner cases. Their task is a complex one. Considerable diagnostic ability is required of medical assistants, but where are they to learn it? Unfortunately, on really suitable books have yet been written, nor has anybody invented a workable rule-of-thumb diagnostic scheme. The only practical method of teaching them is for the doctor seeing the referred patients to let his medical assistants, and perhaps his dressers also sit in on some of his consultations, and so give them regular in-service training in this way. This provides for the continued correction of terms and should result in a steady increase in competence.

Such sorting systems in which comparatively unskilled people play a major role can hardly be said to be ideal. They are not, but under many circumstances they may be the best if not the only way of managing a really busy department. Any form of sorting system in

AN OUTPATIENT DEPARTMENT

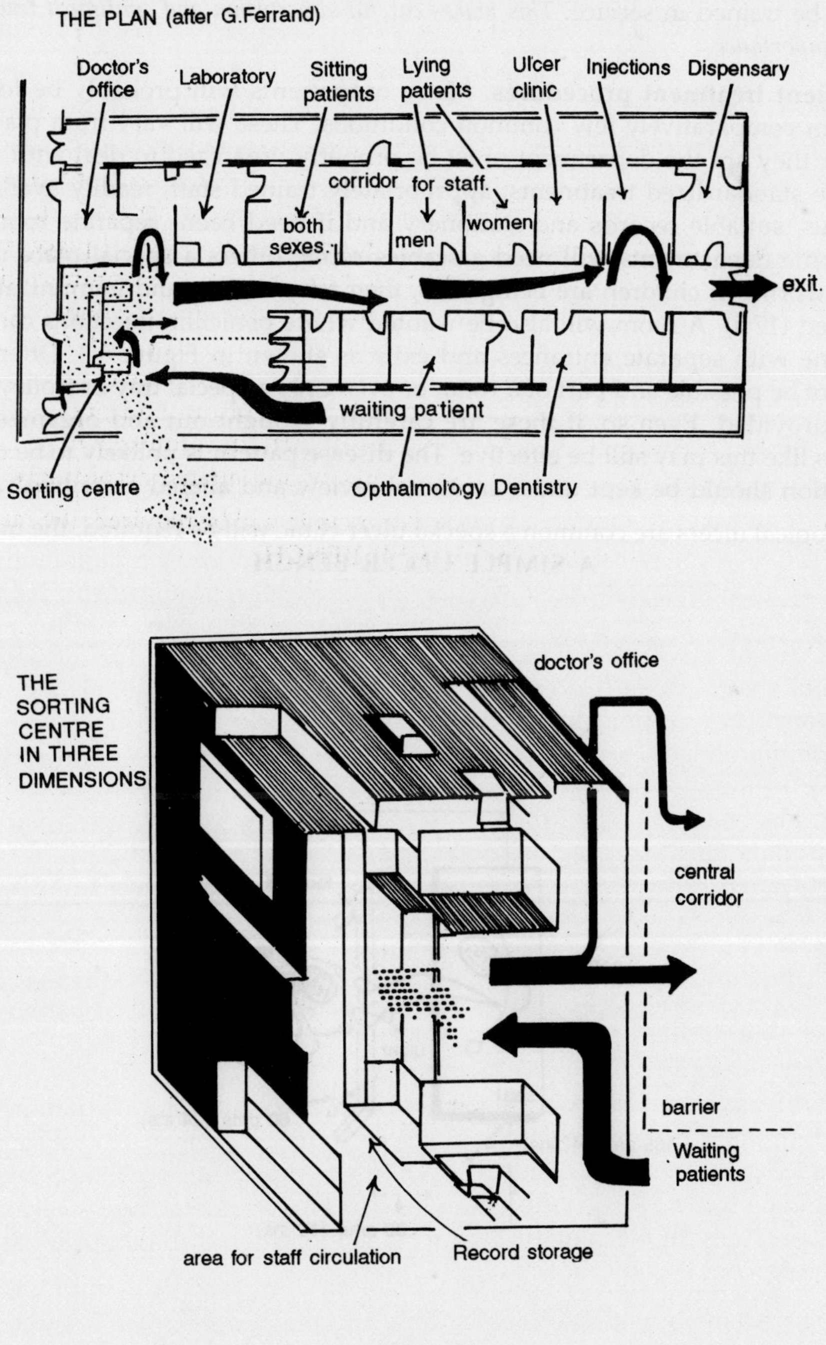

Fig. 6.3

which auxiliaries play a major part inevitably gives them great responsibility, particularly if they have to be trained in service. *This makes careful supervision and continued teaching of the very greatest importance.*

Outpatient treatment procedures. Many outpatients will probably be found to be suffering from comparatively few common conditions. These will vary from place to place but whatever they are the department must be properly organized to deal with them. This means simple standardized treatments, appropriately trained staff, readily available drugs and apparatus, suitable records and stationery and if need been separate room for each condition. Some departments will need a scabies room, others a special place for dealing with guinea worms. If children are being seen, then rehydration and immunization rooms will be wanted (17:5). A room will also be wanted where penicillin injections can be given, preferably one with separate entrances and exits as shown in Figure 6.3. Often, separate rooms will not be possible and part of a room or even only a special tray or trolley will be all that can be provided. Even so, if these are carefully thought out and organized, limited arrangements like this may still be effective. The disease pattern is unlikely to be constant so the organization should be kept under continual review and altered accordingly.

When tropical ulcers are common a special ulcer clinic will be required, the main feature

A SIMPLE ULCER BENCH

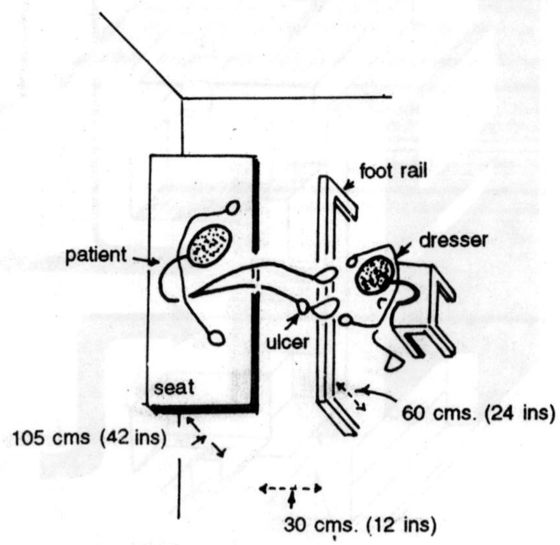

Fig. 6.4

of which should be a high bench where patient can sit while having their ulcers dressed. The one shown in Figure 6.4 has the advantage of being simple to construct and enables several patients to be treated at once.

Some dressings, examinations and treatments have to be given while the patient is lying down, but most of them can be given while patients sit. Sitting patients of both sexes can be attended to in the same room, but lying patients have to be separated. Because of this, big departments may find it practicable to have one big room for the seated patients of both sexes, and two separate smaller ones for the recumbent men and women. This arrangement is shown in Figure 6.3.

No hard and fast rules decide what can be done in an outpatient department and what can only be done in the wards. Some procedures,lumbar puncture for example, are normally thought of as only being done on inpatients, yet it may be very inconvenient to admit the patient for this procedure. When this is so it is very useful to be able to do a lumbar puncture in the outpatient department on young children who might have meningitis. If the fluid is purulent the diagnosis is likely to be straightforward and can be confirmed with a film stained by Gram's method. When the fluid is not purulent Pandy's test and a quick cell count only take a moment and can, if necessary, easily be done by the doctor himself.

Even a rudimentary outpatient laboratory or side room will be found very convenient. Many of the techniques in previous Chapter are likely to be required, and it may be easier to do them on the spot rather than have the patient wait at the main laboratory.

The patient's time. A patient's time is valuable to him, so that anything which will speed the flow of patients through the department is well worth the effort. The importance of reducing the work of the records clerk, the usefulness of patients keeping their own records in ploythene envelopes, the use of rubber stamps albeit in another connection, and the value of a reconized system of shorthand clinical symbols. All these points can save time in the outpatient department, as can the use of prepacked drugs and medicines on the assistant's table, for this makes it is necessary for patients to queue at the dispensary. If fees have to be collected, a cash register is another valuable time saver. A common cause of wasted time is for medical assistants to keep their own record ledgers. As they see so many patients in a day this unnecessary, local work adds up to a significant proportion of their time. This writing should be done by clerks, so that medical assistants can use their scarce skills more profitably.

It is often difficult to get patients to reattend on the correct day. When this is so the use of a set of rubber stamps with the days of the week in the vernacular may be useful, the patients being handed a slip of paper with the appropriate day of reattendance stamped upon it.

Buildings. Because an outpatient department is usually crowded with people who flow all round it and so impede the smooth running of the hospital, it is best sited a little apart from the wards. There are two general approaches to planning it, but both depend on the need to separate the staff from milling crowds of patients.

The first is to let the patients wait on wide verandahs outside the building while the staff remain inside. Under this system patients present at hatches for such things as records and drugs, and are allowed to circulate through limited parts of the building only, preferably through adjacent doors for their easy entry and exit. Such an arrangement is cheap, it is possibly the best system for comparatively small units, and has been termed the 'Fort Plan'. In Figure 6.5 it is shown in two sizes, one, a very small department indeed (A) and the other, a department large enough to provide a central courtyard in which the staff may circulate (B).

The second and more usual method is to keep both patients and staff inside the building, to provide them with separate means of circulation, and to erect some form of barrier to control patient entry. The control point in this barrier is the sorting centre. This system can be arranged in several different ways. One of these is that used in the under fives clinic in. Here the clerks sit behind a desk and let mothers through gates in a barrier. This gives them access to a passage along with they pass to the nurses rooms. The clerks supervise the mothers and weigh the children, but real sorting is done by the nurses.

The relationship of the barrier and the sorting centre to the building as a whole is planned differently in the outpatient department shown in Figure 6.3. This is derived from French experience in West Africa and is very ingenious. The patients arrive, queue on the verandah, and are seen by a medical assistant in a sorting centre. They then pass through a barrier into the central corridor. Some are directed to see the doctor whose consulting room closely adjoins the sorting centre; most however, pass to the several clinics which run the length of the building Staff access is provided down one side of the department by an inter-connecting passage between the clinics, and provision is made for it to grow by the addition of more rooms at one end.

A type of outpatient department which should be mentioned is that built at Bikumbi in Tanzania and shown in Figure 6.5c. Here a long near building has, as it were, been snapped in half and its two halves put together to form an 'A'. This 'A' has then been roofed over, a records department placed at its apex and sliding doors provided along its base. The waiting hall thus formed is of interesting and elegant proportion, it can be blacked out for educational lantern shows and, since no additional walling was required, it was cheap of construct. A feature that is not shown in this diagram is the provision made to post the patients records from one room to another by slots made in the walls. No final conclusion can be given as to which is the best system, but that shown in Figure 6.3 is the most carefully worked out. Its great disadvantage is the large numbers of patients who tend to crowd the central corridor of the building.

Improving an outpatient department. An outpatient department can be likened to a factory or production line for making cured outpatients. Looked at like this, from the point of view of the production manager in a factory, with his emphasis on the work study and job analysis, the faults of a department will become more obvious. Some of the things that might be done to an existing department can be summarized like this:

FURTHER OUTPATIENT DEPARTMENTS

A. THE FORT PLAN

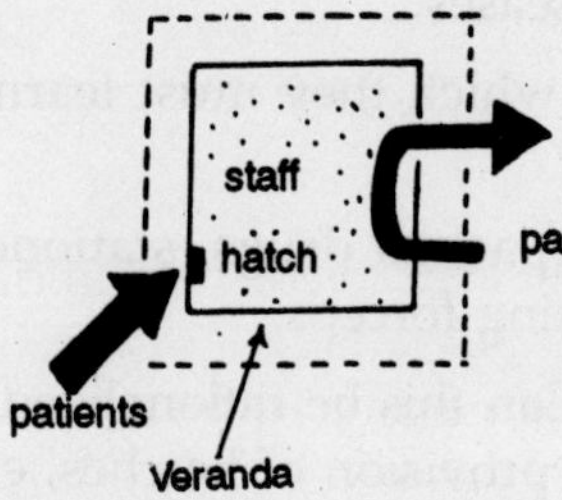

PRINCIPLE: patients stay outside the department as much as possible so letting the staff move around inside it.

B. THE FORT PLAN ENLARGED

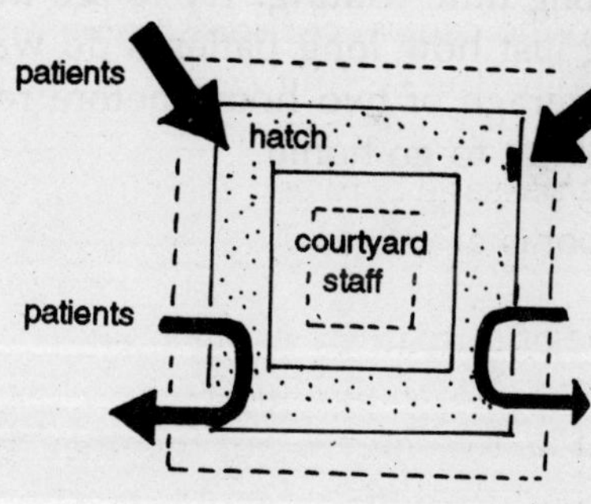

C. THE 'V' PLAN

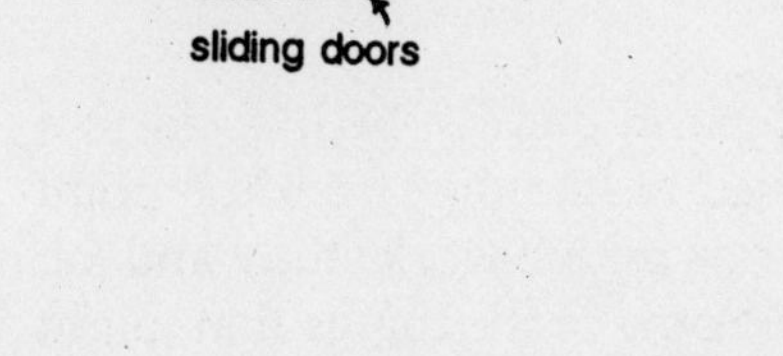

Fig. 6.5

Method: Improving the outpatient department

Analyse the diagnoses of the patients attending, find their six most common diseases.

Determine the samplest, cheapest and most effective routine for treating these diseases. Cut out any unnecessary treatments.

Teach auxiliaries how to diagnose and treat these diseases.

Pay particular attention to more serious conditions which they must learn to distinguish from them.

Provide the relevant equipment, rubber stamps, prepacked drugs, stationery, etc., and especially enough of the simple things like dressing forceps.

Trace the flow of the patients through the building. Can this be rationalized by simple works services such as the alteration of doors, the provision of hatches, etc.?

Examine the queues that form. What is the cause of the delays? Can these be removed by altering the disposition of staff, providing more auxiliaries, reducing unnecessary clerical work or providing additional apparatus?

Where relevant let the auxiliaries listen in on your consultations with the referred cases, so that they may learn continually.

Whatever the success of the above measures, some patients are probably still going to spend a long time waiting. Try to see that they wait in reasonable comfort. It is sometimes surprising just how long patients do wait; in the Mulago Hill Dispensary they are said to wait an average of two hours before registering and to spend a further two houn before finally leaving to go home.

7

The Architecture of Hospitals and Health Centres

The organic nature of a hospitals: Like its patients, a hospital is alive. In Africa some begin as tiny dispensaries and eventually grow to become thriving institutions of several hundred beds. New departments are added, others are adapted and sometimes old wards are pulled down to make room for new. The flux of continued alteration thus complicates the simplicity of mere growth.

Few doctors and not many architects create a whole hospital from scratch. Many however alter and add to them—a new kitchen here, a new mortuary there and an isolation ward somewhere else. But unless this continued creative activity proceeds to some plan, it ends in that untidy and inefficient chaos which so many hospitals demonstrate too well.

The cardinal principle for those planning to build or enlarge a hospital progressively over the years, is to ask an architect with experience in hospital planning to draw out a 'master development plan'—early in the hospital's life. This will make it possible for such expensive and basic services as drainage to be planned with cheapness and efficiency. A master plan is not expensive and saves money in the long run because by his training, an architect is aware of many subtleties that a layman is not.

Although hospitals are the subject of most of this chapter, much of what is said here, particularly that pertaining to cheap methods of construction, applies equally to health centres. Plans for these units are supplied as Figure 11 (3:3).

The adaptation of structure to function. Essentially, the fabric of a hospital is but a box to protect and support the human activities that go on inside it. It must thus be intimately adapted to the needs of both the patients and the staff. What does the tropical villager require when he comes into hospital? This must be uppermost in the mind of the designer, and, had it been better understood, there would not be hospitals in Africa costing millions of pounds where relatives have to sleep on the stairs, because nobody thought about building a hostel for them when the place was built.

The following pages describe some important adaptations to the requirements of the tropical peasant—a mothers' shelter, a hospital garden, benches at the height local people like, the maternity village—these are all adaptations to specific human needs. As they will vary in detail from country to country, careful enquiry into the local preferences must precede any attempt to draw up a plan (Twelfth axiom 1:19).

Space for expansion. No restriction is finally so absolute as a shortage of space. A health centre requires about 3 hectares (7 acres), and a 250 bedded hospital not less than 16 hectares (40 acres). All medical units must thus have a site on which they can grow. Later on the only alternative may be an entirely new structure in another place. This may sometimes be the best course, but so much money is likely to have been invested already that it may be cheaper to go on adding than to rebuild completely on another site.

Not only must all new units have adequate space, but they must also be laid out so that each further addition completes a pre-arranged plan, and be so zoned that shell buildings are kept apart to allow the ordered growth of the central nucleus — it is a pity to have later to pull down a solid useful, but badly sited house to make way for a ward. One point is quite clear in this regard. It is, that, provided the size of a site is adequate and there are no, overwhelming objections as far as the position of the hospital is concerned. It is usually more economical to pull down some of the existing buildings and replan the same site than it would be to build a new hospital of a *similar kind* on another site. If a single storey pavilion style hospital is to be replaced by a multi-storied one this is another matter. But to replace a pavilion style hospital by one of the same kind, albeit better laid out, is likely to be a major waste of resources.

If a new hospital is to be built it should be put up these to the old, for it is certain not to be long before they will both be in use, the new one for the general care of the sick and the old one for a wide variety of other purposes. This is what has happened at Mulago where one new hospital was erected close to the old. The buildings of the latter now form the nutrition rehabilitation unit (14:17), the orthopeadic workshops, the psychiatric outpatient department besides serving many other functions also. The value of making use of old buildings in this way is as great in a district hospital as it is in a national one.

A building can serve a succession of functions during a hospital's life—for example, one which serves both for outpatients and inpatients when the unit is still small can later be adapted for outpatients alone. This flexibility is all important in hospital planning, and is made easier by building to a 'module', such as the commonly accepted one of 100 cms. (40 ins). If the design is drawn wherever possible in units of this length, subsequent alteration will be easier, particularly if the roof is supported on posts and the walls made of panelling which can be modified as required.

Money is often so short that a new building is not put up until it is long overdue, but when eventually it is built, it must be adapted not only to the needs of the present but also to those of the future. It must, as it were, 'leap-frog' today's requirements and be ready for those of tomorrow.

Earlier in the book it was stressed that a health centre is not to be looked upon as an embryo hospital and that these are two distinct units with separate and complementary functions (3:1). The prospect of a health centre growing to become a hospital should not therefore be a common one,but there will be some occasions when a health centre will ultimately be replaced by a hospital, so building must be planned accordingly. An ingenious

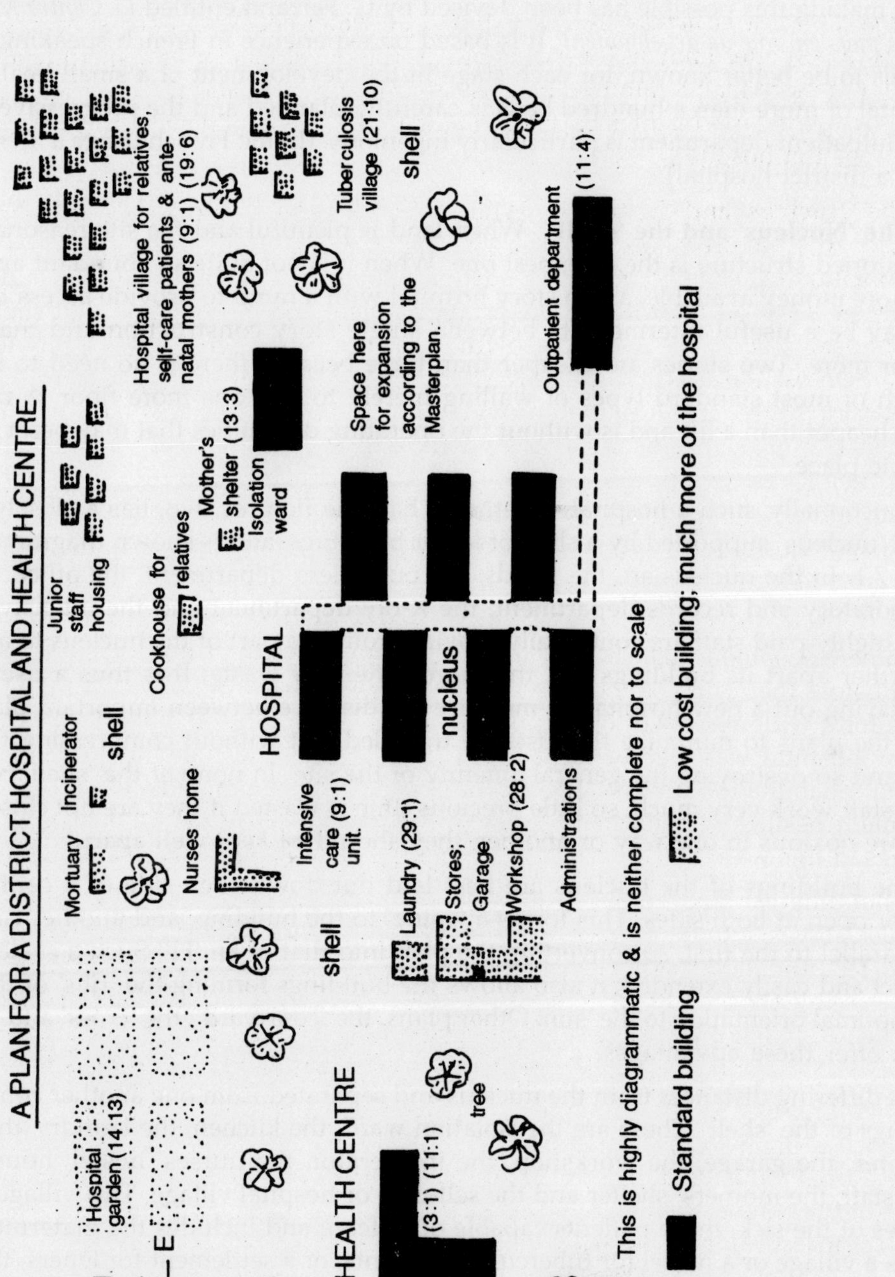
A PLAN FOR A DISTRICT HOSPITAL AND HEALTH CENTRE
N
E
S
W
Hospital garden (14:13)
Mortuary
Incinerator
shell
Junior staff housing
Cookhouse for relatives
Mother's shelter (13:3)
Isolation ward
Hospital village for relatives, self-care patients & ante-natal mothers (9:1) (19:6)
Tuberculosis village (21:10)
shell
Nurses home
HOSPITAL
Intensive care (9:1) unit
nucleus
shell
Laundry (29:1)
Stores; Garage
Workshop (28:2)
Administrations
Space here for expansion according to the Masterplan.
Outpatient department (11:4)
HEALTH CENTRE
(3:1) (11:1)
tree
This is highly diagrammatic & is neither complete nor to scale
Standard building
Low cost building; much more of the hospital

Fig. 7.1

way of making this possible has been devised by G. Ferrand entitled *Le Centre Medical Rural dans les pays en voie de development*. It is based on experience in French-speaking Africa and deserves to be better known, for each stage in the development of a small health centre to a hospital of more than a hundred beds is carefully planned and the progressive adaptation of the outpatient department is particularly ingenious. (In the French usage a *'Centre Medical'* means a district hospital).

The 'Nucleus' and the 'shell'. When land is plentiful and the site reasonably level, a single storied structure is the, cheapest one. When it is not quite so abundant and there is a little more money available, a two story hospital with a ramp to provide access to the upper one may be a useful intermediate between single story construction and that involving three or more. Two stories are cheaper than three because there is no need to increase the strength of most standard types of walling merely to add one more floor. A ramp is also much cheaper than a lift and is without the operating difficulties that may beset the latter in a remote place.

Functionally, such a hospital, whether it has one floor or two, has a closely integrated central 'nucleus' supported by a shell of lesser buildings, and is shown diagrammatically in Figure 7.1. In the nucleus are the wards, the outpatient department, the office, the theatre, the laboratory and records department, the X-ray department and the intensive care unit. Scarce highly paid staff are continually moving from one part of the nucleus to another, and the further apart its buildings are, the more time they waste. It is thus a useful exercise when laying out a new hospital, to measure the distance between important places, and to adjust the plans to minimize the distance travelled, yet without compressing the plan too much and so destroying the general amenity of the site. In none of the 'shell' buildings do senior staff work very much, so little precious time is wasted if they are not close by, and as some are noxious in one way or another, they should be kept well apart.

The buildings of the nucleus are best laid out down each side of a central covered corridor open at both sides. This forms a 'spine' to the building, and another can be added later parallel to the first, so converting the plan into that of an 'H'. Such a system is cheap, compact and easily extended; it also allows the buildings forming the 'ribs' of the spine the same optimal orientation to the sun. Other plans, the 'courtyard', the 'cross' and the 'spider', do not offer these advantages.

At differing distances from the nucleus and separated from one another come the lesser buildings of the 'shell'. These are the isolation ward, the kitchen, the laundry, the mortuary, the stores, the garage, the workshop, the incinerator, the nurses' hostel, housing for the junior staff, the mothers' shelter and the self-care or hospital village. This village houses the relatives of the sick, those patients capable of selfcare and includes the maternity village. If there is a village or a hostel for tuberculous patients, or a settlement for lepers, these should be separate again. One hospital has even built a profitable motel for the relatives of its richer patients. If the relation are expected to cook for the patients, a cookhouse for them has also to be provided among the shell buildings.

There is some difference of opinion on the best position for the outpatient department. If it is too close to the wards it may be difficult to control visitors, yet if it is too far away it is inconvenient for the outpatients to make use of such services as the laboratory and the X-ray department.

The site of the doctor's house is critical. If a doctor visits the hospital four times a day and many visit it more often, he will travel an additional 165 miles each year for every extra hundred yards that separates his home from the hospital. Close proximity thus saves much time.

Orientation. In the tropics east facing windows get the morning sun and those facing west get it in the afternoon; those looking either north or south get almost none. To make the most of this and keep them cool, buildings should therefore be sited with their long axis running east and west letting their corridors, particularly the axial spine, run north and south.

In hot wet cloudy regions, where air movement may be more important than protection from the sun's rays, buildings will be more comfortable if they are turned to catch the breeze as suitable sun screens can always be provided if necessary. Under other conditions there may have to be a compromise between the orientation demanded by the sun and that best for the prevailing wind; this must however always be used to blow away smoke and smells from the kitchen, the mortuary and the incinerator.

Building methods (the editor). The need for really cheap ways of building hospitals and health centres is a recurrent theme in this symposium, for cheap building is one of the keys to making medical care more widely available in developing countries where capital is so critically scarce. This has been discussed under the Third axiom where medical care was considered in the light of the demands of an inter mediate technology. It was pointed out that the amount of medical care that can be provided is determined by the number of medical workers that can be employed, and, that in addition to needing training, each needs the tools of his trade and the buildings in which to work. As far as auxiliaries are concerned training costs are comparatively cheap, so also is equipment. Building are the really expensive item in the provision of a medical job, and thus of medical care. Just how important building costs are is shown in section, where they amounted to as much as 83 per cent of the capital cost of one district hospital.

If the need for cheap buildings is great, how is the cost of buildings compared and what order of difference separates a cheap building from a costly one?

Building costs vary considerably from country to country, and also from one region to another depending on availability of materials and the cost of labour and transport. Also, with the rising standards of living in the developing countries, the cost of building rises steadily, but the present average costs in Uganda are as follows. Expensive buildings cost about 60/- or more a square foot ($72 a sq. metre), and average ones of conventional pattern about 40/- a square foot ($48 a sq. metre). Some mansion hospitals manage to build in burnt brick for as little as 10/- a square foot ($12 a sq. metre). When unburnt bricks, *'pise de rerre'* or 'mud and, wattle-and-whitewash', are used even cheaper buildings can be constructed. Satisfactory structures of this kind can sometimes be built even for as little as 5/- a square foot ($6 a sq. metre). These then are the sort of savings that can be made in building costs, but in being asked to make them the reader must first be convinced that cheap buildings need result in no material diminution in the quality of the medical care going on inside them. What effect does the quality of a building have on the outcome of a patient's illness, either directly or indirectly through its effect on the staff?

There are several misconceptions to be cleared away in attempting to answer this. One is that there are some parts of any hospital which should perhaps be of accepted construction; these include the theatre and possibly the intensive care unit. But cheaper methods can be used for much of the rest of it, especially for the self-care unit, and there is no reason why a hospital or even a building should be constructed to the same standards throughout. A hospital built in several different ways is a break with tradition, but, as the second axiom implies breaks with tradition may sometimes be necessary.

Another is that cheap buildings should necessarily be badly laid out, for cheap building methods need have little effect on the general plan of a single story district hospital, and the conveniences of an efficient and logical arrangement are likely to be obtainable just as easily with cheap building techniques as they are expensive ones. Although short spans are cheaper to build than wide ones, cheap methods of construction are without any great effect on such matters as the closeness with which patients are packed in a ward, or with the width of verandahs and passages, etc. In effect, cheap buildings do not imply lack of space; the necessary number of square feet of floor area can be provided quite as easily in a mud walled building as in one of standard construction.

In most areas the local mud-built buildings have tiny windows, or sometimes none at all, so there is a natural tendency to associate buildings of this kind with a dim interior. Though window frames are more expensive than an equivalent expanse of wall, a mud-built ward can readily be equipped with as much window space as required. This is likely to be cheaper if window frames are of wood rather than metal. Although mosquito gauze may have medical advantages in a warm climate, there is no medical reason for putting glass in a window, providing it can be closed with wooden shutters. If the eaves of the building are wide, as is necessary with mud walls these will seldom have to be closed except in very windy weather. The idea that glazed windows are medically necessary in the this is a convention imported from cold countries where they and needed to retain heat.

The reader will have been thinking about the walls and the floor. A floor that can be sluiced out is essential in many parts of a hospital, but a mud-built ward can well have a concrete floor, though a mud floor may serve the office or the stores quite satisfactorily. Staff housing forms such a large part of a hospital's cost that it may well be justified to reduce the cost of a dresser's house by building it in mud, after all, this is likely to be what he is used to and it will help in making it possible to employ more of them. Mud walls can be plastered with cement and cement can be painted, they can also be plastered with mud, and white washed as often as monthly if necessary.

Lastly, there is the morale of the staff, it benefits nobody to work under conditions of squalor. But mud buildings do not imply squalor, nor do they imply dirt; they can well mean trim wards, frequently scrubbed, patched and whitewashed, and carefully kept in good repair by someone whose special task this is. At the mission hospital from which this section is written there are tin-roofed, unburnt mud brick buildings which look as tidy as they presumably did when they were built fifty years before. Admittedly the squalid tumbledown houses seen in most tropical villages are built by some of the very methods that are being advocated, but the reason for their untidiness is that they were probably badly built anyway, even according to their own standards of construction, and have certainly been badly maintained ever since. Buildings well constructed in unburnt brick, *'pise de terre'*, 'mud-wattle-and whitewash', or whatever other cheap method is used, and roofed with corrugated sheeting, need not be squalid, provided they are well planned, properly put together, and kept in good repair. When this is so they are difficult to tell from brick ones. Maintenance is critical, and it may meat employing extra staff. But there is no difficulty about this, because suitable artisans need not be highly paid. Reckoning that one of them will earn £100 ($280) a year, this sum represents the 5 per cent, interest that might be expected on a capital investment of ƒ2,000 ($5,600). Thus, if this sum can be saved on the capital costs of a hospital, one man can be hired indefinitely whole time to look after it. Even a 7 per cent, reduction in the cost of the hospital building would have freed enough capital in provide man's wages to maintain it. Considering that a 50 per cent reduction may be possible (20/- instead of 40/- a square foot), it will be seen that cheap building methods can both provide for a substantial net saving and take account of increased maintenance costs. When health centres have to be maintained, the staff could well be taught to do at least the simpler aspect of this themselves.

It is for health centres and district hospitals rather than for regional and national ones, that cheap methods of construction are so greatly needed and so very appropriate. Regional and particularly national hospitals become inconveniently spread out if not built in several stories, and therefore they have to be of standard construction. Following from this, it is thus rural rather than urban building that is suited to these methods. Looked at overall, health centres and district hospitals should in aggregate form the largest fraction of the total buildings of a health service. Thus Uganda has one national teaching hospital, four regional ones, about 25 district hospitals (excluding missions), and she should have no less than 400 health centres, even at the rate of one for 20,000 people. But, even allowing for the differing sizes of the units considered, a large fraction of the total volume of building in a health service is suitable for construction by cheap methods.

There is another side of cheap buildings — they can be built by the people themselves, mostly from readily available local materials. In Zambia for instance the local co-operatives regularly entrusted with minor health building in the rural areas. If the local authority want a health centre or a district hospital they could be given plans and manuals 16/- and told to build to a good standard, either all of it, or their share of it, after which the health department would be prepared to complete equip, and staff it. If the local labour can be voluntary, this will be of great assistance in creating capital in the form of building where there was none before.

With the exception of certain mission hospitals, which have of necessity led the way, medical profession and the educated public in developing countries are deeply committed psychologically to the `white corridors' attitude in hospital construction, and any different approach requires radical rethinking. This is enormous impediment to the expansion of district hospital and health centre services in developing countries, to the provision of some services for everyone rather than unnecessarily lavish accommodation for the few.

SOLAR HEATING

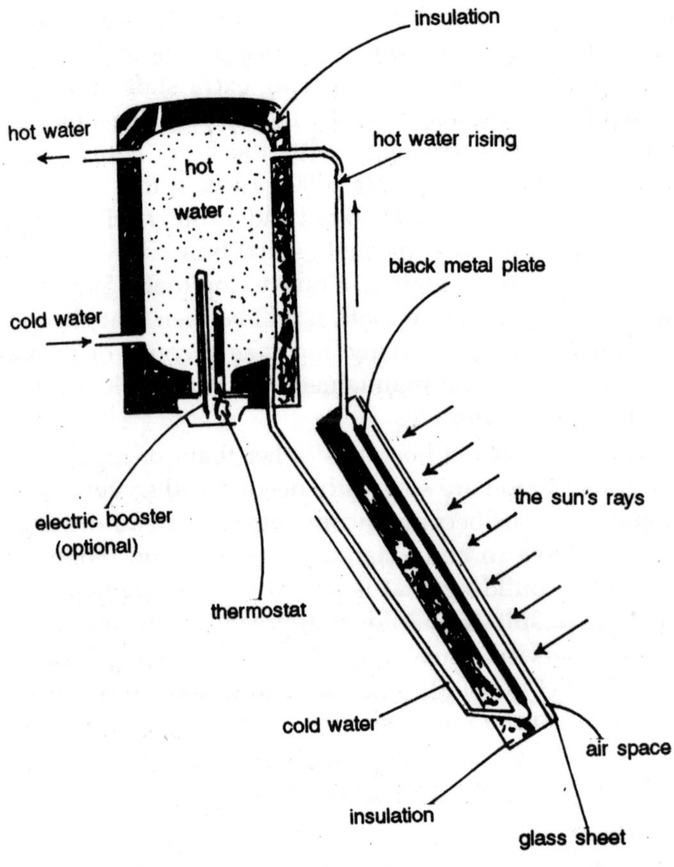

The cheap buildings that are being advocated so strongly are in one sense the very negation of architecture, which is the reason why this section is written by the editor and not by an architect. Yet they are in another sense completely in line with its true spirit — the creation of buildings perfectly adapted to their purpose, which in this case is the housing of medical facilities in the conditions of poverty.

A hospital or health centre is often judged on its look, and though smart buildings may reassure an anxious minister or placate performing electorate, they do not always mean good medicine — this book ends with some better criteria for judging these units than the elegance of their architecture.

Presbrication. Because prefabricated buildings do little to raise employment especially if they are imported and because they are likely to be less economical than the methods that have just been advocated, buildings of this kind should be thought of as being primarily gor emergency use, or for places where local building material are not available fabricated buildings are made by many manufactured but those supplied by one of them (COS) arrive packed in flat crates complete with fittings and a book of easy instructions. They are of heavy gauge aluminum sheets with straight sided 4 cm. corrugations. Such sheets are rigid enough to support the roof without the need for a separate framework, and in the middle of Africa buildings of this type have been erected for as little as 20/- a square foot ($24 a sq. metre)— less than the cost of much traditional construction. A whole hospital can be bought complete.

Only a really solid buildings will keep out noise, but aluminium is a good heat reflector and its thermal qualities can be improved further by lining the building with sheets of expanded polystyrene or other insulation.

Solar water heating. Hot water is perhaps a luxury, but if the sun's rays can be used to provide the heat, it becomes more economic because there are no running costs. Techniques have recently become much more efficient and Figure 7.2 shows how a black-painted metal plate on the roof of a building can, in suitable climates, collect enough heat to provide a useful quantity of hot water (MIR). Such a plate is set at a slight slope, covered by a glass sheet and backed by an insulator. To it is brazed a small bore brass pipe; the water in this pipe collects heat from the plate and rises by convection to be stored in a tank. This device is satisfactory in a wide range of tropical climates and collects heat radiated from the clouds as well as that direct from the sun. Where dull weather might mean a period of cold water an electric booster can be fitted, but this is a luxury. Initial expenses are comparatively low, and a domestic plant costs only about £100 ($280). In Kenya such a plant pays for itself in as little as two years.

The Rural Doctor His Own Architect

Do it self. Most buildings, particularly of those of the nucleus are jobs for an architect, but there are others which need not be, and it may be a choice between not having a building at all or having something which will do. The rural doctor is therefore encouraged to get permission from his superiors, to enlist the help of the local chief, to obtain some money from the local authority and to construct the cheap accommodation that his hospital or health centres need. Volunteers can build very useful structures and all sorts of buildings will probably be required. Housing for relatives or the junior staff, a mothers' shelter and underfives clinics are some of the buildings that are so often in short supply.

One of glories of practice in the rural areas is this 'factotum' quality and a little buildings is an important part of it. Not all doctors are handy out many of the old hospitals particularly those of the missions would not exist at all but for the ingenuity of their staff. In its proper proportion 'the do-it- yourself tradition is thus a valuable one. The doctor's role in it is that of architect or 'clerk of works' and, as in other spheres, it is his task to initiate and organize the work of his helpers.

Methods and Manuals for the Amateur. There is an admirable series of cheap, well illustrated manuals for the amateur builder in the tropics /6/. These are designed for the villager, and, with the classic volume by R.F. Longland /94/, they should enable the novice to start work.

Mud-and-wattle and sun dried brick are both well known constructional methods, but some other simple techniques could also be useful.

'Pise de terre' is carefully selected earth mixed to a stiff paste with a little chopped straw and water. This is then firmly rammed between strong temporary wooden shuttering, like that used for reinforced concrete, and left to solidity before this shuttering is removed. Because no cement is employed, a wall of this kind must, like unburnt brick, be well protected from driving rains by verandahs or deeply overhanging eaves. Both the top and the bottom of these walls also need protection with good damp proof courses.

'Stabilized earth' employs soil mixed to a paste with water and 5.10 per cent of cement. This mixture is then cast into blocks on the site either by hand or machine, in the same way as concrete blocks. The common East African 'murram' and West African 'swish' both serve well, and if well made with sufficient cement, they will support a three story building for many years.

Precast concrete post construction is another useful building method. The posts are used to support the roof, and the panels between then filled in with any of a variety of cheap local materials, such as mud-and-wattle, thatch, 'tin', or asbestos sheeting. Such a building is cheap, the roof stays up, and the panels can be renewed as required.

Not only can several constructional techniques be used in the same hospital but several can with advantage be used in the same building. Thus, the lower courses and the arches of a wall can be burnt brickset in cement mortar rest of it can be sun dried brick set in mud.

Termites. This is an important and complex problem, particularly in cheaper buildings and it is difficult to provide detailed advice. The local pest control firm will probably be the best source of information, but there are some general principles that may be useful.

Termites like moisture and only work in the dark — see therefore that no unnecessary water lies around the building that, waste water is discharged some way away that there are no leaking pipes and that the lower walling is so close that it is difficult for termites to enter. Don't let the builders leave bits of wood lying around in the soil which will attract termites to the buildings above.

If possible, provide a termite proof layer right through the building just above the ground level; a good barrier is made by an 8cm. (3 inch) layer of good concrete which forms the floor of the building and extends across the foundation to project outside them an inch all round. The walls are later built on top of this layer, taking care that they are *exactly* positioned over the foundations.

In areas where the termite is well established, and some of the precautions above are too expensive, treat the foundation trenches, and all the ground on which the building is to stand, with 4½ litres (1 gallon) of 0.3% Dieldrin emulsion per square metre and rake this in to a depth of 15 cms. (6 ins.). To make this even more secure, dig a trench 40 cms. (15 ins.) deep and the same width all round the building, and apply the same solution to the trench at the rate of 2 litres (½ gallon) to each metre (3 ft.) of its length. Replace the soil and treat this with the emulsion in the same way.

`Mud-wattle-Dieldrin-and-whitewash'. Even when untreated good mud walled buildings can last fifteen years and more. Nobody yet knows how long they will last if they are protected from termites by the incorporation of a residual insecticide actually in the mud of the walls and the foundations beneath them. It is likely however that insecticides like Dieldrin have completely changed the economics of cheap buildings, which can now be expected to last very much longer. Not only can Dieldrin be used with mud-and-wattle, it can also be used with *'pise de terre'*. and stabilized earth, etc. The local pest control firm will provide the necessary Dieldrin for these operations, its cost on a new building being only 30 per square foot ($.36 per sq. metre). As it is underneath the floor and the foundations no harm can come from its toxic effects, while it is so stable that it protects the building above indefinitely. Such danger as does occur from its use arises while it is being applied so Dieldrin solutions should be treated with care.

A recent suggestion from Australia for termite proofing concrete with Dieldrin may prove of great practical value in the construction of low-cost housing. It has been shown by the Division of Entomology. Canberra, that a durable barrier is made when the mixing water in both normal and 'no-fines' concrete is replaced by 0.5% emulsion of Dieldrin (i.e. 2.1\2 lbs. of 20% emulsifiable concentrate in 10 gallons of water). It is not yet known how long this will remain effective, but it allows the use of less well compacted concrete for slabs and checks the movement of termites upwards through small cracks.

Not only can new buildings be treated, but old infested ones can also, and their life prolonged indefinitely by piercing holes through the floor and injecting Dieldrin solution into the ground underneath.

Some constructional hints. Use arches to support the roof, for they are both elegant and economical, and can even be incorporated in a mud wall if the arch itself is mortared with cement or, as in West Africa, reinforced with lengths of timber from the fan-palm.

Use tiles for small spans only and make sure that any roof of asbestos sheet is firmly supported, because if this moves, these sheets will crack. Because roof spans are more expensive than mud walls, small buildings of this kind are likely to be cheaper than larger ones.

Be careful about the quality of timber, sheeting and bricks. Timber must be seasoned, free from termites and preferably pressure impregnated. Sheeting should be of a good gauge (e.g. 26 or 29) — if it is too thin it bends easily and if badly galvanized it soon rusts. In default of more refined testing methods, leave sample bricks and blocks in the sun all day, and in a bucket of water all night for at least a week. Accept the batch as fit for the building only if these specimens retain their shape and weight.

Mud walls should be finished with whitewash, either straight on the mud, or on top of a mud and sand or cowdung and sand plaster, which are the best cheap surfacings for these walls. Paint soon flakes off a mud surface. A cement plaster does too, unless it is bonded to the walls, either with a mesh of fine wire netting or, as is commonly done in Buganda with a layer of reeds. The external corners of mud or cowdung plastered walls need protection, so do places where they might be rubbed by furniture, such as hospital beds for example.

Hang cupboards, shelves, equipment and working surfaces on the walls themselves, so leaving the floor underneath free to be swept more easily. This will be simpler if provision is made for their support while the wall is actually being built. Build benches into the brickwork during its construction, by incorporating battens going right through the — to which planks can later be screwed and form a bench either side of the wall. Make these benches 40 cms. (16 ins.) from the floor, the height most villagers prefer, and incorporate them in every suitable wall, particularly those of the outpatient department.

Grace and amenity. Though it is difficult to achieve beauty, it should always be possible to achieve amenity — many small points countries to the comfort of the patients and none are too small to be forgotten.

Provide outpatients with shade in which to wait, something to — on, a supply of drinking water and convenient latrines. If the hospital is a responsible size, see if someone cannot be persuaded to open a shop or canteen to serve them.

Children appreciate amenities as well as adults, so see if space will be found for a playground with a swing and a climbing frame. Such playground will require a latrine, and it may be best to provide one of the deep trench kind specially built for children. This will need a squatting plate containing a hole small enough for there to be no danger of anybody falling through, say 20 x 12 cms.

The graciousness of a building depends as much on the proportions and layout of the spaces enclosed, as it does on the structures which do the enclosing. This 'sculpturing of space' is one of the architectural arts, and while planning, it is well to think carefully about the proportions of any spaces enclosed, be they rooms, courtyards, or merely the spaces between buildings. When laying out a hospital give it some focal point, such as an entrance arch, a waiting hall, or an avenue.

The 'hospital garden' and its usefulness in health education has been stressed elsewhere (6:8). It should be planted with the crops that patients can grow in their own fields or *shambas* to improve their nutrition, as well as that of their families. Because such a garden is an agricultural as well as a medical endeavour, the Agricultural Department may be prepared to help with it as part of their own extension drive. Plant flowers, grow trees for shade and ornament, and so that they may be mature when needed, plant them where the 'master development plan' shows that they will later be wanted. A hospital should be a gay and pleasant place, so obtain educational posters, hang pictures and get someone to paint murals. There may be no money for these extras in the ordinary vote, but it may be possible to find a benefactor. Try approaching a few of the rich shopkeepers of the area, and remind them that their names will not be forgotten.

In the quest for functional efficiency don't forget that a hospital is more than a place in which to cure and be cured, it is also a human habitation — somewhere to be secure, comfortable and content. Hospitals differ greatly in the feeling they impart, their ambience, their general atmosphere, this almost intangible 'something'. Such an emanation is the sum of many things; the loyalty and devotion of *all* the staff contribute most of it, but every little detail plays its part. Near notices, flowers tidy grounds, clean wards and passages all have an effect and are worth striving after, for they add to the lives of those who heal and are healed within a hospital.

8

Medical Records

The importance of good records. To many readers, the title 'Medical Records' will probably bring to mind visions of inky fingered clerks covering in an infinitely laboured hand page after laborious page of a dog-eared ledger; of outpatient forms so grubby, porous and ephemeral that they almost melt in the hand; of queues interminable and of cardboard cartons stuffed record-full lying dusty under tables. Such a state of affairs is highly unsatisfactory for the loss of a record can on occasion mean the loss of a life. At one clinic in Mulago Hospital no less than a third of the patients were considered as 'new cases' merely because their little slips of paper had gone astray. Well adapted records thus require as much careful thought as does any other part of a hospital's work.

There are two sides to a record system. On the one hand, are the patients' own records, which are a summary of their clinical condition to enable the staff to make out at a glance the essentials of an illness; on the other, there are the files and ledgers which record the work of the hospital as a whole, both for its own use and for that of the State. In considering them here frequent reference will be made to the practice of the Wesley Guild Hospital at Ilesha and the records introduced there by Doctor Andrew Pearson and the writer, with the help in one instance of Glaxo laboratories.

Making the most of the record number. On all hospital records, after a patient's age, sex, tribe and village there comes his number. This is usually a six or seven figure serial that started when the hospital first opened. Such a number has its uses, but the writer would like to suggest, though he has never yet had the opportunity to try it out, that this number might be made more useful by making it carry further information—by making it do more 'work'. As well as performing its present task of distinguishing one patient from all others, it could with little extra trouble, be made to contain his birth date and therefore his age. Thus, the first two figures of the number might denote the date, the next, a letter could denote the month; this could then be followed by two more figures signifying the year and finally it could end with a serial number different for each patient born on that day. It would be convenient if every month of the year began with a different initial letter, but as they do not, another would sometimes have to be used, and the third could be chosen whenever the first repeats. The code would thus become JFMAYNLGSTVD for the months from January to December. As an example, the ninety-ninth person registered as born on the 11th August 1964 would be given the number 11G6499. Such a system would mean that the hospital would have to keep daily a list of those born, and give to each of them a different final serial, but this however is easily done.

ALUMINIUM NUMBER TAGS.

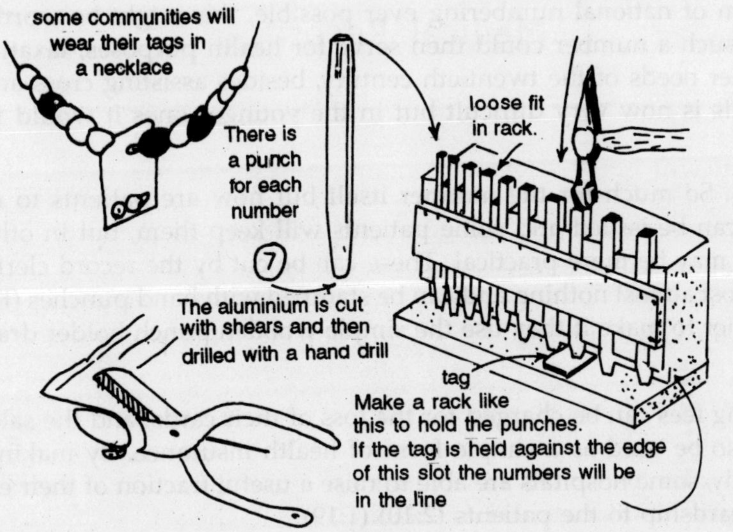

Fig. 8.1

It is critical to system of this that it records the date of a patient's birth and not merely the day be first registers. This is often a matter of difficulty in a rural community, for villagers often do not know the exact date of their birth, it is possible therefore, when a patient does not know his birth date and yet it is required for the records, for the hospital to make a good guess and invent one for him. Under the age of three, it is usually possible for a child's mother to guess it to the nearest week by relating his birth to some fixed event, so all the hospital staff need do is to choose some day within this week.

When a number starts with the birth date, records file automatically in 'cohorts', that is to say, in groups of patients of the same age—a great statistical convenience. Best of all however, a number is easily found if a patient knows his birthday, for the search through final serials is rapid, as only two hundred patients register each day for every million of the population.

Some hospitals use a code for the name of the patient's village and file the record cards by this. But, though such a system is useful epidemiologically, and convenient to the health visitor, who then has all the cards for one village in the same drawer, in Nigeria at least it has one important snag. Here patients are wont to give a fictitious urban address of 'high status', rather than their correct one which may well be in a small hamlet.

A number can also be used which combines both the birth date and the birthplace, but this is cumbersome, and one or other of these two items of information is about all a number will conveniently carry. The point to be made, however, is that a good opportunity is wasted if records are not filed by something more useful than a meaningless serial.

Were a system of national numbering ever possible, this might be worth the effort it would entail, for such a number could then serve for health purposes, taxation, insurance and the many other needs of the twentieth century, besides assisting cross-analysis. In the older countries this is now very difficult but in the younger ones it would be a valuable innovation.

Number-tags. So much for the number itself but how are patients to remember it? Numbered cards can be issued and some patients will keep them, but in other cultures a metal number tag may be more practical. These can be cut by the record clerks from sheet aluminium, they cost almost nothing and can be stamped with hand punches (B & H). Clerks will find them easier to make if they use the simple wooden punch holder drawn in Figure 8.1.

Patients paying fees can be charged for the loss of their cards, and the sale of a card to the patient can also be used as a simple form of health insurance. By making such cards valid for a year only, some hospitals are able to raise a useful fraction of their expenses with the minimum of hardship to the patients (2:10) (1:19).

The value of cardboard. Hospital records have a hard life for they pass through many fingers, and may have to be extracted from the files many times. Records should therefore be made of cardboard, especially as a particular card is much more easily found in a row of others than is a flimsy sheet of paper among a pile of many. No record clerk is therefore to be blamed who cannot locate a flimsy paper from among hundreds of similar ones.

Card may be a little more expensive than paper, but both sides can be both printed and written on, and it lasts much longer. The use of colour helps the illiterate, assists sorting and brightens life generally. Its additional cost is marginal. But colours need to be chosen carefully, for in some societies they have a particular, and even a dreadful significance. Small cards are both economical and easily stored, so records should be made as small as is convenient. Eight inches by five inches (20 cm. x 13 cm.) is a suitable size for outpatient record cards, but before deciding on a size, the printers should be consulted, so as to make sure that the size chosen cuts economically from the standard sheets of card they stock.

The weight chart for the under-fives clinic. This is illustrated in Figure 8.2, and is the most recent version of that devised for this clinic. These charts are now coming into use both in Sierra Leone and elsewhere, and more than a quarter of a million of them have now

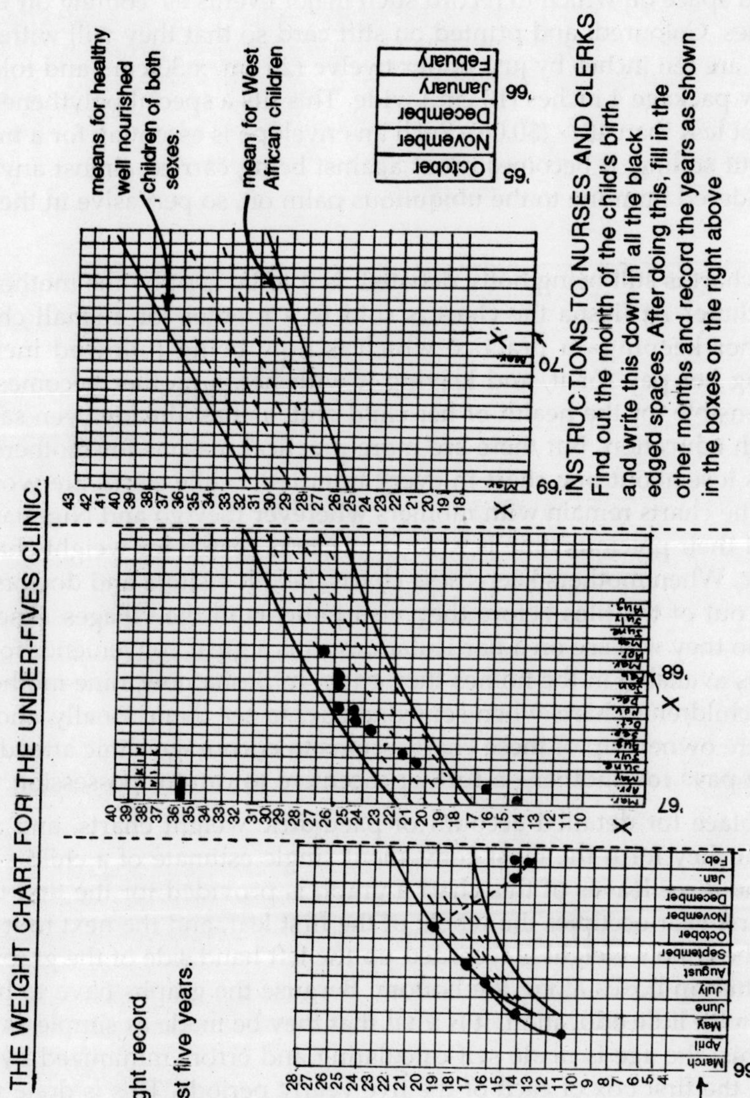
THE WEIGHT CHART FOR THE UNDER-FIVES CLINIC.
Child's weight record over the first five years.
Mojor illnesses and tuberculin state to be entered on this chart
means for healthy well nourished children of both sexes.
mean for West African children
INSTRUCTIONS TO NURSES AND CLERKS
Find out the month of the child's birth and write this down in all the black edged spaces. After doing this, fill in the other months and record the years as shown in the boxes on the right above
March
April
May
June
July
August
September
October
November
December
Jan.
Feb.
October
November
December
January
Febuary
66
65
67
68
69
70

Fig. 8.2

been printed. They are integral with the whole practice of the clinic, for they provide at a glance the child's weight curve in graphic form, a record of his inoculations, some details of his family history and space on which to record such major events as 'coming off the breast' or an attack of measles. Coloured, and printed on stiff card so that they will withstand five years' hard use, they are ten inches by just under twelve (26 cm. x 30 cm.) and fold in three to form a firm narrow package 4 inches (10 cm.) wide. This fits a special polythene envelope and both together cost less than 40/- ($0.06). Such an envelope is essential, for a mother can keep the chart without soiling; it becomes proof against being carried almost anywhere on the person and is rendered immune to the ubiquitous palm oil, so pervasive in the Nigerian household.

The care of this chart is still being hotly debated. Is it to be kept by the mother, or shall it be stored by the clinic? At Ilesha the chart is sold to a mother for a small charge and always remains in her keeping—a practice which is now being followed increasingly elsewhere. By making her pay for it, and leaving it with her, a mother becomes in some additional way responsible for the health of her child and, as has already been said, this is fundamental to health education. But there are more practical reasons for mothers keeping these charts: mothers lose about one chart in every hundred, while clerks are wont to lose five times as many. The charts remain with mothers wherever they go and Nigerian women travel much. None of their precious time is wasted as clerks search for weight charts every time they visit a clinic. When mothers keep these charts, health visitors and doctors have no need to search them out of the files before they visit patients in the villages. And, as they never quite know who they will see on a particular day, it is a great convenience for them to find the charts always available in the homes they enter. In Ilesha now, nine mothers in ten are able to find their children's charts when someone goes to see them. Finally, and perhaps most usefully, the mere ownership of these charts seems to encourage clinic attendance. If a mother loses one she pays for another—a further incentive to careful possession.

This is not the place for detailed account of paediatric weight charts, and it will be taken for granted that they form the most convenient single estimate of a child's nutrition and his health. On the three leaves of this chart a graph is provided for the first five years of a child's life; the first year occupies the whole of the first leaf, and the next four years fill the remaining two. The child's weight is recorded up the left hand side of the graph and his age in months is written in boxes along the bottom. Because the graphs have to be plotted by clerks and nurses with little education, it is vital that they be made as simple as possible. In order to achieve this; the age is made self-calculating and errors minimized by entering the month of birth in the first box of each of the five yearly periods. This is done when the card is first issued, and the appropriate boxes have been heavily outlined and marked 'X' in Figure 8.2. When this has been done the remaining months of each year are inserted in the boxes following. This simple detail is critical to the successful use of these cards, because it means that a clerk does not have to calculate the age of a child at each clinic attendance: he merely fills in the child's weight opposite the box for that particular month. If for instance, the clinic is being held one day in, say March, the clerk weighs all the children and inserts their weights opposite the 'March' boxes on all their charts. These boxes will always be the boxes for March, but they will be in a different position on each child's chart depending on its age. It is probable that the reason why most other weight charts have not been accepted is the difficulty in filling them in, for over the age of two it is not easy, for the average clerk or nurse to calculate a child's exact age in months. By abolishing the need for such, calculation these charts have been accepted much more readily.

A mother is told to bring her child to the clinic every two weeks in the first year of life and every two months thereafter. She is told to keep her child walking along the path on the chart a familiar concept to those accustomed to following paths through the both. The upper line—graph is the mean for the weights of healthy well nourished children of both sexes and the lower—for ordinary West African children. The optimum path is probably some where in between the upper and lower lines for the upper one may well represent the hypernutrition and obesity of more privileged communities. A part from such extremes of mankind as the Watusi giants of Rwanda or the pygmy dwarfs of the ituri forest, such graphs apply to most societies, for it is now becoming increasingly clear that well nourished infants of most human groups follow the same curve in early life. It has now been shown that when well nourished the Nigerian child does so too.

In practice, the position of a child's weight curve on the chart matters much less than the change in his weight, thus if a child continues to gain steadily, he may be flourishing even though his weight is low, while a heavier child who loses weight is likely to be in a worse position and needs examining carefully. The use of these charts makes it possible to see that normal growth is maintained and malnutrition prevented. For example, supplementary feeding, such as the issue of the milk packets advised can be started when a child fails to gain weight as he should. These charts make a positive approach to health possible, which is much to be preferred to merely treating malnutrition after it has occurred.

There is also space on the charts to record a child's tuberculin state and his major illnesses, there being neither time or need for any more detailed records. Because these illnesses often cause dramatic and characteristic changes in the curve, its very shape will often bring a child to mind in a busy clinic, more readily than will his face.

On the back of the card are boxes for the names of a child's father and mother, the date of his birth, the date he was first seen, as well as the name of the house where the family live. Under this is a space for the merest outline of the fate of his brothers and sisters, and overleaf there is a list of the months for the five years of the card's life. These months are ticked off each time the monthly pyrimethamine tablet is given and so form a useful record of a child's malarial suppression. On this leaf there is also a space to record inoculations with small-pox, triple-vaccine, BCG and any other immunizations that may be given Finally, there is room, for some educational slogans.

The successful introduction of these charts into an existing clinic requires careful education of both the mothers and the staff, as well as some additional help in the early stages. This, members of the Red Cross or a woman's voluntary organization may sometimes be able to provide. Both helpers and mothers will have to be taught, and to make this easier a flannelgraph of the weight chart is available for £.2 ($ 5.6) (MOR). As for the charts themselves, it is understood that UNICEF intend to print these on a large scale. Those wanting them should write to their area representative.

Cards for schoolchildren and adults. What happens when the five years are done? This is the time that fortunate children go to school, and a school record card should ideally take over when the clinic card is complete. Height as well as weight needs to be recorded, and, though it has been tried out so extensively, samples of a school record card can be obtained from the writer (MOR).

At Ilesha the adult outpatient record is a simple printed card, eight inches by five, that is filed in the outpatient department, but, unlike those for the under-fives, these cards remain there, because an adult attends hospital so much less frequently that this is the only practical way to keep them. Such cards take little space and can be filed in drawers.

Inpatient records. The quality of a hospital's inpatient records is a good measure of its efficiency. At their simplest they consist of the temperature chart, a card or sheet of paper on which to write the patients' history, and another on which to prescribe his drugs. The many sheets which accumulate are inconvenient in use, and soon become both bulky and difficult to file without comparatively expensive envelope or folder. In order to promote cheapness combined with ease of writing, data correlation and filing. Dr. WIllis of Canada has invented what he calls 'Columnized Medical Charting.

As used at Ilesha this system of medical charting consists of a quarto card and a quarto sheet of paper, which are printed on both sides, pasted for along their edges, and folded over after the manner shown in Figure 8.2. It will be seen that the temperature chart goes down the card rather than across it. Opposite the temperature chart for the day, and going right across both the card and the paper sheet, are spaces to record the patient's pulse, respiration, bowels, and fluid balance, his laboratory reports, the doctor's orders the progress notes and finally the bill.

Nurses quickly get used to charting the temperature down a chart, instead of across it. The time of the observation is left for her to fill in, so, when changing from twice-daily to 4-hourly, or even hourly observations, the same chart can continue. Laboratory investigations are ordered in the laboratory column, the request going to the laboratory on a small coloured slip, six inches by two (15 cm x 5 cm), with space on it at the top for the investigations required, and at the bottom for the result. When these come back from the laboratory, they are folded in half, and stuck to the chart in the laboratory column opposite the day when the test was done (these are not shown in Figure 8.3). The doctor's orders are divided into 'stat.' or 's.o.s.' orders, which are for one occasion only, with a space for the nurse to insert the time a drug was given, and standing, or 'p.r.n., orders, which are to be continued until countermanded. This section is subdivided by dotted lines into several columns. Each standing order begins in a new column, and the time a drug is given is inserted by the nurse in these columns. When the drug is to be discontinued a square is cross-hatched under the last dose given. This column can then be used for another drug if required. In Figure 8.3 it will be seen that procaine penicillin has been prescribed once daily, and has been given at 10.00 on the first and second day of admission. Sulphadimidine has been prescribed 6-hourly, and the time each dose has been given is written in—10.00, 16.00, 22.00 etc.

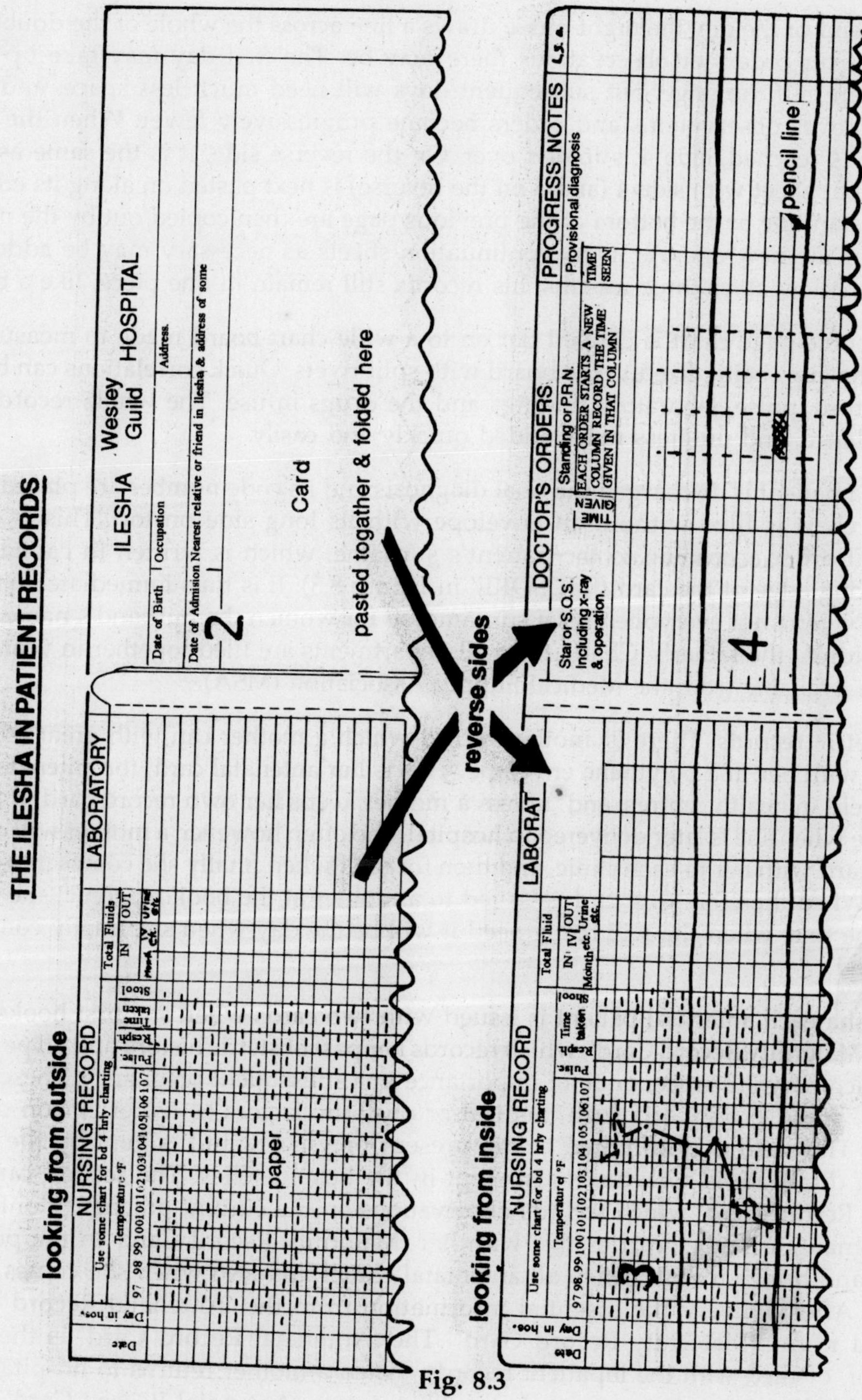
THE ILESHA IN PATIENT RECORDS
looking from outside
NURSING RECORD
LABORATORY
ILESHA Wesley Guild HOSPITAL
Card
pasted togather & folded here
paper
reverse sides
looking from inside
NURSING RECORD
LABORAT
DOCTOR'S ORDERS
PROGRESS NOTES
Provisional diagnosis
pencil line

Fig. 8.3

At the end of the day the night-nurse draws a line across the whole of the double page, below whatever orders or observations there may be. The first day may take up several lines, or even half the page, but subsequent days will need much less space, and, as the patient improves observations and orders become progressively fewer. When the bottom of the page is reached, side 4 is folded over. On the reverse side, it is the same as side 3. Another paper sheet with side 4 (and 3 on the reverse) is next pasted on along its edge, and orders still standing at the bottom of the previous page are then copied out by the nurse on to the top of the new one. As many continuation sheets as necessary may be added, and, even it the patient stays three months, his records still remain in one piece, like a book.

The double-page chart is clipped flat on to a wide chart-board made to measure from plywood, the clips being fixed to the board with split rivets. Ouick correlations can be made of temperature, pulse, laboratory findings and the drugs in use. The whole record can be seen at a glance, and progress notes added quickly and easily.

When a patient is discharged the final diagnosis and its code number are placed on side 2, and the chart is filed without an envelope with its long side on top. This is done in alphabetical order according to the patient's surname, which is written in capital letters along the long edge of the card ('MUSOKE' in Figure 8.3). It is thus immediately visible in the file. In Nigeria not everyone uses a surname, so for women the husband's name is used, and for children, the father's. Charts from all departments are filed together in years. These records are available from the Medical Supply Association (MSA).

Obstetric records. There is another record which a mother can with great advantage take home with her in a polythene envelope. This is her antenatal card, for antenatal clinics are often held in health centres, and, unless a mother keeps her own record card, it may not be available when she is later delivered in hospital. Too often however, a mother will carefully bring this card with her to each clinic, and then forget it when finally she comes into hospital in labour. When therefore this card is issued to a mother at the booking clinic, she must be told that the time when she will really need it will be the day when she finally comes in to be delivered.

At Ilesha each antenatal patient is issued with two cards when she first books in. The first is the 'Maternity Record Card', which records her past obstetric history and all permanent factors which may influence, or be of importance in a subsequent pregnancy. These include her height, blood group, and such medical or obstetric factors as hypertension or pelvic deformity. This card is not limited to the present pregnancy and is kept by the mother, although a duplicate is sometimes also kept in the hospital files. The second card is the 'Antenatal Record Card' which records observations on the current pregnancy only. While she is pregnant, a mother carries this with her 'Maternity Record Card' in the polythene envelope, and brings it with her to all antentatal clinics and also when she comes in to be delivered. After delivery the essential information from the 'Antenatal Record Card' is transferred to the 'Maternity Record Card'. The 'Antenatal Record Card' is then either disposed of, or filed with the inpatient records. When a mother returns to hospital for her second and subsequent pregnancies she is given a new 'Antenatal Record Card', but the original 'Maternity Record Card' is retained, so her previous obstetric history does not have to be written out again. A great advantage of this system is that a mother holds her own 'Maternity Record Card' on which an accurate obstetric history is built up unencumbered by excessive detail. If she travels to another part of the country, this valuable record goes with her.

Hospital data. There is comparatively little to say about the second side of the system—the ledgers and files that record the work of the hospital. It is however worth looking at that dog-eared ledger and the laborious clerk who fills it. Just what is he recording? Is it worth while? At some hospitals clerks merely write down the patient's identification number and use the time saved more profitably. Many hospitals are however beset by daily, monthly or yearly returns and the complex forms that they are required to send in. Much valuable time is wasted recording this information which is mostly useless, and a more rational and economical system is often required. It should be a duty to educate those who demand such forms to make them simpler and at the same time more valuable. There is excellent manual on this subject /82/.

Ministries of health need to know the prevalence of diseases in a country, but much of the data sent into them in the form of hospital outpatient returns is valueless. They would obtain more correct information. If they were to depute some competent person to examine a random sample of those attending an outpatient department—say one patient in every twenty. A full examination, including, X-rays and laboratory investigations, could then be done on this limited number and the data obtained would be of much greater value.

When the diseases to be reported have code numbers it may be found useful for the clerks to have a board with numbered nails corresponding, and for paper slips to be impaled upon them for counting at the end of the week—foolproof perhaps, but time consuming.

Disease notification. This is often a farce, as was proved at one hospital when more cases of measles were found in one town than were notified during a similar period from a population of nearly twenty million. If notification is to be done, it is worth doing properly, and in the under-fives clinic or general outpatient department it may be found useful for nurses or medical assistants to have duplicated sheets on their tables with boxes in which to mark off the notifiable cases they see. If particular information is required, such as the age or address of the patient, these duplicated sheets can be designed with special boxes so as to make this information easy to collect. Each week these sheets can be collected for analysis and will provide some of the information required for making the community diagnosis. Epidemiologic tables can be constructed and the relevant information entered on maps of the defined area. (Samples of these sheets can be obtained from the writer (MOR)).

Taking notes and the use of shorthand.(Written by the editor). Well designed stationery makes good records possible, but the notes that are written on it are what really matter. This final section is therefore devoted to certain ideas on record taking that deserve wider use. But, before discussing them further, there is an important principle to be made clear as to the occasions on which clinical records are made, and the notes appropriate to them.

The classical approach to a clinical diagnosis requires a lengthy history, a detailed physical examination, some tests on the urine, and the ordering of further investigations, the complete process taking about three-quarters of an hour. At the other end of the scale are cases in which experience enables a snap diagnosis to be made and treatment prescribed in a minute or two. The classical approach is that by which students are trained, but the method of snap diagnosis is the one which doctors in developing countries have inevitably to use for most of the patients they see. The classical method requires extensive notes, the snap diagnosis almost none. It might seem therefore that to discuss any form of complete clinical record is unjustified, when there is so little time to spend on each patient. The point to be made, however, is that a detailed history and examination on a limited number of cases is of great value in maintaining and developing a doctor's clinical skills. Occasional cases should therefore be examined completely, and for this purpose as well as for student use, some rational system of note taking and 'clinical shorthand' is required. Most doctors employ some form of shorthand and, though a few symbols are more or less standard, practice varies from one school to another and differs even more from country to country. Because clinical shorthand is not private to the writer but has to be interpreted both by other doctors and by the nursing staff, some standardization is clearly desirable. A recognized list of abbreviations will also be useful to doctors trained on the continent of Europe when they come to practice in developing countries whose medicine is based on the English pattern.

TABLE 8.1

SOME CLINICAL SHORTHAND

OE	On examination.	IM	Intramuscularly.
CO	Complaining of.	SC	Subcutaneously.
PH	Previous history.	PCM	Protein calorie malnutrition.
FH	Family history.	SBE	Subacute bacterial endocarditis.
SH	Social history.	PTB	Pulmonary tuberculosis.
HPC	History of present complaint.	PA	Pernicious anaemia.
POGH	Previous obstetric and gynaecological history.	PUO	Pyrexia of unknown origin.
		URI	Upper respiratory infection.
CNS	Central nervous system.	GC	Gonorrhoea.
URT	Upper respiratory tract.	CA	Cancer.
RS	Respiratory system.	NG	New growth.
CVS	Cardiovascular system.	CCF	Congestive cardiac failure.
GIT	Gastro-intestinal tract.	LVF	Left ventricular failure.
UGT	Urogenital tract.	RVF	Right ventricular failure.
KJ	Knee jerks.	MS	Mitral stenosis.
AJ	Ankle jerks.	MI	Mitral incompetence.
AB	Apex beat.	POP	Plaster of Paris cast.

MCL	Mid-clavicular line.
JVP	Jugular venous pressure.
HS	Heart sounds.
BP	Blood pressure.
RVH	Right ventricular hypertrophy.
LVH	Left ventricular hypertrophy.
SOB	Short of breath.
PN	Percussion note.
VR	Vocal resonance.
VF	Vocal fremitus.
BS	Breath sounds.
RUL	Right upper lobe.
RLL	Right lower lobe.
MCH	Maternal and child health.
ROA	Right occipito-anterior.
LOP	Left occipito-posterior.
FHH	Foetal heart heard.
FHS	Foetal heart sounds.
FIND	Full term normal delivery.
FINL	Full term normal labour.
BBA	Born before arrival.
BID	Brought in dead.
PM	Post mortem.
TCU	To come up.
TCA	To come again.
PR	Per rectum.
PV	Per vaginam.
PU	Per urethram.
IV	Intravenously.
SPC	Suprapubic cystotomy.
EUA	Examination under anaesthesia.
DSM	Dried skim milk.
FCM	Full cream milk.
EBM	Expressed breast milk.
PAM	Penicillin alluminium monostearate.
PPF	Procaine penicillin forte.
SM	Streptomycin.
INH	Iso-nicotinic acid hydrazide.
PAS	Para-amino-salicylic acid.
TB 1	Thiacetazone.
TCE	Tetrachlorethylene.
ATS	Antitetanus serum.
WBC	White blood count.
ESR	Erythrocyte sedimentation rate.
HB	Haemoglobin.
BS	Blood slide.
AAFB	Acid and alcohol fast bacilli.
HW	Hookworm.
MT	Malignant tertian.
BT	Benign tertian.
CSU	Catheter specimen of urine.
ECG	Electrocardiogram.
NR	Not relevant.
NAD	Nil ad demonstrandum,`nothing to show'.
b.d.	*Bis die*, twice daily.
t.i.d.	*Ter in die*, thrice daily.

Before proposing a table of abbreviations there is one convention that could be used more often. This is the 'plus notation'. It runs like this: '—' negative',± doubtful, '+' mild, '++' moderate '+++' severe, '++++' gross. This notation is often applicable, whether it be the size of the spleen that is being described, the degree of a patient's anaemia, the amount of albumen in his urine or the number of acid fast bacilli in his sputum. It is better than the vague adjectives that are usually the only other alternative. Thus, 'Pus cells+' is preferable to 'scanty pus cells' and avoids the use of such terms as 'a few', 'some', or 'present'. '+' and `+ + + +' are easily defined, `+' meaning definitely positive but minimally so, and '+ + + +' meaning maximal, 'it could hardly be larger' or 'there could scarcely be any more'. `±'

meaning doubtful is also straightforward. The symbols '+ +' and '+ + +' are less easily defined, but represent useful degrees in between '+' and '+ + +'.

Figure 8.4A largely explains itself but there are certain points in it which are worthy of note. One is the use of a larger bracket like those after 'cough' or 'pain', in which all the features distinguishing a symptom or sign can be grouped together. Another is the practice of putting all the symptoms and signs that have been inquired after, or searched for and found absent, in brackets on the extreme right of the page with the symbol 'o' after them. The convention of putting the presenting symptom in capitals is a good one; as is that of underlining other symptoms that have been volunteered by the patient. Symptoms that have to be elicited by direct questioning are distinguished by being written in small letters without underlining.

At the bottom of Figure 8.4B a prescription is shown for penicillin which was started on March 6th and stopped on March 10th. It is cancelled with a large 'Z' which is dated and signed, a practice that is to be commended because if makes the subsequent analysis of case notes very much easier.

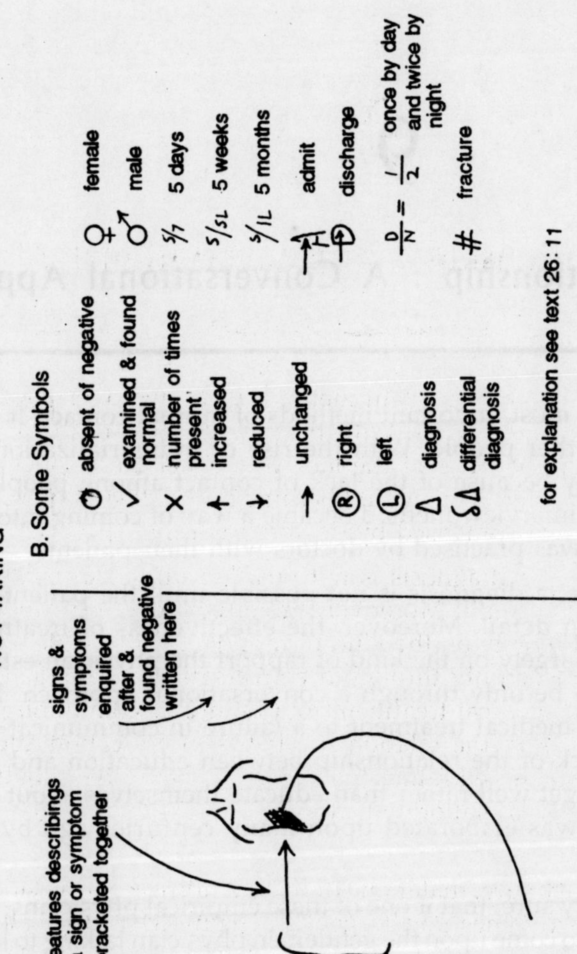
A. Clinical History ♂
features describing a sign or symptom bracketed together
signs & symptoms enquired after & found negative written here
NOT TAKING
Capitals
B. Some Symbols
absent of negative
examined & found normal
number of times present
increased
reduced
unchanged
right
left
diagnosis
differential diagnosis
female
male
5/7 5 days
5/SL 5 weeks
5/IL 5 months
admit
discharge
D/N = 1/2 once by day and twice by night
fracture
for explanation see text 26:11

Fig. 8.4

9

Doctor-Patient Relationship : A Conversational Approach

Conversation is one of the most important methods of mutual contact. It enables us to understand the inner life of other people. With the rise of industrialization, life turned difficult and complex primarily because of the lack of contact among people. Hence the conversational approach or the interview method became a way of coming into contact with the people. The same method was practised by doctors with their patients.

In the practice of medicine, a diagnosis is not possible until the patient's problem is communicated to the doctor in detail. Moreover, the effectiveness of treatment and the cooperation of patient depend largely on the kind of rapport the physician establishes with the patient. And a rapport can be only through a conversational approach. Most doctors accordingly attribute failure in medical treatment to a failure in communication. It is then very important not to lose track of the relationship between education and medical care because most patients want to get well rather than educate themselves about diseases and their consequences. This fact was elaborated upon many centuries ago by plato in his dialogues:

"For of this you may be vary sure, that if one of these empirical physicians, who practise medicine without science, were to come upon the gentlemen physician talking to his gentlemen patient and using the language almost of philosophy-beginning at the beginning of the disease, and discoursing about the whole nature of the body, he would burst into a hearty laugh he would say that most of those who are called doctors always have at their tongue's end: foolish fellow, he would sav. you are not healing the sick man, but you are educating him; and he does not want to be made a doctor, but to get well". Thus especially keeping these vital roles and reasons of failures in view, the present research study had been initiated to identify the positive and negative aspects of the conversational approach adopted by the varied categories of medical professionals in selected departments of Medical College Hospital, Rohtak in Haryana, a State of India.

Material and Method

The conversational approach used in this study has its genesis in the Guidance—Co-Operation Model that usually underlines the doctor patient relationship when the circumstances are less desperate than that of activity—passivity model. It applies to most acute disorders and especially to those relating to infections. Although the patient is sick, he is keenly aware of what is going on, is capable of taking instructions and of exercising judgement, and has to be taken into account as a person. In essence, in this situation, the patient is expected to recognise that the doctor knows best, that is why he is there and he wants to be told what to do so that he can follow instruction and get better. This is the type of relationships most writers assume when discussing doctorpatient interaction. It is compatible with the 'rational' conception of the sick role.

The adoption of this model necessitates the selection of doctors in Medical College Hospital Rohtak. On the whole 40 doctors representing different departments, namely, psychiatry, medicine and orthopeadics were selected. The criterian of selection was based on the availability of the doctor at the time of interviews, his co-operation and qualifications. The professional qualification of the doctors was laid down as M.B.B.S., M.D. who should either be lecturers or below of the rank of lecturers; since the category was closer to the patients on the one hand and had a wider orientation of the other medical fields on the other. The group of selected doctors were interviewed with the help of interview guide which covered three dimensions of diseases: the quality, location and duration. The overall approach was the conversational approach.

Results and Discussion

Of the 40 doctors interviewed 13 were females and 27 were males. The age group of the doctors were as follows: 25 were below the age of 25 years and 15 were between the age of 25 to 34 years. The thirty four of the selected doctors had MBBS degrees, five were M.D's and the qualification of one doctor could not be ascertained; of the total doctors selected 4 were Lecturers, one was a registrar and the remaining 35 were either interns or house-surgeons.

The orientation of the selected doctors towards various dinensions of diseases which fall under the purview of the conversational approach while treating rural patients, it was discovered that all of them were aware of the important domensions of disease, that is, type, location and duration. The importance attached to each of these vary from doctor to doctor. A majority, that is, 40 per cent of them believed that the type of disease was the most-important aspect, whereas 25 per cent of them gave equal importance to all the three aspects. Duration as an important dimension was stressed by 20 per cent of them followed by 15 per cent of the doctors who pointed to location as the most important dimension of disease treatment.

In this context, it can be said that doctors are well versed with dimensions of diseases used for treatment of the patients, since variation in importance of each aspect varies from kind and qualities of diseases (Table 9.1).

Generally speaking the tool need by most doctors to treat patients was the conversation or the case history method. Variations did occur when it was adopted with a combination of other tools, for instance, it was used with investigation by 65 per cent of the doctors and with observation of examination by 45 per cent of them and 42.5 per cent of them respectively. This made us realize that since the conversational approach is used by all the doctors the problem of failure can be delineated to the procedure adopted in conversation, which would be reflected in the following findings (Table 9.2).

Regarding the general problems faced by the doctors while treating rural patients, especially in their out door patient clinics where the conversational approach is used the most majority, that is, 94.2 per cent of the doctors reported a lack of familiarity with local accent. A large number of patients attended the outdoor patient clinics as compared to the number of doctors was attended. They were from different socioeconomic backgrounds and 5 per cent of them were from the backward classes whose ignorance of diseases precluded the conversational method from becoming a success.

The fact that the conversational approach was found to be useful to all the doctors is demonstrated by the findings of Table 9.3 which depicts that 40 per cent of the doctors had found it very useful while 60 per cent had found it useful. None spoke of its negative impact.

A further analysis of the conversational approach's usefulness revealed following: 92.5 per cent of the selected doctors expressed that it helped in making diagnosis along side its other functions; 47.5 per cent opined that it helped to phychologically boost the patients alongside its other functions followed by another 42.5 per cent who felt likewise. The rapport establishment lunction of the coversational approach was underlined by a small per centage of doctors that is 20 per cent of doctors who also highlighted the othe functions of this approach.

In the present context, the cause for the failure of the conversational approach can be attributed to the minimal use of this approach in rapport establishment which in fact forms the base of further use of conversational approach in treating the patients (Table 9.4).

A probe into the specified technique preferred by doctors to check the symptoms of diseases revealed that a majority, that is, 17.5 per cent of the selected group of doctor respondents prefered checking with clinical records alongwith other techniques or simply with another technique alone. Another 35 per cent respondents favoured *Verbitein.* Direct questioning by itself in combination with other techniques was also adopted by 30.0 per cent followed by direct questioning by 22.5 per cent of the group of doctors.

The findings, especially the lack of preference for the verbitem method and the use of direct questioning for checking the symptoms of diseases facilitates the conclusion that there are procedural problems in treating the rural patients, or in other words, this adds to the failure of the conversational approach (Table 9.5).

Similarly, in the preference of techniques for checking out the location of diseases while treating the rural patients, the majority that is, 57.5 per cent of the chosen group of respondents showed a preference for relating the site (location) of the disease to other parts of body, either alone or by combination of other techniques followed by others. (Combination of techniques depends upon the kind of disease). The use of verbitem technique alone or in combination with other technique/techniques was preferred by 28 per cent of the selected respondents followed by the technique to continue the interview after making him understand the purpose of he gets upset. Once again, the lack of preference for the verbitem method alone or that in combination with other techniques for checking the location of the disease add to methodological problems in treating the rural 'patients. The verbitem method helps in identifying the location of the disease on the one hand and provides moral strength to patient on the other. It also enhances the following of instructions and ultimately helps in treatment (Table 9.6).

Once again for checking the duration of illness to treat the rural people a low preference was shown for the verbitem as a technique either by itself or with other methods. Doctors support the aforesaid fact of procedural problem involves conversational approach (Table 9.7).

Of the total number of doctors 25 per cent of them found the environment to be responsible for infectious and parasitic diseases excluding waterborne diseases followed by 22.5 per cent of the doctors who attached importance to the environment in treating infections both parasitic and water borne diseases. Another 17.5 per cent of the selected respondents attached importance to the environment for treating waterborne diseases only, whereas 15 per cent recognised the importance of environment in treating psychiatric rural ailments (Table 9.8).

The findings thus reveal that the doctors are aware of the importance of environment in treating the rural patients. The varying importance accorded to environmental conditions can be delineated to the types of diseases and the persons, knowledge of its causes. This reflects a positive dimension of the conversational approach adopted by the doctors of this group.

Similar positive trends with regard to the use of family history and personal history for treating rural patients have been revealed in (Table 9.9. Table 9.10).

Conclusion

It has been found that different socio-cultural problems, varying languages, lack of understanding of a particular culture, different socio-economic orientation and a woeful lack of doctors are responsible for the ineffective implementation of the conversational approach.

With regard to the methodological impediments in the adoption of the conversational approach, the lack of attention to rapport establishment, the limited use of the verbitem technique and the use of direct questioning where checking the symptoms and the location and duration of the diseases have been found to be negative features.

This highlights the need for a sociological orientation of the doctors, especially in the use of the conversational approach and the need to educate the rural patients, especially in getting rid of the psychological complexes which are embedded in their socio-economic and cultural backgrounds.

This study has made way for further such studies/surveys on primary health centre doctors and private doctors who treat the maximum number of rural patients.

References

1. Lasanga, L., *Principles and Techniques of Research and Therapeutics*. Futuro Publishing Company, 295. Main St. P.O.B.O. 260. Mount Kisco, 10549, 1976.

2. Mayerson, E.D., *Putting the III At Ease*, Harper and Row, Hygerstows, Maryland, 1976.

3. Tuckett, D. *An Introduction to Medical Sociology* (ed.). Tavistock Publications, 1976.

4. Yong, P.V., *Scientific Social Surveys and Research*, Prentice Hall of India. Pvt. Ltd., New Delhi, 1972.

Table No. 9.1: Doctors Opinion on the Dimensions of Diseases

	Dimensional aspects of diseases				
	Type of diseases	*Location*	*Duration*	*All the three*	*Total*
Number of doctors	40	40	40	40	40
Number of doctors given importance	16	6	8	10	40
Percentage	40%	15%	20%	25%	100%

Table No. 9.2: Doctor's Opinion on the Tools for Treating the Sick

	Category of tools			
	Case History	*Examination*	*Investigation*	*Observation*
Number of doctors	40	40	48	40
Number of doctors used	40	17	26	18
Percentage	100%	42.5%	65%	45%

Table No. 9. 3: Conversation Approach as a Tool for Treating the Sick

	Category of use		
	Very useful	*Useful*	*Total*
Number	16	24	40
Percentage	40%	60%	100%

Table No. 9. 4: Functional Aspects of the Conversational Approach

	Functional Categories				
	Repport	*Mental preparation*	*Moral tools*	*Diagnosis*	*Treatment*
Number of doctors	40	40	40	40	40
Number of doctors accept it	9	17	19	37	3
Percentage	22.5%	42.5%	47.5%	92.5%	7.5%

Table No. 9. 5: Structural Orientation of the Doctors towards Conversational Approach

	Techniques prefered to check symptoms				
	Verbitem	*Direct questioning*	*Indirect questioning*	*Checking clerical records*	*Others*
Number of doctors	40	40	40	40	40
Number of doctors prefered	14	9	12	19	11
Percentage	35%	22.5%	30%	47.5%	27.5%

Table No. 9. 6: Techniques Preferred for location of Disease

	Verbitem	*Relating disease with other parts*	*Stopping Inquiry upon patients' getting upset*	*Continue for purpose*	*Others*
Number of doctors	40	40	40	40	40
Number of doctors prefered	10	23	1	6	11
Percentage	25%	57.5%	2.5%	15%	27.5%

Table No. 9. 7: Techniques Prefered to Check Duration

	Verbitem	*Relating events*	*Combination 1 plus 2*	*Others*
Number of doctors	40	40	40	40
Number of doctors prefered	8	26	1	5
Percentage	20%	65%	2.5%	12.5%

Table No. 9. 8: Awareness of Environmental Hazards in the Conversational Approach

	Categories of diseases need use of environmental care				
	Water born diseases	*Other infectious diseases*	*Combination (1+2)*	*Psychatric*	*Combination (1+2+4)*
Number of doctors	40	40	40	40	40
Number of doctors stated the need	7	10	9	6	8
Percentage	17.5%	25%	22.5%	15%	20%

Table No. 9. 9: Family History Details Revealed in the Conversational Approach

	Diseases Requiring Probe into Family History					
	Multiple pregana-ncies	*Infectious parasites; circulatory/ respiratory problems*	*Combination 1-2*	*Combination 2-Psy*	*Psychiatric*	*Total*
Number of doctors	40	40	40	40	40	40
Number of doctors stated the need	1	21	1	16	1	40
Percentage	2.5%	52.5%	2.5%	40%	2.5%	100%

Table No. 9. 10 : Role of Personal History in Conversational Approach

	Diseases which require a check into personal history							
	Abortions	*IVGR*	*Addition and related diseases*	*Combination 1+3 normal prg.*	*Combination 1+2 Psy.*	*Psychiatric*	*All illnesses*	*Total*
Number of doctors	40	40	40	40	40	40	40	40
Number of doctors used this tech.	1	1	23	2	7	4	2	40
Percentage	2.5%	2.5%	57.5%	5%	17.5%	10%	5%	10%

10

Administration of Primary Health Care

A. Need. Meaning and Scope of Primary Health Care

Need

Two-thirds of the world population is living only on 4th income of the world. Such a situation is politically unstable, morally untenable and psychologically unsound. "On the face of our planet today." World Bank President, George D. Woods has said, "two billion people out of three billion live in countries that are still facing the travail of economic and social transformation. These people account for two-thirds of the world population but share only one-sixth of its income, one-third of its food production and less than one-tenth of its industrial output."[1] In spite of the efforts made to improve the living standards, two-thirds of the world's population is still beyond the reach of even the most minimal health, nutrition, education and social services. The greatest sufferers are the 80 per cent people living in rural areas, slums and shanty towns and the nomads. The world has the capacity to provide the health care services to all the people and this can prevent the high rates of morbidity and mortality from diseases to people living in these areas. It is worth enumerating some of the characteristics of underdeveloped rural areas.

"economic stagnation;

cultural patterns that are unfavourable to development;

agricultural unemployment and lack of alternative employment opportunities;

poor quality of life because of the scarcity of essential goods, facilities and money;

isolation caused by distance and poor communications and unfavourable environment predisposing to communicable diseases and malnutrition;

inadequate health facilities and lack of sanitation;

poor education opportunities;

social injustice including inequitable land tenure systems and a rigid hierarchy and class structure;

inadequate representation and influence in national decision-making."[2]

According to Dr Manuel Carballo. "Rural communities the world over have tended to share a common predicament, namely that relative to urban areas they have been underserved and, in many respects, have experienced a quality of life and health inferior to that found in large towns and cities. In terms of overall national investment directed towards them or of the self development they have been encouraged to generate, rural areas have historically been at a disadvantage and have enjoyed less well-developed communication infrastructures, educational facilities and health related services."[3]

It is estimated that more than half of the world population, inhabiting mostly rural areas, does not enjoy proper health care. This gross inequality particularly between developed and developing countries as well as within countries is not desirable and acceptable. Let us review the situation in the developing countries. Ghana reported to the First International Conference on Primary Health Care, "In spite of huge infusions of resources, there has been little improvement in the general health status in the last 15 years... The basic problem is that the present system, based on passive service delivery points—hospitals, health centres and posts—is not doing the job. Seventy per cent of Ghanians had difficulty in making use of the Static system because of inaccessibility."

The implementation gap can be reviewed from the following statistics:

(i) Less than 10 per cent (203 million) of the rural population of developing countries, (2032 million), is within walking distance (10 km) of a national health facility of any kind.

(ii) WHO sources estimate that 3 per cent of approximately 10 million of children under five years in developing countries suffer from severe protein calorie malnutrition and a further 80 million from moderate level malnutrition.[4]

(iii) A WHO study of 91 less-developed countries indicated that 85 per cent of the rural population has no access to safe drinking water.

(iv) Nutritional deficiency[5] diseases affect large number of persons; goitre 400 million; anaemia 300 million; xerophthalmia 100 million.

It appears that the benefits of modern medicine would accrue to only a small population. The Regional Director of South-East Asia Region affirmed that most of the governments in the Region recognise that despite every effort to extend the provision of basic health services to the population, during the last three decades, the achievements have not been impressive. In view of this situation systematic health planning and country health programming have, in some countries, resulted in the formulation of primary health care projects as integral part of the basic health services.[6]

Thus, the health care administration in developing countries has failed to meet the minimum health care needs of its people. Dr. N.R.E. Fendall has nicely explained the short-falls of health care system: "If I were asked to compose an epitaph on medicine throughout the twentieth century, it would read: brilliant in its discoveries, superb in its technological breakthrough but woefully inept in its application to those most in need. Medicine will be judged, not in its vast and rapid accumulative of knowledge *per se*, but on its trusteeship of that knowledge. We are now experienced and all that remains is the problem of translating what is common knowledge and routine medicine and hence practice, to the world. The implementation gap must be closed."[7]

The basic question which needs to be answered is: What model of administration on health care can meet the health care needs of all the people in the developing world? What are the constituents of such a model? Past experience has amply made clear that by adoption and uncritical transfer of the model health systems from the developed to the developing world, the basic health needs of the people in the developing world cannot be fulfilled. Henry R. Labouisse, Executive Director of UNICEF, vehemently held while submitting to the First International Conference on Primary Health Care, "The developing countries have come to realise that the conventional approach inherited from industrialised countries was hopelessly inappropriate when it came to meet, within a reasonable period of time, the health care needs of these vast populations. And the industrialised countries themselves after making spectacular advances in the field of medicine and building up services with expensive facilities, sophisticated technology and highly specialised personnel, are now finding themselves burdened with ruinous medical care systems with which they are unable to provide proper health protection to their own very numerous people. So, there has to be change everywhere."

It has been recognised and accepted that the health care services which exist in most parts of the world have not been meeting the basic needs of very large groups of the population especially in the developing countries.

Meaning and Strategy

The most effective and acceptable form of health care delivery system for the people in the developing world has to be evolved by the community itself. Development is indigenous to each society and builds primarily on a country's resources—mainly land and people. Each country must develop its own model to social fulfilment. This will enlarge the capacity of individuals and communities to create and innovate. The mobilisation of the energies and resources of the people especially the rural poor themselves emerges as the key factor in increasing their productivity and self-reliance. Such mobilisation assumes the formation, adaptation and strengthening of community structures. Since each country differs from others in its resources and needs, the concept of Country Health Programme (CHP) must be proctised by every country. It is a pragmatic approach which tailors the services precisely to the national situation. In his Preface to the Annual Report for 1975 Dr. Mahler said that, "Such programming is a long-term process, not a one-time intensive planning effort. In order to attain the systematic development of health programmes and services, countries that have not already done so well need to set up permanent mechanism for formulating health policies and translating these policies into operational programmes. This implies a continuing process of planning, implementing, monitoring, controlling, evaluating and re-planning—a truly new approach for most countries and the need for appropriate mechanism to launch the venture and maintain its dynamism which well continue for the foreseeable future." Community Health Programming would give high priority to the needs of the undeserved. Thus, the developing countries must design their own health care delivery models to provide primary health care to all its people. Let us now define the meaning and essential features of such care commonly known as Primary Health Care.

Nature of Primary Health Care

The WHO defined Primary Health Care as "essential health care made universally accessible to individuals and families in the community by means acceptable to them through their full participation and at a cost that the community and country can afford. It forms an integral part both of the country's health system of which it is the nucleus and of the overall social and economic development of the community."[8]

The first International Conference on Primary Health Care defined it as "essential health care based on scientifically sound and socially acceptable methods and technology made universally acceptable to individuals and families in the community through their full participation and at a cost that the community and country can afford to maintain at every stage of their development in a spirit of self-reliance and self-determination." There are many different ways of defining primary health care. The 28th World Health Assembly accepted the working definition of primary health care. According to this definition primary health care is taken to mean, "A health approach which integrates at the community level all the elements necessary to make an impact upon the state of health of the people. Such an approach should be an integral part of the national health care system. It is an expression or response to the fundamental human needs of how a person can know of and be assisted in the actions required to live a healthy life and where a person can go if he or she needs relief from pain or suffering. A response to such needs must be a series of simple and effective measures in terms of cost, technique and organisation which are easily accessible to the people in need and which assist in improving the living conditions of individuals, families and communities. These include preventive, promotive, curative and rehabilitative health measures and community development activities."[9]

In short, we can say that primary health care is an approach which integrates at the community level all the elements necessary to make an impact upon the health status of the people.

Primary Health Care should not be understood as primitive care. In uses simple administrative structures, procedures and operates within the community but "it is an essential frst level in a scale of services and is in no way inferior." It is providing the benefits of modern medicine to the community through better methods based upon the socio-economic conditions prevalent in each country. It was mentioned by a delegate from Switzerland: "To wish to promote primary health services does not signify the establishment of two parallel or juxtaposed systems of which one is for the poor and the other, the classic system, more complex, more sophisticated, is reserved for the rich. The goal is to set up a system where primary health care forms the base of a structure accessible to all, upon which other levels of care can be grafted and can develop."

Jagdambi Prasad Yadav, in his presidential address delivered at the Twentieth Convocation of IIPA (Bombay, 15 July 1978) defined the philosophy of the Primary Health Care as: "The philosophy of the community health workers' scheme is to place people's health in people's hand. It is well-known that in most parts of rural India even rudimentary public health facilities are lacking from times immemorial. The CHW's scheme is designed to take health care to door-steps of people. It is hoped that the community health workers will bridge the gap between rural community and health care—preventive, promotional and curative."

Speaking on the new health policy, Shri Morarji Desai, former Prime Minister of India, said, "Whatever development we want to do in the country depends upon the capacity of the people to do their work efficiently and to go on increasing their productive capacity in any field of work, that they can take up. And if this is to be done,health becomes a very primary condition. Unless a person enjoys fairly good health, it will not be possible for him to do work efficiently. It is, therefore, necessary for us to see that the people of the country are enabled to maintain their health in a fairly good manner, so that they are able to follow their work and profession efficiently and live also a health life."

Essentials

1. Primary Health should be shaped around the life styles of the people to be served.
2. The local people should be actively involved in planning health care so that it suits their needs and priorities.
3. The health care offered should make maximum use of community resources.
4. Primary Health Care should not only deal with the prevention and cure of disease but also promote health, in the community, in the family and in the individual.
5. All health interventions should take place in or as near as possible to the patient's home and be carried out by the worker most simply (but adequately) trained to give the treatment in question.
6. Other services, in particular supplies, supervision, and referral and technical support, should be designed to support the needs at the local level.

Basic Concepts

I.*Availability of Health Services*

The availability of health services is a major factor of the accessibility of services, and is taken to mean the physical presence of a health service provider who constitutes a primary entry point to the health service system, either providing the service directly, or providing referral to another health care provider at an appropriate facility level.

II. *Accessibility of Health Services*

"Accessibility" is taken to mean the composite of the characteristics of health services which facilitate or obstruct their utilization by potential consumers. Accessibility also incorporates such factors as the availability of needed drugs and supplies; affordable costs to consumers who seek and receive services, including service cost, transportation cost, and cost in time, and social factors relating to the consumer provider interaction, such as the service provider's attitude towards and rapport with consumers.

III.*Acceptability and Acceptance of Health Services*

The proof of accessibility and acceptability of health services is "acceptance" of health services that is the actual *utilization* of health services or the expressed demand for services by consumers.

We must, however, be clear that Health for all does not mean that in the year 2000 nobody will be sick or disabled nor does it mean that in the year 2000 doctors and nurses will provide medical repairs for every body in the world. It does mean that health begins at home, in schools, and in working places. It does mean that the people will use better approaches than they do now for preventing diseases and reducing unavoidable illness and disability and better ways of growing up, growing old, and dying gracefully.

B. General Principles of Primary Health Care while development of Primary Health Care is likely to be:

(1) Increasing involvement of the community in all aspects of programming.

(2) Adaptation of local health service personnel to Primary Health Care.

(3) The closer links of health with general development.

(4) Need of national resources and political will to support Primary Health Care.

Increasing Involvement of the Community

"Participation means self motion."[10]

It gives the ordinary citizen "a chance to show his willingness to carry out constructive public work and to demonstrate his good citizenship by other means than periodically exercising his right to vote."[11]

It means the full involvement of the community in the planning, implementation and control of Primary Health Care. People's involvement has to be understood in the following four senses:

(i) Participation and decision-making, such as in the identification, development priorities and planning of development programmes, projects and activities;

(ii) Participation in monitoring and evaluation of development programmes and projects;

(iii) Participation in implementation of development programmes and projects; and

(iv) Participation in sharing the benefits of development.[12]

Such participation can be mobilised if the community is properly educated. This education would help them pinpoint the obstacles to development. In the field of health, this would enable them to diagnose their health problems and to deal with their problems in the most effective way. When the community is enlightened, every man and woman would become a secret teacher. Man's energy is the most powerful tool of health and socio-economic development.[13] "It does not tally with reality to view the political and administrative environment solely in terms of a Central Government acting upon an inert periphery."[14] According to Professor Ramalingaswami, Director General ICMR:

> "An indigenous health system based on community health derived personnel is needed in which the services are economical, acceptable, continuous and belong to the people."[15]
>
> Community participation must not become an amorphous and abstract slogan like all other socio-political entities; a community comprises different and often conflicting interests. Community participation will only have real meaning when a democratic and genuinely participatory system prevails political power must be in the hands of the people and not in those of interested groups, such as local chiefs and property holders. The poor individually cannot stand up or speak up for their rights and privileges and remain meek spectators in the development process. So, participation by the majority is possible only if they are mobilised. Mobilisation should be done tactfully. To gain the confidence of the poor, we must guard against the strong opposition by the power group in the village.

Adaptation of Local Health Service Personnel to Primary Health Care and their Utilisation

The Primary Health Care envisages the provision of health care through trained personnel indigenous to the community. This worker is chosen from the village and by the village and trained to deliver elementary integrated health service. Such workers properly trained through well-designed short-term courses can provide effective, acceptable and inexpensive health care to the community. According to WHO; "Primary Health Care is likely to be most effective if it employs means that are understood and accepted by the community and applied by community health workers at a cost the community and the country can afford. These community health workers, including traditional practitioners where applicable, will function best if they are properly trained socially and technically to respond to the community's expressed health needs. The skills that community health workers require and their consequent training will vary widely throughout the world. But whatever their level of skill, it is important that they understand the real health needs of the communities they serve and they gain the active confidence and backing of the people." Professor. V. Ramalingaswami while receiving the Leon Bernard Foundation Award stressed that this system of community based health services employing auxiliaries must not be understood by the people as "providing inferior medicine to the rural poor." He went on. "An Auxiliary is a health educator, a rudimentary physician, a social worker and a preventive person, all in one... The education and training of auxiliaries is the most challenging task that medicine faces today. Auxiliaries served to bridge the catastrophic separation between hospital-based, fragmented, episodic medicine and mass public health. The principles of educational science and technology must diffuse into their training programmes. It is on our willingness and ability to experiment with auxiliary training programmes that the chances of success will depend. The moment modern medicine penetrates the social veil in developing countries, that it is the moment of triumph of modern medicine. Here is medicine in the raw, medicine rooted in the reality of rural life."[16]

The Closer Links with General Development

Community health actions cannot be effective in isolation. These must be linked with the effort of total community development. These should be supported by a community based organisation. As WHO has stated "since Primary Health Care is an integral part both of the community's health system and of overall economic and social development without which it is bound to fail, it has to be coordinated on a national basis with the other sectors that contribute to a country's total development strategy."[17]

Need of National Resources and Political Will to support Primary Health Care

National resources are needed to support primary health care. We have to find resources partly from the community and partly from the national exchequer. We have to change priorities of investment in the interest of the poor. The responsibility of the state must be there to provide continuous support in terms of technical knowledge, guidance and supervision, training, supplies and maintenance, the solving of specific problems, and the care of patients referred to other levels of the health system. The presence of a supportive health service infrastructure is essential for primary health care. Political leadership must also understand and appreciate the needs and aspirations of the rural poor. We are sure to provide an acceptable level of health to all the people by the year 2000 if each government has the political initiative, courage boldness, innovation to reorient for the population, its health priorities according to their socio-economic conditions.

Health Information System in Relation to Primary Health Care and Community Development

Information is the planner's raw material, forming the basis for the diagnosis structuring his objectives and permitting him to evaluate the programme's efficiency and effectiveness which have been planned. The degree to which a planner can be successful in terms of the provision of primary health care services will depend upon the degree to which he is able to obtain information about them which is valid and reliable. The term system has been defined as a coherent, integrated whole, being a combination of a number of entities or elements. Similarly, in the information area there are a number of elements which have to be considered in an integrated manner, as components of one system so that they are viewed in totality as means of providing the health administrator with required formation in the appropriate form and at the appropriate time. These elements are:

Input (data)
Analysis and Processing
Storage and retrieval
Output
Flow

In order to improve the information for Primary Health Care, the following essential steps should be taken into account:

(i) *Analysis of System's Requirements*

It analyses in depth the system's requirements. Such an analysis will require answers to questions like:

— What are the objectives of Primary Health Care?

— What are the activities to be carried out?
— What type of evaluation is required to assess the impact of primary health care?
— Who will collect the data?
— How will the data be collected?
— Where, how and by whom will the data be processed?
— How accurate and reliable should such data be?
— What will be the frequency and timeliness of the report?
— Who will use the information generated and how will it be used?

(ii) *Design of Information System*

The next step is the actual design of an information system covering all its five elements already mentioned, in such a manner that it fulfils with minimum cost and delay and in the required form, the information requirements of the health care administrator. The following points may be kept in mind:

(a) The data generated at the primary health care level should correspond to that actually needed for management of primary health care services.
(b) The necessary links between the various sub-systems of the national health information system and the information systems of the other health related sectors on the one hand and with the primary health care sub-systems on the other, should be provided.
(c) An appropriate method for the processing and analysis of basic data by the supervisors of primary health workers should be designed. The primary health workers may be trained to understand the meaning and the value of the data so that they can play an active role rather than passive transmitters of data.

(iii) *Procurement of Necessary Material*

The third step is the production of necessary material and the provision of required facilities so that the system could be put into operation, *e.g.*, for a manually operated system the formats have to be produced.

(iv) *Installation*

The information system should be set up keeping in mind, to retain as far as possible, the existing procedures and system. It may replace the other components which require change slowly.

(v) *Operation and follow-up*

The output of the system is examined against the objectives for which the system was designed. It should be the endeavour to continuously improve upon the system taking into account the changed situation.

This information in primary health care may be supplemented with the case studies carried out by the community. The system of community case study implies a form of popular participation and thus would enhance the utility and scope of primary health care.[18]

C. Experiments of PHC in Different Parts of the World

In this section we would review (on the basis of case studies conducted by the health experts in different parts of the world) the progress of the implementation of primary health care in different parts of the world. After this we shall discuss the progress of primary health care in India.

Experiment of the Soviet Union (Kazakhstan)[19]

Before the Russian Revolution of 1917, Soviet Kazakhstan was one of the most backward and neglected provinces of Tsarist Russia. Not more than two per cent of the total population could read and write. In the field of health, there was not a single medical institution and the number of medical personnel was negligible.

Today, this region enjoys all the health facilities. Five medical schools and 26 junior medical colleges have helped to train some 40,000 doctors and more than 130,000 intermediate level medical workers. The bed-population ratio is 12:4.

After the revolution, primary health care formed the basis of the health system. It provided service through out-patient clinics and posts staffed by midwives and fieldscher

PRIMARY HEALTH CARE SYSTEM

A Conceptual Model of the Health Information System with special Emphasis on the Local Community Level

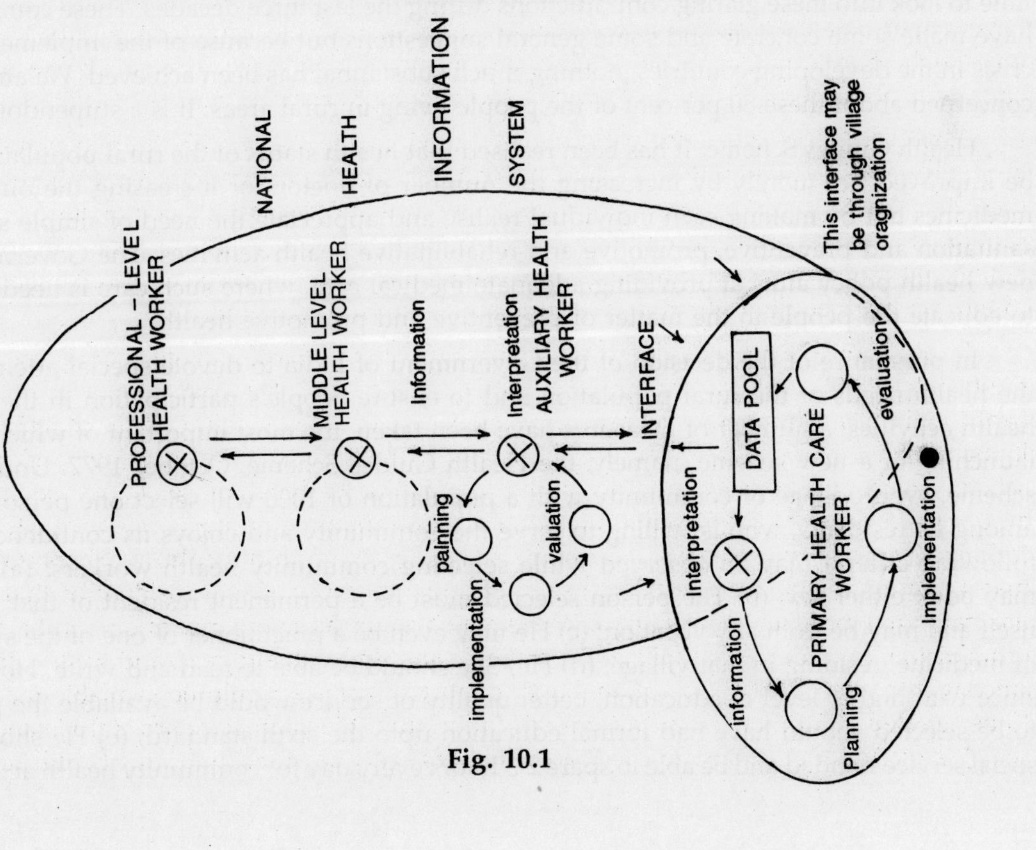

Fig. 10.1

(medical auxiliaries). Each post is staffed by a nurse as well as a fieldscher and a midwife and covers about five hundred people. Those posts enlist the support of continuous and persistent efforts of their governments and especially the health departments. All these countries may learn from each other's experiences and improve the mechanism of primary health care programmes. If such programmes are successful, it is sure that the health care would be available to all the people in the world by 2000 A.D. without exception.

Primary Health Care in India

The problems of providing adequate health care to 670 million people is a challenging task. The Government has been trying to provide health care through primary health centres, dispensaries and mobile units.

The quality and quantity of medical care available is extremely variable—ranging from organised, sophisticated and advanced in urban areas to the most primitive in rural areas. The Fifth Five-Year Plan emphasised that the correction of the regional disparities and heavy concentration of health infrastructure and manpower in the urban areas is the imperative of the social justice in the health sector. With the objective a re-orientation of the health programmes and policies was planned an envisaged in the Master Plan considered by the Health and Family Planning Conference held in Delhi in December, 1970. The consensus was that a minimum infrastructure for the entire country particularly in the rural areas should be set up with the resources available. Many expert committees were appointed from time to time to look into these glaring contradictions during the last three decades. These committees have made some concrete and some general suggestions but because of the implementation crisis in the developing countries, nothing much substantial has been achieved. We are much concerned about these 80 per cent of the people living in rural areas. It is a stupendous task.

Health Guides Scheme: It has been realised that health status of the rural population can be improved not merely by increasing the number of doctors or increasing the output of medicines but by making each individual realise and appreciate the need of simple steps in sanitation and preventive, promotive and rehabilitative health activities. The Government's new health policy aims at providing adequate medical care, where such care is needed and to educate the people in the matter of preventive and promotive health.

In pursuance of the decision of the Government of India to devote special attention to the health needs of the rural population and to ensure people's participation in their own health activities, a number of measures have been taken, the most important of which is the launching of a new scheme, namely, the Health Guides Scheme, October 1977. Under this scheme, every village or community with a population of 1000 will select one person from among its residents, who is willing to serve the community and enjoys its confidence. The following criteria may be observed while selecting community health workers: (a) CHW may be of either sex; (b) The person selected must be a permanent resident of that village itself and may be from any vocation; (c) He may even be a practitioner of one of the systems of medicine, residing in that village; (d) He/She should be able to read and write. However, since with higher level of education, better quality of service would be available the person to be selected should have had formal education upto the sixth standard; (e) He should be social service minded and be able to spare 2-3 hours every day for community health activities;

(f) He should be physically active and willing to serve at least for 3 years as community health worker; (g) He should be acceptable to all sections of the community; (h) He should not belong to any group, faction or political organisation of the village which may limit his acceptability.

With these guidelines, the village community is requested to recommend 2-3 persons considered suitable by them to be Health Guides. The final selection may be made by the medical officers of the Primary Health Centre jointly after consulting the Block Development Officer and the field staff of various government organisations. The Health Guide a given training in simple and basic health services for three months at the Primary Health Centre to which he belongs. During training, the Health Guide is taught the fundamentals of health and hygiene, treatment of common ailments, maternity and child health care, first aid, etc. After training, the Health Guides go back to the village to serve the community. He is provided with a kit containing medicines and also a manual. The kit consists of common remedies belonging to the modern system of medicine, besides remedies under the traditional system in vogue in that part of the country. The worker is expected to work in his spare time for two to three hours daily. During the period of training he is paid a stipend of Rs. 200 per month for three months. After training he is given an honorarium of Rs. 50 per month for working with the community and also Rs. 50 worth of medicines per month.

In the first phase, the scheme has been introduced in the 28 districts in which the training of multipurpose workers has been completed and in one of the primary health centres in each of the remaining 364 districts in the country.

States and Union Territories of Gujarat, Chandigarh, Dadra and Nagar Haveli, West Bengal, Maharashtra and Himachal Pradesh have been fully covered under the scheme. Haryana, Madhya Pradesh, Manipur, Orissa and Tripura will be fully covered by 1982-83. Bihar, Punjab and Rajasthan which had discontinued the scheme have agreed to re-introduce the scheme.

Out of 5484 PHCs functioning as on 1.4.1980, 674 PHCs of Jammu & Kashmir, Kerala, Tamil Nadu and Arunachal Pradesh are covered by alternative scheme and the remaining 4810 are to be covered by Health Guides Scheme. By the end of September 1983 4247 PHCs had been covered and 2,51,030 Health Guides had been trained.

From 1977-78 too 1978-79, the scheme operated as 100 per cent Centrally-sponsored scheme while during 1979-80 the scheme was converted into category II Central Scheme as 50:50 basis, as a result of which States like Punjab, Rajasthan and Bihar discontinued the scheme. However 100 per cent financial assistance is again being provided for implementation of the scheme since 1.12.1981. As a result, Punjab, Rajasthan and Bihar have now agreed to implement the scheme again.

Multipurpose Workers' Scheme

The Multipurpose Workers' Scheme aims at establishing a Health Delivery System in the rural areas through a team of Multi-purpose Workers; one male and one female for every 5,000 rural population. Implementation involves (a) intensive training programme to train unipurpose workers in the technical concepts and skills of the Multipurpose Workers at all levels and (b) employment of additional workers.

Training

(a) The seven Central Training Institutes conduct training programmes for the Key Trainers and for the District Level Medical Officers.

(b) The forty-seven Health and Family Welfare Training Centres impart training to the Medical Officers and the Block Extension Educators (BEEs) of the Primary Health Centres (PHCs).

(c) Trained MOs and BEEs organise training at their own PHCs/at the selected PHCs for their para-medicals.

Achievements

The MPW Scheme is being implemented in the country in a phased manner and it is envisaged that the entire country will be covered under the scheme by March 1984. Upto 31st March, 1983, training was complicated in 326 districts and as on 1st October, 1983 another 7 districts have completed the training and it is going on in 40 districts. The States of Gujarat, Karnataka, Meghalaya, Haryana, Sikkim, Maharashtra, Himachal Pradesh, Uttar Pradesh, Punjab, West Bengal, Rajasthan and Orrisa have completed the training in all the districts of the State.

Dais Training Programme

It has been envisaged to train at least 1 dai for each of the 5.80 lakh villages in the country by the year 1984-85 so that MCH vices available in the country could be improved and she will be the key person to propagate the small family norm to the community members. After the training, each dai is given Midwifery Kit to conduct safe and hygienic delivery.

During the year 1982-83, 42,473 dais were trained against the target of 80,591. The target fixed for 1983-84 is 75,000. Total number of dais trained during the years 1974-83 is 4.5 lakhs.

ANM/Health Workers: Till 1983, there were 339 Auxiliary Nurse Midwives Health Workers (F) training schools in the country with an annual admission of about 15,549. However, under the multipurpose workers scheme, based on the duties and responsibilities of Health Workers, the curriculum has been revised and the duration of the training has been reduced from two years to 1½ years. The entrance educational qualification of the ANM training used to be VIIth class pass and at present an entrance qualification for Health Workers Training has been raised to Matric pass. For hilly and tribal areas where there is a dearth of eligible candidates it has been decided that the basic qualifications for admission to the training course may be relaxed from X class to 7th class pass. However, training in these courses will be for 2 years.

LHV/Promotion/Training Schools: Till 1983, there was 35 LHV Schools in the country with an annual admission capacity of 253. Under the multipurpose workers scheme, the posts of the Supervisors/Health Assistants (F) will have to be filled by giving promotion to ANM/HW (F) after giving 6 months training. Therefore, at present the regular LHV training programme has been discontinued and these schools are being utilised for promotional training. According to the norm prescribed, there should be one Health Assistant/Health Supervisor for every 4 ANM/HWs.

Community Health Officers Training Scheme

This is a new scheme to be implemented in rural areas on a 100 per cent Centrally-assisted basis. As per recommendation of the Working Group on Health appointed by the Planning Commission, one Community Health Officer is to be appointed for each of the New Primary Health Centres and subsidiary health centres established during the 6th Plan period and thereafter.

A committee appointed by the Ministry of Health and Family Welfare worked a detailed training programme for the Community Health Officers. The report was considered and recommended for implementation by the Joint Meeting of the Central Council of Health and Central Family Welfare Council.

These Community Health Officers, selected from the supervisory staff at PHCs and District Level, would be provided training for a period of 6-9 months. CHOs would be responsible for providing supervision, support and guidance to all Health Personnel and Community Health Level Workers in implementation of Health, Family Welfare and MCH Programmes.

It has been decided to start the training of the Community Health Officers in the following Training Institutes on an experimental basis.

1. All India Institute of Hygiene and Public Health, Calcutta.
2. Family Planning Research and Training Centre, Bombay.
3. Rural Health Training Centre, Najafgarh.

A total number of 21 candidates have already been trained for a period of 6 month in these three training centres during the year 1983. Next training is to start in March, 1984.

Reorientation of Medical Education: Under the scheme of reorientation of Medical Education the Government of India has introduced from 1977-78 the scheme of reorientation of medical education, based on the plan of Action on the Report of Group of Medical Education and Support Manpower. The scheme envisages involvement of medical colleges in the delivery of health care in three selected community development blocks through a referral service system linking the medical college with district/tehsil/taluk hospitals and the peripheral units like Primary Health Centres. The scheme is to be extended to further blocks in a phased manner and an entire district would be covered within a period of 4-5 years. The Government of India has decided to give Central assistance to the tune of Rs. 4.79 lakhs per medical college for the purpose of providing infrastructural facilities. Under the scheme, medical colleges have so far been given financial assistance for implementation of the scheme. In addition, the Government of India has given three mobile clinics per medical college.

Critical Appraisal of the Health Guide Scheme in India

Health Guide Scheme in India has not made much impact so far. It was initiated to provide health care for the people and by the people. A seed can flourish and develop into a full-fledged plant only in a congenial soil and environment. Similarly, Health Guide Scheme can be successful if a sound organisational set up is provided for its growth. Let us analyse the reasons which are responsible for its failure in the areas where the scheme was introduced. If we want to put the scheme on a sound footing, we may keep the following facts and suggestions in mind.

Lack of Commitment on the Part of Health Experts and their Associations

There persists widespread negative and unhelpful attitude among health personnel towards the health care of the poorest strata in the rural and urban population. They are not aware of the social responsibility to the society. If the doctors at the primary level are not mentally convinced of the scheme, changes at the grassroots are unimaginable and impracticable. Most of the doctors and health experts contacted by the writer pointed out that, "Such schemes are unworkable as the community health workers cannot learn much during such a brief training. Instead of being an asset to the health care system, they may reverse the trends and these may create more problems than solutions". Others remarked. "They are already too busy with their routine functions. They are already over worked. They do not find any time to have intimate contacts with the community". A few remarked that "the present health care system cannot meet the needs of the society. The new system may be given a trial but the care may be taken to plan the scheme effectively before its introduction". The Medical Association has been vocal enough and described this scheme as a "cruel joke". The major hurdle is the opposition to change. Established health associations, institutions and organisations and it difficult to come out from their ivory towers and adjust to change and accept new challenges and responsibilities. Their resistance may be an attempt to defend their false prestige or traditions. Thus, there is a need to convince and train the health experts and their organisations before launching such schemes. We may cultivate a change in their attitudes in the interest of the programme.

At the recent Golden Jubilee celebrations of the Indian Medical Association, its President, Dr. J.V.R. Sarma, said that the IMA had not been consulted by Planning Commission in the matter of evolving an effective pattern of rural health care and a national policy on health. He complained that various Governments had instead devised schemes arbitrarily to "suit the fancies and philosophies of changing personalities". If the entire medical manpower could be involved through their professional organisations he was confident that it would be possible to achieve the objective of the scheme. There is an element of truth in this criticism.[23] The Government should not only consult experts before formulating any scheme but should also be able to energize, enthuse and develop a rapport with the professional organisations and, through them, their individual members to take an active part in the community health programmes.

Opposition from the Personnel of Traditional System of Medicine and Local Allopathic Practitioners

The scheme is being opposed by the established personnel of traditional system of medicine and local allopathic practitioners. They view this scheme as an encroachment on their authority and prestige. Most of the community health workers interviewed by the writer remarked, "practitioners of all the systems of medicine are making a lot of money by exploiting the illiterate poor in the villages. They think that if the scheme becomes successful, their future existence is uncertain. Besides, they have a strong hold on their clients and through them they spread propaganda against the utility of this scheme". One of the workers went on to the extent, "These practitioners would warn community that those people who would consult the community health workers would be in trouble as they knew nothing". Thus there is a need to educate these practitioners properly and associate them in the planning and implementation of the scheme.

Insufficient Training to Community Health Workers

The training imparted to the community health worker is quite inadequate. He has a very weak educational base. Dr. C. Parkash, Senior Medical Superintendent, Medical College, Rohtak remarked about this scheme to the *Tribune*. "The scheme is conceptually sound.... Since the success of the scheme will largely depend on the quality of personnel chosen for the job.. A bare three months training to a person who had schooling up to sixth standard is not likely to adequately, equip him for the job."[24] The same opinion was expressed by Prof. S.P. Gupta, Professor of Medicine in Medical College, Rohtak.[25] The Indian Medical Association suggested that the qualification for a CHW should be matriculation and that he must undergo at least 15 months training to acquire the fundamental knowledge needed for his work. He is to be trained in medicine, art of communication, leadership, etc. The people pointed out that the community health workers do not have much education and training to discharge the responsibilities entrusted to them. The success of the scheme would depend upon the confidence of the community in these workers. There is need for screening these workers so that we retain only those workers who can really be effective. Besides it has also become apparent that the process of retaining is essential in order to fill the gaps in the initial training or to refresh the health and medical knowledge imparted on a poor educational base.

Absence of Rural Bias in Medical Education

There is national commitment to reorient medical education profession and health services, so as to serve the needs of rural people. All the expert bodies have agreed to modify the syllabus of under-graduate medical education so as to produce a basic doctor who would have the ability to cater to the needs of the rural area. It is necessary to make the medical colleges act not as ivory temples in majestic isolation but take on the responsibility for providing total health care for specified segments of the rural population.[26] The aim of medical education should be to promote happiness through better health of most of the deprived hundreds of millions of human beings. With the contemplated changes in the contents of the undergraduate course; the students would be in a position to appreciate the problems of rural people and would develop proper motivation to help them.

Lack of Proper Health Education of the Village Community

Rural people lack functional literacy which is *sine qua non* for any endeavour towards community development. This requires a great effort on the part of the State governments; voluntary institutions and the health administrators should properly educate and enlighten the people. Properly planned programmes of health education would go a long way in propagating the ideals of a primary health care. It was observed by the writer that no regular efforts are being made to educate the public either by the health department or by the CHW. CHW devotes most of his time in providing curative care rather than laying much emphasis on educational approach. We must provide elementary and simple health education to the community. It should be based on indigenous technology. According to Dr. Mahler, the required new type of health education should be, "neither oversophisticated nor condescending but that against the confidence of the individuals and communities by explaining health technology in a language they can understand so that they can participate genuinely in taking decisions concerning their health. In short, a replacement of passive health education by active health learning". Besides, the beneficiaries should be asked to contribute to the cost of Primary Health Care. Everyone should realise his responsibility towards the health coverage of the community. When the rural people would be contributing, they would like to participate and take interest in its functioning. Some nominal contributions may be taken from the people themselves depending upon their income.

Absence of any Mechanism to Involve the Community

Community participation is the way to development but how to go about it? In the field of primary health care, it was pointed out by the workers that, "It is impossible to educate all the people by them. They have to carry out their own work, and this is only their part time duty. At present, there is no system to involve the community." It is suggested that we may involve teachers, Panchayat members and other influential men and women to diffuse the health education in the community. The constitution of Youth Clubs, Mothers Clubs, etc. as has been done in USSR, DRK, may be set up to promote functional literacy and health education among the community.

Exploitation by Community Health Workers

Community health worker is the pivot of the whole scheme. The success or failure of the scheme would depend to a great extent upon the attitudes, perception and ethos of the workers. It has been mentioned that, "These workers are not being selected properly. The selection of a Community Health Worker has become a political patronage". Such a scheme would have no chance to grow and ultimately survive if we do not find workers who are committed to bring about a social change in the villages. They must have missionary zeal. Their enthusiasm should not be dampened by unfavourable local conditions. They must have zeal and perseverance to reorient the attitudes of the people, otherwise the whole scheme would be a failure. Some people went to remark, "These community health workers have become the agents of the political parties. They are making a lot of money. They want to pose as doctors. They are not easily accessible. They are exploiting the poor people." A section of medical practitioners apprehends that, "half-baked and semi-literate persons masquerading as barefoot doctors will play havoc with the health of the masses". What is the difference then between the private practitioners and CHW workers. It is high time that we select, train and develop our community health workers properly. We must get a system by which we must be able to assess the work of these workers. The *Tribune* editorial dated 17 July 1975 had rightly commented that, "If picking good men is the most important of them all, dumping the bad one is the next most important". We know that even poorly devised machinery may be made to work if manned with well trained, intelligent, imaginative and devoted staff. On the other hand, the best planned organisation may produce unsatisfactory result if it is operated by mediocre or disgruntled people. So, we must find out workers who are committed, willing to accept hardships and prepared to work in a spirit of dedication.

Absence of Political Support/Interest in the Problems of Rural Areas

The political elite in the country are not sensitive and responsive to their duties. They are busy with manipulation of politics and find hardly any time to look into the problems of the people. Because of instability in politics, there is no continuous, concerted and consistent effort to weed out the obstacles in the path of development. What is required is a strong political will and determination to make these schemes successful. Political elite at all levels must support the cause of the rural poor and help them to enjoy the good standards of life which were promised to them at the inception of independence. Political powers and wisdoms are constantly required in a democratic set up to resolve any problem arising out of the policies and implementation of the scheme. The political elite may have to take bold and unpleasant steps to re-allocate the resources between urban and rural sectors.

No Sound Administrative set up to Implement the Politics of Community Health

A revolutionary scheme of this type can be successful only if there is proper administrative set up to implement it. Most of the health experts are of the view that the scheme has been rushed through without examining its requirements. It is suggested that some experts in Public Administration may examine the organisation and procedures which are being used to implement the scheme. They may also examine the problems of coordination, control, supervision and headquarter-field relationships. In the light of the suggestions, the existing scheme may be modified to suit requirements and the scheme in new areas may be set up according to new recommendations. One of the very important problems is the poor quality of supervision of the scheme. Multipurpose health workers who are supposed to be their immediate supervisors lack proper orientation and training themselves. It is suggested that the multi-purpose workers may be given refresher courses to discharge their duties efficiently.

Absence of Proper Evaluation

Evaluation is one of the most important components of any scheme. The good evaluation is to measure the impact of this scheme on health, the process of operations and scheme replicability. When the writer contacted the health experts, they pointed out many difficulties. Most of them observed, "No evaluation machinery has been designed. No methodology has been designed to measure the output. There is no simple information system by which the assessment of the scheme implemented so far can be made". This situation leads to failure in taking timely decisions and lack of feedback. Without an appropriate feedback, the health workers of the PHC level feel frustrated and their function as agents for information becomes meaningless to them. This lack of feedback is probably one of the most important problems in the development of primary health care which needs solution. It is suggested that a simple information system may be designed to suit the conditions prevailing in a particular area.

Problem of the Supply of Drugs

The drugs are very costly. Most of the workers mentioned that "The amount of Rs. 600 per year for drugs is too small to meet the demands of the people". It is suggested that:

(a) The Government must strengthen the drug industries in the public sector and manufacture essential drugs at cheaper prices.

(b) The indigenous medicine may be standardised and used to provide cheaper services.

(c) Beneficiaries may be asked to contribute two to five rupees per head per year to make the scheme viable and effective. This would also encourage more participation.

(d) Researches to exploit local flora and fauna as medicine may be encouraged.

(e) More treatment may be suggested through the control of diet and naturopathy which would lead to better health.

(f) The supply of drugs may be made in time to keep the morale of the workers high and win confidence of the people.

Conclusion

The experimental of Community Health Workers Scheme in India has not gone on long enough to reveal all the problems inherent in it. Besides, it has not acquired the sophistication and expertise that one associates with already existing health programmes. There has been great opposition from many quarters. They consider this system as inferior and primitive. But their opposition is based on superficial thinking. There is not substitute for a poor country like India where the people cannot afford the costly medical care system. It may be noted here that even highly industrialised societies as in USSR are depending upon such schemes to provide effective health care to the community. There is no denying the fact that this is theoretically sound and can help the unprivileged people and deprived communities to take care of their health problems which otherwise would remain unattended to because of financial and professional constraints. The scheme is a vital link in the country's health schemes. The weakness of the scheme is because of the poor design of the implementation machinery which may be streamlined to provide the health facilities for all.

References

1. Isenberg, *The Developing Nations: Poverty and Progress*, New York, 1969, p. 13.
2. UNICEF/WHO Study - *Alternative Approach to Meeting Basic Health Needs in Developing Countries* by V.D. Juleanovic and E.P. March, 1975.
3. WHO, *World Health*, May, 1978, p. 26.
4. WHO, *The State of World Nutrition* (NUTP/73).
5. UN, World Food Conference: E/CONF/65/4, pages 502-04.
6. WHO, SEARO: Annual Report of the Regional Director (1966-77) p. 5 SEA/RC30/2).
7. WHO, "The Role of Frontline Workers" *WHO Chronicle*, Vol. 29. No. 1 (January, 1975).
8. WHO, *World Health*, "Primary Health Care", May 1979, p. 6.
9. WHO: SEARO: SEA/RC 30/Sept. 1977, p. 38.
10. Giovanni, Sartori "Concept Misformation in Comparative Politics", *The American Political Science Review*, Vol. LXIV, No. 4, December, 1970, pages 1050-52 (Pluralism, integration, participation, mobilisation).
11. M. Soysal "Public Relations in Administration: The Influence of the Public on the Operation of Public Administration, Excluding, Electoral Rights", *General Report to the XIII International Congress of Administrative Services*, Paris, 1965, Brussels 11 AS, 1966, p. 47.

12. P. Yadav Ram "People's participation: Focus on Mobilisation of the Rural poor", U.N. Asian and Pacific Institute, *op. cit.*, p. 6.

13. Mahler, H., "Further Thoughts on WHO Mission" *WHO Chronicle*, 29, 253-56, 1975.

14. Lucan Pye, *Aspects of Political Development*, p. 64.

15. Ramalingaswami, *op. cit.*, p. 12.

16. WHO, *World Health*, July, 1976, p. 12.

17. For details refer to Chapter 1.

18. See figure 1.1 to understand the intricacies of Health Information System in relation to Primary Health Care System.

19. Based on the article "A land transformed" written by Prof. T.S. Sharmanov, Minister of Health of the Kazakh Soviet Socialist Republic, and corresponding member of the Soviet Academy of Medical Science, in *World Health*, May 1978, pp. 4-6.

20. Based on the article "Building a Bridge" by Paul Harrison, British journalist and photographer in *World Health*, May, 1978, pp. 7-11.

21. Based on the article "Medicine Man" by John Lofus, a journalist, *World Health* Oct. 1976, pp. 17-19.

22. Based on the article, "Generating Self-confidence" by Manual Carballo, a member of the unit of maternal and child health division of Family Health, WHO Headquarters in Geneva, *World Health*, May, 1978, pp. 26-29.

23. *Sunday Standard*, oct. 1, 1978.

24. *The Tribune*, Oct. 25, 1978, Chandigarh.

25. *Ibid*.

26. *India: National Plan for Health Care Services in the Rural Areas*.

11

Administration of A Primary Health Centre Complex

A. Genesis, Growth and Functions of Primary Health Centres

Genesis

The concept of the PHC as an institution to provide both curative and preventive services can be traced to the report of the consultative council on Medical and Allied Services, held in 1920, in England under the chairmanship of Lord Dawson of Penn[1] In this region, the PHC was established at Kalutura, Ceylon, in 1926 with the assistance of Rockefeller Foundation.[2] Provision of Rural Health Services through Rural Health Centres was recommended by the European Conference on Rural Hygiene of Geneva in 1931 under the Health Organisation of League of Nations.[3] It defines the 'Rural Health Centres' as:

An institution for the promotion of the health and welfare of the people in a given (rural) area, which seeks to achieve its purpose by grouping under one roof or coordinating in some other manner, under the direction of a health officer, all the health work of that area, together with such welfare and relief organisations as may be related to the general public health work.

The concept gathered momentum in socialist countries. The inter-governmental Conference for Eastern countries, convened at Bandung under the auspices of League of Nations recommended the integration of preventive and curative services and preference to curative services. Similar developments took place in the Eastern European countries that have come under the influence of socialism.[4]

This concept spread to other countries after World War II. Let us discuss in detail about the development of this concept in India. The Bhore Committee (1946) recommended that a Primary Health Centre should be set up to serve as the focal point for providing comprehensive, curative and preventive health services in the rural areas. In 1962, the Mudaliar Committee suggested that Primary Health Centres may be set up in all 5,000 "blocks". Each centre should serve a population of 60,000 to 1,00,000. This concept spread to all the Asian and African countries and a little later to Latin America.

Functions

The functions of a PHC have been enumerated in a publication from India as [5] : (1) Medical Care; (2) Maternal and Child Health Services; (3) School Health Services; (4) Family

Planning; (5) Control of Communicable Diseases; (6) Environmental Sanitation; (7) Health Education; and (8) Vital statistics. The staff to provide these services would comprise: a medical officer, a woman physician, a public health nurse, a health educator, a statistical clerk, a clerks-stenographer, a midwife, a health inspector (Sanitarian) a laboratory technician, and several family planning field workers, with health assistants to assist the staff members. Similar range of health services have been mentioned in a "Guide to rural health centre work" issued by the Government of Burma.[6]

Growth

The scheme was launched in India in 1952. Till March 1983, 5,959 PHCs and 65,643 sub-centres have been established in 5,258 blocks.

Progress Achieved and Targets for Sixth Five Year Plan (1980-85).

(A) *Sub-Centres*

The sub-centres will be established on the basis of one sub-centre for every 5,000 population in general and for every 3,000 population in hill, tribal and backward areas. The additional sub-centres to be established during the 6th Plan period will raise the number to about 90,000 against the estimated total requirements of 1,22,000. Their progress is as follows:

(a) Functioning on 1.4.1980	47,172
(b) Established during 1980-83	18,471
(c) Target for the 6th Plan period	37,940
(d) Target for 1983-84	9,010

(B) *Primary Health Centres*

The additional Primary Health Centres will be established in places where the existing Primary Health Centres cater to a larger population, so as to reduce the work-load on existing Primary Health Centres for providing better services.

(a) Functioning on 1.4.1980	5,484
(b) Established during 1980-83	475
(c) Target for the 6th Plan period	756
(d) Target for 1983-84	405

(C) *Subsidiary Health Centres*

It is proposed to convert the Rural Dispensaries into subsidiary Health Centres.The ultimate object is to involve all the rural dispensaries at present providing only curative service, in providing the package of promotive, preventive and curative services:

(a) Functioning on 1.4.1980	2,056
(b) Established during 1980-83	1,126
(c) Target for the 6th Plan period	2,270
(d) Target for 1983-84	804

(D) *Upgraded PHCs*

It is proposed to establish rural hospitals by upgrading the existing PHCs. Each of the upgraded PHC will have 30 beds to meet the need of the rural population.

(a) Functioning on 1.4.1980	218
(b) Established during 1980-83	253
(c) Target for the 6thPlan period	315
(d) Target for 1983-84	70

A study of the Pilot-Project in Nurpur Bedi Community Development Block in District Ropar (Punjab)

The State Health and Family Welfare Department launched a pilot project to deliver primary health care to the rural masses in Nurpur Bedi block of Ropar district with effect from 1 August 1979. The district of Ropar was carved out as a result of reorganisation of the erstwhile State of Punjab on 1 November 1966. Nurpur Bedi is one of the 6 Community Development Blocks in the district, comprising 110 villages and is inhabited by 57,021 people as per 1971 census. The present population of this block has risen to 62,000. Topographically, the Nurpur Bedi contains sub-nontane and plain areas. The summer in the block is a little hotter than in other parts of the State whereas the winter makes the climate too cold. The annual rainfall during the year 1971 was 137.4 centimetres. The average rainfall for the last five years works out to 93.85 centimetres.

The object of the project is to provide curative, preventive and promotive health care through MCH, family welfare, environmental sanitation, maintenance of vital statistics, health education and health functionaries.

Organisation and working of the project. Under the project, Nurpur Bedi has been divided into 12 subsidiary health centres including the PHC. Each subsidiary health centre serves 5,000 population and has been further divided into five units i.e., each having a population of 1,000 (approximately) and a unit may consist of one or two villages. In case a unit consists of more than one village, the biggest village serves as the headquarter of the unit. The health team consisting of a medical officer incharge of subsidiary health centre, multipurpose workers (male and female), an indigenous trained *dai* and a Class VI employee visit each of these headquarter's main villages in its area on Monday, Tuesday, Wednesday, Thursday and Friday, respectively. The health team remains at the main village located at the headquarters of the unit of the subsidiary health on Wednesday. Saturday has been kept reserved for visiting the missed beat during the week due to holidays, leave, etc., or for completing the pending work of the week. In this way the health team is to visit each unit (village) once in a week. The health team maintains up-to-date record of each household in the area in the family folder. The family foiders would contain a complete health record of all members of the household and all the vital events, i.e., birth, death, marriage, sickness, immunisation, etc., recorded as and when these occur, during the visit of the male and female worker as per programme. The important information from the family folders are to be transferred into a master register by the worker.

The health team has selected a fixed place as venue of their routine visit and work for three hours daily at each headquarter of the unit from 8 to 11 a.m. in summer and 9 to 12 a.m. during winter with prior intimation to the village concerned. A steel almirah or a steel box containing basic medicines, dressing material and family folders of the village has been provided in every village (in the house selected for the purpose). The Medical Officer is to intimate the community, while on tour, to visit the service-cum-education camps and MCH clinics in the main unit villages on the day fixed for their health requirements.

In order to ensure mobility of the Medical Officer of the subsidiary health centre, the department has provided a motorcycle to each Medical Officer in the block, to help him to extensively visit all the villages falling in his area of duty to provide comprehensive health care to the community as well as to give necessary support to the multipurpose worker and the local village health functionary. The Medical Officer conducts medical check-up of school children and gives treatment for minor ailments to the sick students on the spot and the students requiring specialist treatment to the nearest primary health centre\hospital. He also arranges the immunisation of student against DT, etc.

The health team is supposed to give special attention to the promotion of the community health and prevention of communicable diseases through health education. In order to ensure that health education is effective, the department had planned weekly rosters for the year 1979-80 for the subjects to be taken up during the week by all the personnel of the Health and Family Welfare Department in the State.

Multipurpose Health Workers

(a) *Female.* The M.P.H.W. (F) has a calendered tour-diary for noting down all the needy cases to be visited on her next visit after consulting the family folder. After finishing need-based service, she does her routine home-visits depending upon the time available at her disposal. She plans her home-visits in such a way that all the families in her area are visited at least once in two months on the one hand but with provision of the maximum services to the needy mothers and children. She will take the active cooperation\involvement of the Mahila Mandals, trained indigenous Dais, CHWs, and the Gram Sevikas, besides supervising and taking the cooperation of Anganwadi staff for health education and nutrition supplementation. In case of a unit consisting of more than one village, she is to cover all the other villages in the unit on fixed visit-days.

(b) *Male.* The M.P.H.W.(M) visits the same unit as mentioned in the schedule for the health team. He visits all the villages in the unit in such a manner that he contacts every family in his area at least once in a fortnight. He notes down the births and deaths and other changes of circumstances required to be entered in the master register and respective family folders. He is also responsible for detecting needy persons to be attended to be the MPHW (F) and intimates her the same day. The calendered tour-diary is to be kept up-to-date, showing the work to be done on the visit and the work done on that visit. Male workers are also instructed to collect the sputum slides of the suspected TB cases during the field visit and get the slides examined at the subsidiary health centre.

Both the male and female MPHWs are to post the entries in the family folders and the master register on the same day, legibly and correctly.

Health Assistant (Male and Female) (See Table 2)

Health Assistants (Male and Female) have separate headquarters and work separately. They are not supposed to issue any instructions to the multipurpose health workers but report weekly to the BHO\MO who in turn, issue necessary instructions to the multipurpose health workers. In MCH clinic, ante-natal and postnatal clinics are attended by the health assistant (female) and concerned multipurpose health worker (female). The number of such clinics under the supervision of health assistants (female) has been increased to 20 clinics in a month instead of 4 earlier. The worker (female) attends the clinic and the pregnant and other female patients and children in the village. In the clinic, all the women in the area are to be given TT irrespective of the fact whether they are pregnant or not. The children are given immunisation against six deadly diseases namely, diphtheria, pertussis, tatanus, tuberculosis and poliomyelitis. The health assistants (f) are to supervise the Anganwadis and ensure that children are being given protected water and clean food supplements.

Laboratory Science

Special arrangements have been made at all the subsidiary health centres for laboratory services. A laboratory assistant has been provided in the subsidiary health centre with a microscope and other reagents for examining the blood slides for malaria, sputum for tuberculosis and other routine urine and stool examinations.

It is hoped that under the pilot project, the objectives of delivering primary health care to the community will be achieved.

Critical Appraisal

We have described the pilot project. It appears that the Department of Health, Punjab, has taken great pains to design a sound setup for the implementation of this project. The Director of Health Services is personally interested and involved to make the project a success. It is very difficult to assess the impact of the scheme during such a short period. However, we have examined the scheme by our personal visit, discussions with officials and experts interested in the project and people for whom the scheme has been designed. We give some of the facts and suggestions which can help in improving the performance of the project.

1. *Lack of Coordination Among the Developmental Agencies.* There are a large number of developmental agencies working at this block and the villages under its jurisdiction. We have already discussed that health affects and is affected by all other sectors of development. We find no coordination among these agencies. It is suggested that all the developmental agencies in a particular area must promote the problems of development simultaneously to produce sustained impact on the population inhabiting these areas.

2. *Absence of Organised Structures Among the People.* We do not find any organised structure in this block at any level to involve the beneficiaries and utilise their potential energy profitably. It is very difficult for the government to contact all the individuals\families through their paid employees. There is a need for some structures or groups of people to help themselves under the guidance of the expert

advice offered by the government. We have already witnessed the failure of the Community Development Programmes as we could not associate the people with our programmes. It is suggested that the Health Department, Punjab, may try to set up voluntary organisations of the people in collaboration with other developmental agencies to ensure effective communication and understanding.

3. *No Provision for ISM and Homoeopathy.* The scheme in the block provides only allopathic system of medicine which is costly and beyond the reach of most of the people. It is suggested that out of 12 subsidiary Health Centres manned by one Medical Officer trained through allopathic system of medicine, 6 may be manned by doctors trained through ISM and Homoeopathy. In this way, the people would get opportunity to get treatment through these systems as well.

4. *Absence of Linking with Cultural, Social and Religious Institutions.* We know that the success of health programmes depend upon their acceptance by the people. It was found that the health personnel do not try to go into the cultural, religious and social factors affecting the health of the people. These are very subtle factors which need our attention and care. The health personnel must try to enlist the cooperation of informal leaders who can help in accelerating the acceptance of these programmes. Customs and conventions of the area must be studied which can throw light on the behaviour of the people. It would be very easy to help the people provided we understand their attitudes and preferences.

5. *Absence of Political Will and Direction.* We already know of the political crisis in the country and absence of rationality among the political leaders at the block and the lower levels. There is a need to create political will and sensitivity towards development. The Department of Health, Punjab, should motivate the local political leaders to associate them in the developmental tasks.

6. *Absence of Missionary Spirit Among the Health Personnel.* The problems of public health are challenging as can be gauged from the statistics already enumerated. It is very difficult to solve these problems with bureaucratic and inhuman attitudes. It requires hard work, sympathy, and tolerance on the part of the health personnel engaged in this arduous and challenging task. It was told by most of the people that the personnel working are fulfilling only their legal duties reluctantly. We do not need highly specialised people in these areas. We, however, require dedicated people with missionary zeal to serve the people suffering from abject poverty. We must ensure that the health personnel assure the people of their full involvement in their own welfare. Dr Mahler, Director General of the WHO in his article "Health For All-Everyone's Concern" in *World Health* (April-May 1983) has rightly said that no longer should health workers act as minor deities, expecting mortals to behave in certain predetermined ways and, when the outcome is not what they expected, putting the blame on culture, apathy and illiteracy. Illiteracy is not an unsurmountable obstacle to health education, it is only used, too often, as a handy excuse for nonacti... So is apathy. But what are its real causes: a lack of concern or the consequence of frustrated efforts ? And when we invoke cultural barriers, we

Table No. 1: Job Responsibilities of Multipurpose Health Workers

Duties of Female Worker	*Joint Duties (both) for Male and Female*	*Duties of Male Worker*
1. M.C.H. Care-Pre-natal care; Natal care; Post-natal care; Infant care; Pre-school child care	1. Multipurpose Health Survey	1. N.M.E.P
2. Care at clinic	2. Family Planning	2. N.S.E.P
3. Assistance in Dai training	3. Minor ailments	3. Environmental sanitation
4. Immunisation Pregnant mothers and children T.T., D.P.T., Polio	4. Control of communicable diseases	4. Immunisation, small-pox, primary and revaccination
	5. Vital statistics	
	6. Maintenance of Record & Returns	
	7. Health Education	
	8. Referral General and M.T.P.	
	9. P.H.C. staff meeting sub-centre	
	10. T.B. Control Programme	
	11. Nutrition	

Table No. 2: Job Responsibilities of Multipurpose Health Assistants (Male & Female)

Duties of Male Health Assistant	*Common duties of both Male and Female Health Assistants*	*Duties of Female Health Assistant*
Supervision Concurrent and Consecutive	Supervisory Supervision of Joint M & F M.P.H. Ws' duties	Supervision Concurrent & Consecutive
M.P.H.Ws (Male) Specific duties School Health	Weekly visit to every S.C.	M.P.H.Ws (Female) Specific duties Attend weekly Sub-Centre M.C.H. Clinic
Containment measures of communicable diseases outbreak	*Administrative* Supplies, indent, procurement and distribution of equipment, medicine, vaccines etc.	Attend emergency calls from M.P.H.Ws (Female)
Ensure Malaria Radical Treatment Spray of insecticides	Ensure Consolidation and Submission of reports; ensure proper records maintenance Hold regular staff meeting	Contact pre-natal mothers to be delivered, during ensuing week, last week post-natal mothers Dai's Training
Dog destruction, rodent control including antifly measures	Attend P.H.C./Block meeting Attend referred cases Assist M.O. in F.P. Camps Assist M.O. in Special Health Campaigns Participate in Health Education. Any other duty assigned by M.O. I/C	

invoke another escape mechanism. For culture is ever changing and it is our duty both to conform to culture, to understand it, and to accelerate its evolution in the right direction.

7. *Absence of the Involvement of the Universities/Colleges of the Area in the Planning and Implementation of the Programme.* It is a matter of great regret that no attempt is being made to associate the faculty members of the universities and colleges to involve them with these programmes. The teachers through their knowledge and influence can help a lot in this direction if they are given due status. Some of them can take up such studies as research projects or encourage their research students to undertake such problems. Such studies can be of great use in improving the implementation and the future planning.

8. *Absence of Informal Supervision Through Medical Colleges Institutes.* There is no involvement of the medical colleges/institutes in the area. There must be a regular dialogue between these institutions and the persons responsible for the planning and implementation of the programme of primary Health Care. Student doctors may be encouraged to take interest in such projects. This would ensure the quick success and the future benefits in other areas.

9. *Absence of Research in the Flora and Fauna of the Area.* The health department is providing allopathic medicines to the people. These medicines have side effects and are costly. No attempt is being made to encourage research in the flora and fauna of the area which can provide cheap and effective medicine without side effects. The flora and fauna of the area is full of promise. This would encourage the development of the area also indirectly. We may extract medicines from plants and animals available in the area. This would be possible only if our research in the medical colleges/institutes is relevant to the area rather than only of theoretical significance and utility.

B. Need and Object of the study

Need of the study

The efficiency of the health services in rural areas being provided through Community Health Workers, Multipurpose Workers, Health Assistants, Sub-centres, Subsidiary centres, would depend upon the role of PHCs. PHCs would be able to serve the people if they are housed in good buildings, equipped with all facilities—laboratory and general sanitation, provided requisite staff, ensured regular supply of medicine etc. Besides, the officer looking after the PHCs and the institutions and functionaries under him should be professionally sound and possess administrative competence. However, it has been observed that these centres are not serving the purpose for which they were set up. A seminar report observed that:

> In most of the states, there were bitter complaints about Government-run hospitals and PHCs.It was mentioned in the consolidated reports from various states that hospitals are disgustingly dirty, patients are lying on the floors, there is even lack of elementary articles like spirit, hot water and cotton sheets are drenched with blood.

Comprehensive Health Care Delivery System
Nurpur Bedi, CDB Ropar

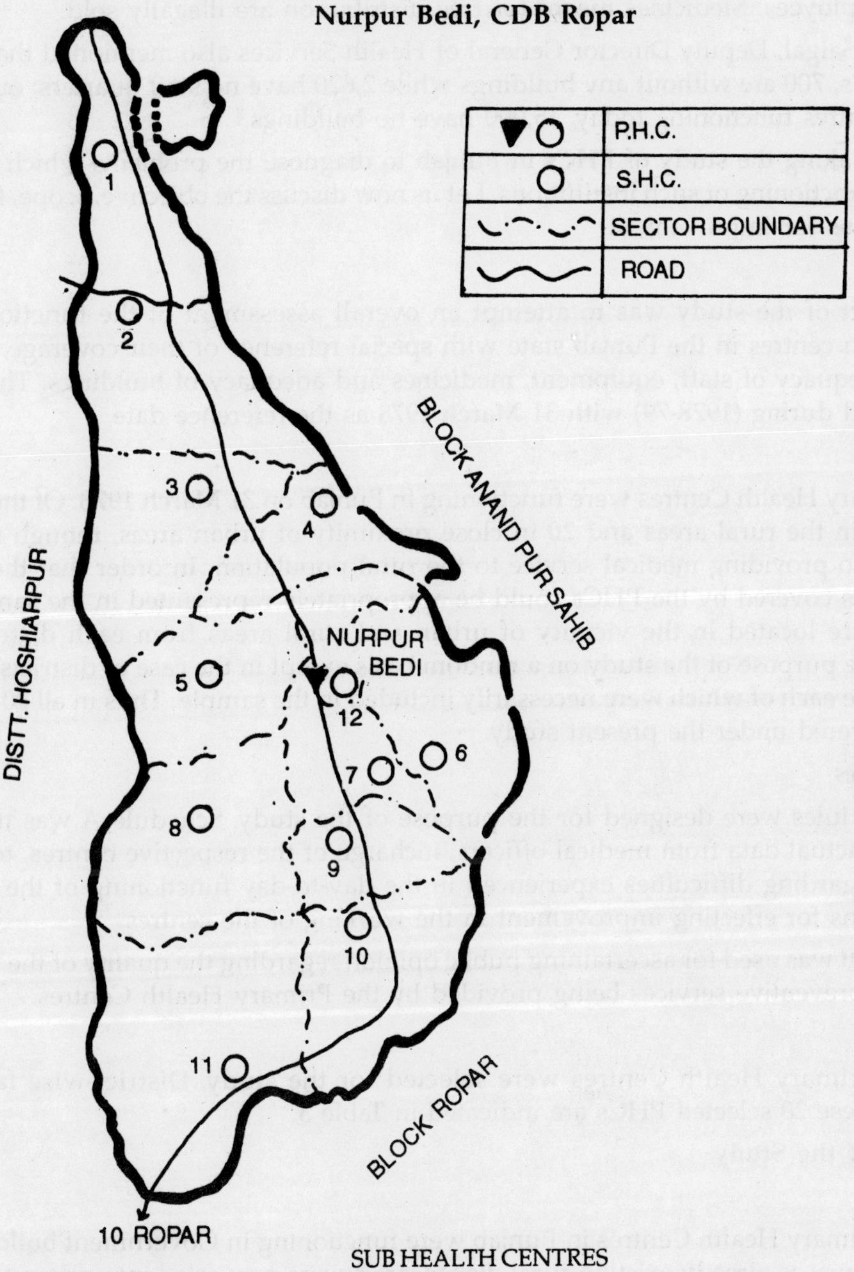

SUB HEALTH CENTRES

1. Khera Kalmos	2. Khanpur Khuds	3. Jhaj
4. Thana	5. Nurpur Khurd	6. Chanoli
7. Lalpur	8. Chandpur	9. Tahkatgarh
10. Sarhali	11. Tiba Tarion	12. Nurpur Bedi

> There were complaints about the corruption and indifference of doctors and class IV employees. Medicines meant for free distribution are illegally sold.[7]

Dr. M.D. Saigal, Deputy Director General of Health Services also mentioned that out of the 4,500 PHCs, 700 are without any buildings while 2,620 have no staff quarters; out of the 39,000 sub-centres functioning today, 15,000 have no buildings.[8]

We are making the study of PHCs in Punjab to diagnose the problems which impede the effective functioning of such institutions. Let us now discuss the objective, scope, findings and suggestions for improvement.

Object

The object of the study was to attempt an overall assessment of the functioning of primary health centres in the Punjab state with special reference of their coverage, quality of service, adequacy of staff, equipment, medicines and adequacy of buildings. The study was conducted during (1978-79) with 31 March 1978 as the reference date.

Sampling

128 Primary Health Centres were functioning in Punjab on 31 March 1978. Of those, 108 were located in the rural areas and 20 in close proximity of urban areas, though most of them were also providing medical service to the rural population. In order that the urban and rural areas covered by the PHCs could be appropriately represented in the samples at least one centre located in the vicinity of urban and rural areas from each district was selected for the purpose of the study on a random basis except in the case of districts having only one centre each of which were necessarily included in the sample. Thus in all 20 centres have been covered under the present study.

Survey Schedules

Two schedules were designed for the purpose of the study. Schedule A was used for collection of factual data from medical officers, incharge of the respective centres, to solicit their views regarding difficulties experienced in the day-to-day functioning of the centres and suggestions for effecting improvement in the working of the centres.

Schedule B was used for ascertaining public opinion regarding the quality of the various curative and preventive services being provided by the Primary Health Centres.

Coverage

The 20 Primary Health Centres were selected for the study. District-wise facilities available in these 20 selected PHCs are indicated in Table 3.

C. Findings of the Study

PHC Buildings

All the Primary Health Centres in Punjab were functioning in Government buildings at the time of survey as already existing rural dispensaries were converted into primary health centres. The limited space available in these buildings could not be sufficient to cater to the needs of the people. As many as 35 per cent of the centres reported this difficulty. The remaining 65 per cent which had been newly established had sufficient accommodation but need more additions to make room for new facilities.

Public Health Facilities

The PHCs are supposed to provide health education to the people. This would be possible only if the premises of the PHCs are clean and well-equipped. It was found that only 60 per cent of the centres had public health facilities, like flush latrines, piped water supply and electricity while 40 per cent did not possess such facilities.

Residential Accommodation

Non-availability of residential accommodation in remote rural areas is acting as a great deterrent in motivating medical officers to work in such areas.

The residential accommodation for officers has been provided in 55 per cent of the centres. The problem was not less acute in the case of para-medical, clerical and class IV personnel.

Medicines and Equipment

The supply of medicines and equipment was inadequate in 55 per cent of the selected health centres due to the paucity of resources. Besides, there was no regular supply. The stock of medicines was inadequate in all the centres.

Laboratory Facilities

Each Primary Health Centre in the State had been provided a laboratory under National Malaria Eradication Programme for the examinations of malaria cases. But many of these laboratories were not equipped to handle cases for investigation of general diseases.

Sanitation and Preventive Function

It was found that the sanitation was neglected since 50 per cent of the villages covered under the study were having poor sanitation.

Control of Communicable Diseases

Communicable diseases take a heavy toll of human life, especially in the rural areas. The study revealed that disease control programmes were implemented satisfactorily. Regular vaccination was being carried out by 80 per cent of the PHCs. However, arrangements for clearance and disinfection of stagnant water were lacking badly because of the lack of people's cooperation and involvement.

Administrative Training

No Medical Officer under study has undergone any administrative training. There is no arrangement of coordination between the private practitioners and the PHCs. The indigenous system of medicine is not being administered through the PHCs. Beneficiaries are very little involved in the health care administration. The frequency of visit by the PHC staff to the fields is very low.

Health Education

Dissemination of health education among the masses is an important function of the health workers. It was found that health education of the people was not being done scientifically since the villagers were found ignorant about the basic health and hygienic practices.

Table No. 3: District-wise various facilities available in selected Primary Health Centres in Punjab (percentage)

Sl. No.	District	No. of Selected Primary Health Centres		Building Accommodation		Public Health Facilities		Residential Accommodation			
								Medical Officer		Para-Medical Officer	
		Urban	Rural	Adequate	Inadequate	Available	Non-available	Available	Non-available	Available	Non-available
1.	Amritsar	1	1	70	30	90	10	75	25	75	25
2.	Jalandhar	1	1	60	40	90	10	75	25	75	25
3.	Ludhiana	-	1	65	35	90	10	75	25	75	25
4.	Kapurthala	-	1	60	40	75	25	50	50	50	50
5.	Ferozepur	1	1	60	40	70	30	50	50	50	50
6.	Bhatinda	1	1	65	35	50	50	50	50	40	60
7.	Faridkot	-	1	65	35	40	60	50	50	50	50
8.	Patiala	1	1	70	30	50	50	50	50	60	40
9.	Ropar	1	1	65	35	40	60	50	50	60	40
10.	Sangrur	1	1	70	30	50	50	50	50	50	50
11.	Gurdaspur	-	1	60	40	40	60	50	50	40	60
12.	Hoshiarpur	1	1	70	30	40	60	50	50	50	50
	Average	8	12	65	35	60	40	55	45	60	40

Table 3 (contd.)

Sl. No.	District	Supply and stock position of medicine: Stock of medicine — Adequate	Inadequate	Supply of medicine — Adequate	Inadequate	Vacancies of medical para-medical staff: Medical Officer	Para Medical Staff	Sanitation arrangement: Good	Bad	Opinion survey regarding doctors' behaviour: Courteous	Callous	Preference of rural people for medical treatment: PHC & private physician	Pr. PHC		Administrative training of PHC doctors: Training received
1.	Amritsar	-	100	40	60	30	15	60	40	80	20	50	50		
2.	Jalandhar	-	100	40	60	25	20	60	40	75	25	50	50	-	100
3.	Ludhiana	-	100	40	60	30	15	60	40	80	20	50	50	-	100
4.	Kapurthala	-	100	50	50	40	20	50	50	80	20	40	60	-	100
5.	Ferozepur	-	100	45	55	30	15	40	60	70	30	40	60	-	100
6.	Bhatinda	-	100	50	50	35	20	40	50	70	30	30	70	-	100
7.	Faridkot	-	100	45	55	40	20	40	60	80	20	20	80	-	100
8.	Patiala	-	100	40	60	30	15	50	50	70	30	40	60	-	100
9.	Ropar	-	100	50	50	35	20	50	50	80	20	30	70	-	100
10.	Sangrur	-	100	50	50	40	20	40	60	65	35	20	80	-	100
11.	Gurdaspur	-	100	40	60	40	25	40	60	75	25	20	80	-	100
12.	Hoshiarpur	-	100	45	55	35	20	40	60	70	30	20	80	-	100
	Average	-	100	45	55	35	20	50	50	75	25	30	70	-	100

Opinion Survey

With a view to ascertaining the response of the people towards rural health services an opinion survey was carried out by inter-viewing members of panchayats/municipal committees located in the areas covered by the selected primary health centres.

Majority of the people were appreciative of the functioning of the PHCs. In all 40 members of panchayats/municipalities were interviewed. Most of them (75 per cent) were satisfied about the performance of the PHCs. A few cases of unsatisfactory behaviour of staff especially at lower levesst awards the patients were observed. Besides, 70 per cent of the people interviewed indicated preference for Rural Health Centres in comparison to private practitioners due to ready availability of expert medical service, free service and free medicines. They were very sore about the non-availability of medicines. Besides, 80 per cent wanted the institution of indigenous system of medicine at the PHC (additionally; 80 per cent respondents mentioned that the PHC staff did not visit the community. Sixty per cent of the interviewed were very sore about the fact that performance is given to influential people.

D. Suggestions for Improvements

The study suggests the following for improving the functioning of the primary health centres:

1. There is an urgent need of providing adequate building accommodation in each centre to provide good environment for service. Besides, the construction of houses for the staff should be taken up as it will increase the morale and efficiency of the personnel working there.
2. It is essential to provide adequate basic public health amenities, like piped water, sewerage, flush latrines and electricity in each centre to provide full facilities to the patients. This would also create better image of the PHCs.
3. Immediate steps may be taken to fill up the vacant posts of doctors and other para-medical staff to provide health care to the people. One lady doctor may be posted in each Primary Health Centre, since rural women generally prefer to be examined by a lady doctor. Besides, the PHCs may be put under the control of medical colleges to make the services more effective. This would also provide opportunity to undergraduate medical students to ascertain the health needs of the population.
4. Steps may be taken to ensure adequate and timely supply of medicines and equipment to health centres. They should maintain adequate stock of at least life saving drugs. This will raise the confidence of the people in PHCs and the people would not rush unnecessarily to city hospitals. Medicine may not be provided according to quota system but should be given according to the needs of the people.
5. For efficient discharge of curative functions, the Primary Health Centres should be provided sufficient equipment like refrigerators, X-ray and laboratory facilities, oxygen cylinders, operation tables and surgical instruments. It may also be ensured that X-ray plants and laboratories remain in working condition. The existing laboratories should be suitably strengthened with equipment.

6. The study revealed that indoor beds in PHCs generally remain unutilised. It would be worthwhile if some of these beds were transferred to the nearest referral hospitals and reserved for patients referred to it by the Primary Health Centres. These beds may be utilised for other patients in case these remain unutilised. This arrangement would serve a dual purpose of reserving beds for the PHCs and also increasing the bed-strength in referral hospitals.
7. While opening a new Primary Health Centre care may be taken in selecting such a site which should be easily accessible to the largest number of villages in the block as it was revealed that only those people visit frequently who are within 2-3 kms of the PHCs. A study of the patients coming to PHCs at Najafgarh indicated that among people living more than 2 miles from the health centre, the utilisation rate is very low. The people outside the radius of 2 miles accounted for only 19.8 per cent while 80.2 per cent were from the radius within two miles.
8. For efficient functioning of the centres, the administrative powers should be decentralised. The Medical Officer of the PHC is supposed to be the planner, the manager, the supervisor, the coordinator as well as Public Relations Officer, besides being a technical expert. Is he well equipped to discharge all these functions entrusted to his care? At present, all the incumbents possess no administrative competence which is essential to administer the PHCs complex. It is suggested that the officers of these PHCs may be got trained in health administration either at NIHFW or some special course may be arranged for them at the State headquarters.
9. In order to supervise and inspect sub-centres, transport facilities should be provided.
10. The auxiliary-nurse and midwives posted in sub-centres were engaged in the tasks of family planning, maternity and child health services only. They could be trained in elementary curative services for treatment of common diseases. This step would go a long way in meeting the emergent medical needs of rural population and fuller utilisation of the staff.
11. PHCs have no information regarding the extent and coverage of patients by private practitioners. It is suggested that the coordination between PHCs and private practitioners may be encouraged to provide efficient health care.
12. The opinion survey indicated that the services of indigenous system of medicine including homoeopathy should be made available in the PHCs. This would encourage fruitful relations among the various systems of medicine. Besides, the cost of health care administration can be controlled by using indigenous system of medicine. Such a system is cheaper, provides complete care, is easy to administer and is devoid of side effects.
13. The survey indicated that there are very poor linkages between the PHC staff and the community. The staff rarely find time to visit the community and diagnose its problems to ascertain its needs. The Medical Education Committee appointed by the Government of India observed that medical education should produce a basic doctor. The Committee defined: "A basic doctor is one who is well conversant

with the day-to-day health problems of the rural and urban communities and who is able to play an effective role in the curative and preventive aspects of the regional and the national health problems."[10] It is suggested that the PHC staff must visit once a week to provide health education through well arranged lectures in school building/panchayat ghars or arrange exhibitions. This would lay the foundation of health care administration.

The Fifth Plan (Approach Papers) also emphasised that the main thrust may be directed at making up the deficiencies in building, staff, equipment and drugs and medicines in a coordinated way.[11] Such studies and evaluations may be encouraged by the Health Department on institutional basis to provide clues for the effective functioning of PHCs. There is a need to invest funds to evaluate the functioning of these centres. If inadequate funds are invested, the entire effort may well be wasted whereas properly designed and supported research may yield the answer to this important question.[12]

The purpose of the study should be to ensure that PHCs and sub-centres are giving the best possible coverage in preventive and curative services within the resources available.

References

1. England and Wales, Ministry of Health, Consultative Council on Medical and Allied Services (1920). *Interim Report on the future of Medical and Allied Services*, London, H.M. Stationary Office.
2. Wickremesingh, W.G., *The Premier Health Unit in Ceylon*, Colombo, 1951.
3. League of Nations Health Organisation, European Conference on Rural Hygiene (1931), *Recommendations on the Principles Governing the Organisation of Medical Assistance, the Public Health Services and Sanitation in Rural Districts*, Geneva.
4. Veinerman, R.R., *Social Medicine in Eastern Europe*, Cambridge Mass, Harvard University Press, 1969.
5. India, Department of Community Development (1960), *Primary Health Centres*, Faridabad.
6. Burma (1962), *Guide to Rural Health Centre Work in Burma*, Rangoon, Govt. Printing and Stationery.
7. Gandhi Peace Foundation, *Problems, Programmes and Actions: Women's Point of View*, New Delhi, 1979, p. 52.
8. *Indian Express*, Chandigarh, 28 August 1978.
9. India, Rural Health Training Centre, Najafgarh (1964), *The Service from a Primary Health Centre*.
10. Govt. of India (1969), *Report of the Medical Education Committee*, Ministry of Health, New Delhi.
11. Govt. of India, Planning Commission, *Approach to the Fifth Plan* (1974-79), p. 10.
12. WHO, *Public Health Papers*, 48, p. 38.

12

Management of Primary Health Care

After the Conference held in Alma Ata, U S S R, in 1978, on Primary Health Care, many member countries of the World Health Organisation declared "Health for all by the year 2000 A.D., as their national policy objective. As a consequence these countries made increased budgetary allocations for progressively extending the scope and extent of essential health services provided to their people. Buildings were constructed for health centers and health workers were trained in large numbers. Results of health effort were more evident and effective in settings, where primary health care activities were properly planned, compared with those health care projects, in which healthcare services were expanded without due planning and preparation. As outlined earlier, primary health care should meet people's essential health *needs*. It should be *effective* in achieving the desired health objectives, so that the people can be motivated to actively participate in the health programs. Without proper planning and resources primary health care may soon become equated with inexpensive or

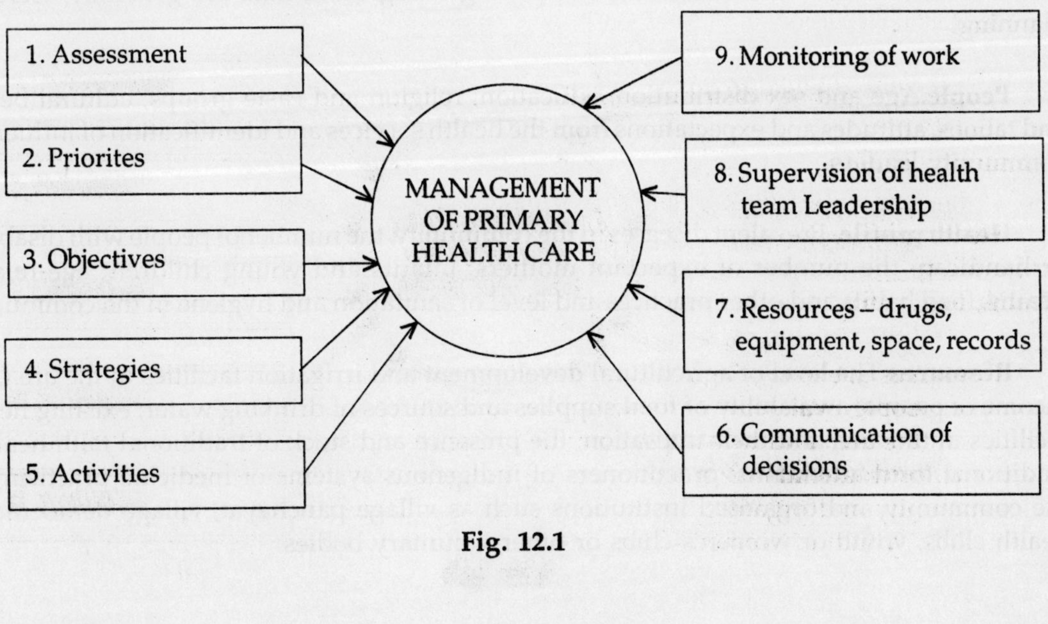

Fig. 12.1

inferior type of health care with minimum of health inputs for the underprivileged people, with which a country can get away with. Therefore, primary health care system should be *backed by all levels of health care delivery system* to ensure that the maximum benefits are derived from the investment made in primary health care. In the initial flush of enthusiasm, some countries built a large number of health posts, but did not train enough health workers to man these. Provision for housing of the staff was not made. Referral services were not developed concurrently. Logistics for supply of drugs and other supplies were irregular and inadequate. Means of communication between different levels of health care were non-existent. The people soon lost faith in the effectiveness of the health posts. The services provided there, were not fully utilised. The people travelled long distances to seek medical aid from the better equipped and staffed hospitals and clinics in the nearby large towns and cities. Where adequate transport facilities were not available, the people relied on folk remedies or indigenous practitioners.

Since anticipatory preparation, planning and good management procedures are crucial for getting a job well done ensuring maximum effectiveness with the given resources, some vital management techniques necessary for implementing primary health care programs in the community are discussed below.

1. ASSESSMENT OF THE SITUATION

Before embarking on a program, it is essential to make an objective evaluation of the health needs and available resources. Before the primary health care program is started, the health situation in the proposed area should be reviewed, especially with respect to the people and their health profile. Availability of community resources should be assessed and information on other characteristics of the population in the catchment area of the proposed health facility should be obtained. The following background data are generally useful in planning.

People. Age and sex distribution, education, religion and caste groups, cultural beliefs and taboos, attitudes and expectations from the health services and identification of influential community leaders.

Health profile. Prevalent diseases in the community, the number of people with disability or handicap, the number of expectant mothers, infants and young children; age-related deaths, food habits and other practices and level of sanitation and hygiene in the community.

Resources The level of agricultural development and irrigation facilities in the area, the income of people; availability of food supplies and sources of drinking water; existing health facilities in the area and their utilisation, the presence and stock of traditional faith healers, traditional birth attendants, practitioners of indigenous systems of medicine practising in the community and organised institutions such as village panchayat, village democracies, health clubs, youth or women's clubs or other voluntary bodies.

Catchment area. The geographic terrain of the catchment area, its climate, roads and means of communication.

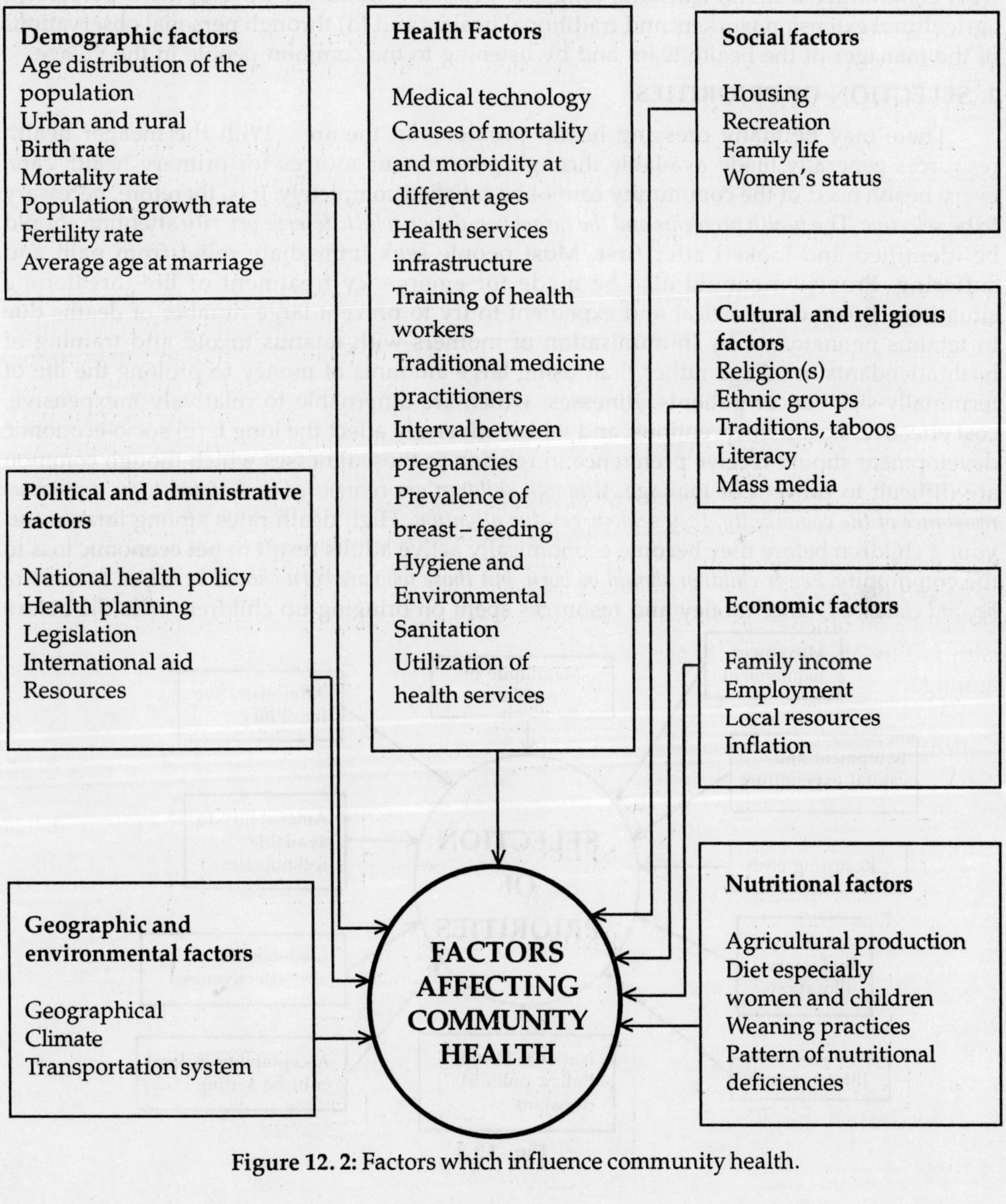

Figure 12. 2: Factors which influence community health.

How to Obtain this Information. This information obtained by (a) studying any published government reports such as the census figures, survey data or national health policy documents, area maps and annual reports on the health problems or health needs of the area (b) scanning the health center or clinic records for the last few years (c) discussion with community leaders, teachers, religious priests, community development personnel, agricultural extension workers and traditional healers and (d) through personal observations of the manager of the health team and by listening to the common people in the village.

2. SELECTION OF PRIORITIES

There may be many pressing health problems in the area. With the meager health resources generally made available through government sources for primary health care, every health need of the community cannot be satisfied completely. It is, therefore, necessary to be *selective*. The *health problems and the target population which deserve priority* attention should be identified and looked after first. Most people seek immediate relief from pain and suffering. Provision should also be made for emergency treatment of life-threatening situations. It is more practical and expedient to try to prevent large number of deaths due to tetanus neonatorum by immunisation of mothers with tetanus toxoid and training of birth attendants in village rather than using large amounts of money to prolong the life of terminally-sick cancer patients. Illnesses, which are amernable to relatively inexpensive, cost effective, health interventions, and which adversely affect the long term socio-economic development should receive preference in relation to those illnesses which though common are difficult to prevent or manage.*Although children are recognised and stated to be a precious resistance of the community, they seldom get due attention*. High death rates among infants and young children before they become economically active adults result in net economic loss to the community. *Fewer children should be born, but those who are born should be helped to surrvice beyond childhood*, since money and resources spent on bringing up children, who die before

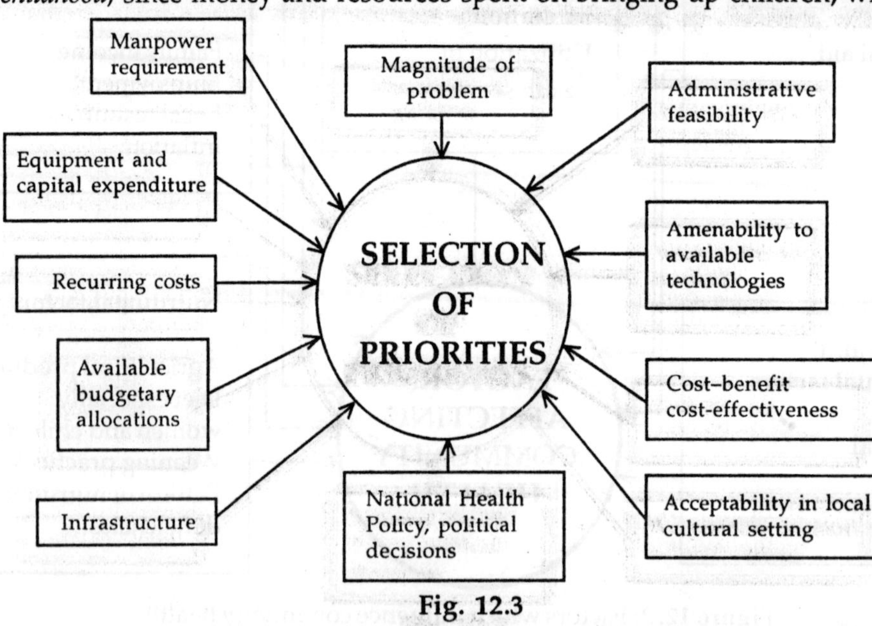

Fig. 12.3

becoming economically -productive adults are wasted. Health of the fetus, infant or young child is intimately related to the health of the mother. There is urgent need to control the spiralling rise in population so as to conserve the national wealth and to ensure equitable social justice for the people. Thus efforts for providing services for women,children and family planning deserve greater consideration in any primary health care program.

The *target population* to which health education should be specially directed to achieve the desired results should also be identified. Health education of the mother leads to better health care of children resulting in improvement of their health status. Family planning services are more often accepted by mothers, if the working husbands and mothers-in-law of young women are also concurrently motivated to limit the size of the family.

3.Defining Objectives

After the health priorities of the community have been identified health objectives or what is proposed to be achieved through health care should be defined. It is not always necessary that the health objectives should appear to be idealistic. It is more important to be realistic and set the objectives which are feasible, and can be achieved within the given time, with the use of available resource. The objectives should however always be relevant to the country's national health policy and needs. It should be possible to measure the results of health interventions so that their cost-bendtion cost-effectiveness can be evaluated. Thus a health objective mayaim at reducing the birth rate in the country to 25 per 1000 of population in a period of 5 years, to reduce the infant mortality rate to less than 60 per 1000 live births within a period of 3 years.

4. Considering Possible Stratfsies to Accomplish the Objectives

An objective may be achievable by the use of several alternate strategies. Some methods may be very effective in achieving the desired results, but the cost may be disproportionately high, being beyond the available resources. Other strategies may be relatives less expensive,but the anticipated end results may be of doubtful value. If the activity does not result in the desired impact on the health situation such as reduction of morbidity or mortality within a given frame of time, the community may become dissatisfied and all the investment made on primary health care may be wasted. The advantages of the proposed health care activities should be carefully evaluated in relation to the available manpower and other financial and material resources. As a general principle, the relatively inexpensive strategies should be adopted for the management of commonly prevalent health problems, for which there is a large popular demand. For relatively less common problems, requiring more effective methods, it may be expedient to use more costly approaches. The management approaches should always be flexible in that one should be willing and ready to respond to the new thinking and knowledge with an open mind. Let us consider an example. In several countries three doses of live attenuated oral poliovirus vaccine are given at age 3,4 and 5 months. Studies in India showed that about half to two third of infants who had received all the three doses did not develop humoral antibodies against all the three strains of vaccine virus. A few cases of paralytic poliomyelitis in the previously immunised infants were also reported. It become necessary to review the strategies for polio immunisations. Various possible alternatives were considered, such as (a) infants should receive 5 doses of OPV instead of 3 doses for primary vaccination, (b) inactivated poliovirus vaccine (Salk) should be given along with the triple antigen by injection, (c) and the vaccine should be given from the existing health posts, as at present, with periodic reinforcement or pulsing by mass immunisation of most children in the community at specified intervals by special immunisation teams working intensively. The questions that needed consideration were the cost of the vaccine, assurance of continuous supplies, logistics, especially reliability of the cold chain, attitudes of the people towards injectable vaccine and the scientific aspects of local tissue immunity *vis-a-vis* humoral antibodies and the duration of protection achieved with the different vaccines.

BCG vaccination was reported to be ineffective in reducing the incidence of pulmonary tuberculosis in a study at Chingleput in South India. This is currently under intensive review to find the possible reasons for the poor results and devise practical solutions.

5. Making Correct Decisions about activities to be undertaken

After carefully reviewing and considering various alternate strategies, their advantages, disadvantages, cost-effectiveness, scientific soundness and cultural acceptability, decision should be made about the activities that should actually be undertaken in accordance with the expressed national health policy. The decisions should be technically sound and correct. Possible constraints and obstacles in implementing these activities should be carefully looked into. Adequate prior planning should be done by interaction between the community, members of the health term and the administrative officers in the Department of Health.

6. Communication of Decisions to Appropriate Levels.

After the decisions about the health—care activities to be undertaken in the community are finalised these should be communicated to the health workers in the field, who are required to implement the programs. All instructions should be detailed, explicit, clearly worded, avoiding ambiguities and always given in writing. These should be conveyed promptly to the concerned officials, so that the programs are implemented promptly within the proper time frame.

7. Mobilisation and Development of Resources

It is not enough to make a decision to undertake a specific health activity. There should be resources to implement it. Staff needs to be recruited and budgetary provisions for their salaries and other perquisites, such as housing, medical services, education of children, social security obligations like pension and gratuity should always be made. Materials such as common drugs, agents for prophylactic immunisations, food supplements, vitamin capsules and hematinic tablets, surgical dressings, and other equipment for minor surgical work, instruments for delivery of pregnant women and resuscitation of preterm or asphyxiated babies, simple diagnostic apparatus, laboratory stains, besides the furniture for the staff and racks and cupboards for storage of drugs and supplies are required. There should be adequate working space at the health post for members of the health team to operate from a base. Means of communication with the referral centres should also be easily available.

All these activities require money and this has to be mobilised, either from the government, community, non-government-voluntary agencies or recognised United Nations agencies such as World Health Organisation, United Nations International Children's Fund, Food and Agriculture Organisation and United Nations Fund for Population Activities. Some foreign foundations in Europe and USA disburse large sums for specified projects in some countries. It is advisable to rely only on those funding agencies, who assure help on a long term basis and who create a permanent infrastructure, so that the projects aided by them can become self reliant in the long run.

Good budgeting involves a balanced allocation of resources for different groups of activities. Overhead administrative costs should be kept at a minimum, consistent with efficiency. Actual benefits to the target population should be maximised. Preventive services and those activities which promote positive health should receive more or at least as much consideration as the demand of drugs for curative activities.

A proper accounting control over the expenditure, prevents the meager resources being frittered away for furthering personal interests of some members of the health team or of the influential members of the village community.

7.1. Drugs

Drugs, immunising agents, vitamins, hematinics and food supplements are needed for primary health care. People have faith in the efficacy of drugs and often demand these. Drugs are useful, but these should be used with adequate knowledge and proper skill. Most drugs are potentially dangerous, if these are given for inappropriate indications and if prescribed in large doses. These may result in permanent disability or even death of patients in some cases. Most drugs should be kept out of the reach of children. Being expensive, the drugs should be used judiciously. If some drugs are expended at an unusually fast rate, some needy patients reporting later in the year might be deprived of their benefit, if stocks are depleted soon. In primary health care setting in the most countries, the drugs are generally in short supply. It is, therefore, improper to use drugs wastefully. Excessive consumption of drugs can be curtailed by (i) using a minimum number of drugs for one patient (ii) minimising the use of placebos (iii) withholding drugs from patients without a correct diagnosis or indication (iv) not forcing use of drugs on unwilling patients, who do not have faith in their efficacy (v) not stocking more than what is actually needed (vi) proper storage of perishable drugs and (vii) preventing their pilferage. The cost of drugs can be reduced considerably if these are ordered by their generic names, rather than by their brand names, since the popular-brand-name drugs are generally expensive. Perishable vaccines and drugs should not be indented and stocked, if a refrigerator or cooling arrangement is not available. If the power supply in the village is erractic, chances of drugs being spoiled should be kept in view. Even kerosene-operated refrigerators have become impracticable in the rural health posts, due to erratic supply and high cost of kerosene.

The health workers should be properly instructed about the correct use of drugs, their appropriate doses and side effects. The patients should receive proper guidance about the correct dose, mode of administration, need for regularity of therapy and the duration of full course of treatment especially for chronic illnesses, such as tuberculosis and leprosy, which require drug therapy of prolonged periods.

Standard List of Drugs

The scarce resources available for the purchase of drugs can be most effectively employed if a standard list of drugs, which are likely to be needed most for the health problems, which prevalent in the region or drugs which are most often prescribed, is made. However, the health team should be permitted to exercise some flexibility in the choice of drugs so that it may be able to respond to an unforeseen change in the health situation. A provision should be made for contingency purchase of some urgently required drugs.

The standard list of drugs is generally prepared from an analysis of the prevalent diseases and health problems, availability and cost of drugs, their effectiveness, risks of toxicity and facilities for proper storage. It may not be possible to give complete guideline on the standard lists, but the following indications are generally useful in most developing countries.

Antibiotics and chemotherapeutic agents for specific infections and infestations

Benzyl pencillin for injection, streptomycin for injection, sulphadimidine (with the rapidly reducing cost of co-trimoxazole, it may become competitive and more cost-effective in some situations), chloramphenicol capsules, tetracycline eye ointment, isoniazid, dapsone, chloroquine, metronidazole, mebendazole, piperazine, terrachlorethylene.

Pain relieving

Asprin, codein tablets, lidocaine for injection.

Antihistaminics

Only one or two antihistaminics may be stocked, chlorpheniramine or promethazine are recommended. An injectable preparation may also be kept.

For skin infections

Gentian violet lotion and benzyl benzoate emulsion for scabies.

For asthma

Adrenaline hydrochloride injection aminophylline injections and tablets.

For convulsions

Tablets of phenyl-hydantoin, phenobarbitone and diazepam injections.

For delivery work

Ergometrine maleate

Vitamins and hematinics

Vitamin A and D capsules, iron tablets and folic acid tablets.

For dressing of traumatic wounds

Tincture of iodine, vaseline, cetrimide lotion (Cotton wool and dressings).

Logistics of Drug Supplies

A primary-health-care post should periodically get its supplies of drugs at prespecified intervals according to the administrative convenience. The worker incharge of the health post should be aware of the sources of supply of drugs and procedure for ordering these. He or she should have a catalogue giving the correct generic names of the drugs, contents of each unit of the drug packing and the approximate price. The requirements of drugs may be estimated by multiplying the expected number of patients who are likely to be treated during the period by the full course of drug needed for each such patient. Accordingly, an indent of drugs is made. The indent generally provides for about 10 to 15 per cent in excess of the estimated quantities to provide for unforeseen excessive demands or possibility of delay in receiving the next installment of supplies.

Indent should always be scrutinised by a senior medical officer and then forwarded to the agency responsible for the supply of drugs. The procedure for the despatch of drugs should be streamlined for minimise avoidable delays. When drugs are received from the supply agency, these should be duly inspected and checked before these are stored in the primary-health-care post.

As general principle, the drugs should be best stored in a cool-dry place away from direct sunlight. These should not be exposed to damp atmosphere, since the quality of drugs may deteriorate or coating of tablets may become unsightly. The drugs should preferably be stocked in air tight tins or screw capped jars. Perishable drugs should have clear written instructions on the package, about optimal storage conditions. Drugs with a recent date of expiry should be used early. These should be stored in such a way, that they are easily identified from those with longer shelf-life. The former should be issued for use in the health post before the latter. Dangerous, habit forming and very expensive drugs should be stocked separately in a locked cupboard with a different accounting register.

In order to prevent unexpected shortage of drugs, the store keeper should make an estimate of drugs needed in the interval between the time of next indent and the expected time of their receipt, in a separate store shelf or bundle. He should generally issue these for use only after the stocks are replenished, or in emergency situations.

The drugs should be issued by the storekeeper to the dispenser against a specific *issue voucher* and an entry should always be made in the stock book. Only the minimum essential quantity of drugs required for use on that day or week should be issued at a time, to prevent excessive wasteful use and to minimise the possibility of pilferage.

In accordance with the established policy of the administration, the dispenser should be asked to issue drugs for the specified number of days for which prescribed to the patients, preferably in already prepared small paper or polythene bags or pill boxes. It is desirable to include a slip of paper in the package itself giving instructions for the use of the drug. These may be written in the local language either by hand, during the spare time of the dispenser or alternatively a cyclostyled or printed instruction slip may be used. The stocks of drugs should always be replenished well in time to avoid discontent among the community.

7.2 Equipment and Stores

Just like drugs, equipment and stores are also essential resource needed for primary-health-care posts. Non-expendible stores such as furniture weighing scales, bed pans, screens, surgical equipment, microscopes and motor vehicles are not easily damaged, if these are properly handled, and can be kept in use for several years. These should be maintained in working order by regular and timely repairs when needed. On the other hand, drugs, food, paper, syringes, laboratory reagents, kerosene, petroleum, candles, match boxes, torch cells, cotton wool and surgical dressings etc. are actually expended and hence these are called extendible stores. Logistics of supply and procurement of stores should be established on the same lines as described for drugs.

Non-expendible stores should be handled carefully. A proper inventory should be made. Issue vouchers should show details of their distribution, with the signatures of the persons responsible for their use, also indicating the place, where the equipment will be used. The person using the equipment should be held responsible for keeping it in good working condition. He should undertake judicious and economic use of the equipment and arrange for its timely repairs. Equipment kept in dusty and damp atmosphere deteriorates rapidly.

7.3 Space

It is advisable to build the health post for primary health care at a site which is easily accessible to the people living in the catchment area. Its construction should be functional, not extravagant. Architecturally the space within the building should be so arranged, that it facilitates srnooth and orderly work and does not inconvenience or obstruct the movement of staff or the patients. The patient should be able to move without obstruction from the registration desk to the room of the health worker. The latter should have the facility to record the relevant clinical observations and advise the necessary health measure. The patient should then be able to move forward to the laboratory area if necessary and to the dispensary for collection of prescribed drugs etc. without difficulty. A reverse flow of patients or a

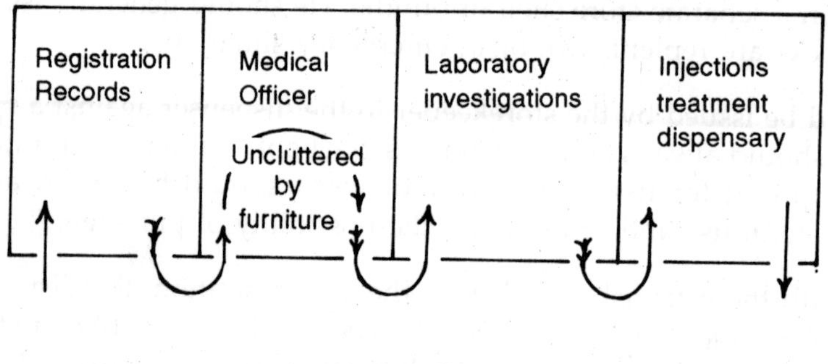

Fig. 12.4

common entrance and exit are not conducive to good working arrangement. A patient should preferably not leave the health workers, room through the same door, from which other patients are entering. Furniture and equipment within the rooms should be so placed that it helps the staff in the efficient discharge of their duty, while assuring complete privacy to the patient. Security of the equipment is also an important consideration when arrangements are being made.

7.1 RECORDS AND PAPER WORK

In a primary health care setting some paper work and records are essential and unavoidable. It is necessary to record patients' health status and the treatment prescribed on printed forms. Stock books and ledgers have to be maintained and general correspondence needs to be attended to. Periodic reports of work have to be submitted to the higher authorities. Well-kept records are the best objective criteria of efficient management of the primary-health-care facility. Poorly maintained and disorganised record books indicate poor management, inefficient patient care, inadequate supervision, mishandling and wasteful use of resources. Printed forms look neat and are easier to work with. It printed forms are not available, cyclostyled sheets may be used only for a short period. Cyclostyled papers are generally difficult to handle and more expensive in the long run. The use of thick cards is preferable in situations where a particular record is likely to be used for a long period extending over years. Laboratory forms should be kept bound in pads, since loose sheets get scattered and are wasted. Proper forms should be used for each investigation. It is inappropriate to use a different printed form made for a specific purpose in place of a form or printed stationery, which is temporarily in short supply. In such cases, it is advisable to use plain sheets of paper in place of regular printed form, which is not available.

For the record of patient's illness, the following stationery is needed: An outpatient registration card, a treatment sheet, forms for referring the patient to the referral center, laboratory and x-ray requisition slips, special cards for antenatal delivery and postnatal work for women, growth (road to health cards) cards for children, immunisation records and cards for follow up of special diseases such as tuberculosis and leprosy. If the primary-health-care post has some maternity or general beds, in-patient admission forms, record forms and discharge summary will also be needed. The health-care forms should be so designed, that these can be easily used by the health staff. Paper should be used economically, but there should be large enough space for writing the data. A badly printed form may be used badly, making if difficult to retrieve useful information and thus it may be a total waste of effort.

8. HEALTH TEAM

The sick individuals in the community seek relief of pain and suffering from a variety of health worker and facilities available in the village or from other persons according to the prevailing cultural practices. In some tribal communities the illness is attributed to the curse of evil spirits or a divine retribution for sins in the past life. The tribals seek the help of a *priest, faith* healer or exorcit in the village to propitiate the evil spirits or gods and goddessess, to whom sacrificial offerings are made and witchcraft, branding or other rituals are performed. Elders in the house often use herbal-folk remedies which were known to be useful for some common ailments, traditional birth attendants, who learn their trade by apprenticeship in the family, help the expectant mothers during delivery. *Practitioners of indigenous or traditional systems of medicine,* such as Aurveda, Sidha or Unani provide back bone of health-care system in the rural areas of India. Old Chinese or Egytian traditional systems of medicine are practised in those countries. These practitioners may often be untrained, or semi trained. They learn their trade as apprentices. India and some other countries are now organising their training through schools of traditional medicine. *Dressers and dispensers* after having worked with a qualified doctor for a few years set up practices in rural areas.*Since these persons do not work as a team in an organised system they do not constitute the health team.* Some of these health personnel have recently been drafted to help the health team on voluntary basis in some countries according to the local circumstances.

Many countries have taken up the responsibility of primary health care by providing the essential health *services to the people in an organised manner, through a set of specially trained personnel who collectively provide the medical relief and supporting services.*

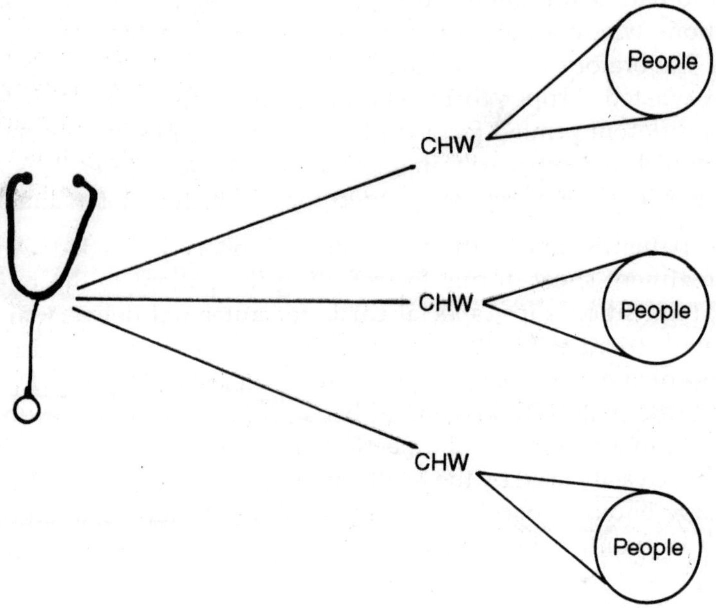

Fig. 12. 5: To increase the outreach of the physician to the people in the community, it is desirable to use health workers or volunteers from the community to perform simpler health related activities.

8.1 Definition

By definition the *health team* includes all personnel working in the primary health care post, subcenter or center. It does not refer to the staff concerned with the patient care only. Health team also comprises other supporting personnel as well, such as the driver of the vehicle, clerk, storekeeper and peon working in the health post. Smooth and effective functioning of the health team need motivation, cooperation and coordination of all members of the health team.

The health team has a leader. The leader should inspire confidence in the consumers or the community who need and seek medical care. The leader should be able to induce colleagues and team mates to work to their best capacity in cooperation with all members of the team, so that the efficiency and output are high and the work is interesting, satisfying and rewarding. Because of the nature of his training, education and status, the primary-health-center doctor has to assume the role of a natural leader of the primary-health-care team. Public-health nurse or another senior paramedical worker may assume the local or limited leadership role in the absence of the leader.

8.2 The Leader of the Health Team

The leader of the health team, should recognise, that the health team consists of individuals, who have feelings, their personal interests, anxieties, stresses, conflicts, likes and dislikes, just like any other people. Persons can think, react to favourable or unfavourable situations with enthusiasm or hostility and openly express their opinions. Human beings cab be easily frustrated or discouraged. They do not feel at ease, if they are not allowed to feel important and are not heard before decisions concerning their work or welfare are taken. They appreciate encouragement, praise and approbation by their leader for their achievements, howsoever minor these may appear to be. This induces them to work harder to get greater recognition from their manager. People like to be useful. Their emotional needs are better satisfied, if they are given the responsibility and authority to carry out the jobs assigned to them. Their efficiency and work output improves, if their working conditions are congenial, peaceful and relaxed with the least tensions and conflicts. The efficiency of a worker declines if he or she is unhappy about personal needs, such as lack of housing close to the place of work, long hours of work, want of personal security, financial worries, inadequate facility for children's education, poor health or perfunctory personal medical care. It is distressing to them if their salaries are not paid in time. Monetary incentive by itself is not adequate for motivating a health worker to do his work more conscientiously. Monetary reward should be judiciously combined with recognition and approbation for his good work. As the workers mature in course of years, they desire to upgrade their knowledge and skills and ascend in position to the higher level in the team. They are frustrated, if they stagnate in a job for many years and visualise few avenues for their self-advancement. The leader of the health team should try to *satisfy emotional needs* of the workes, and *inspire* them to do better work. He should zealously guard his own *credibility for fairness, impartiality, honesty and integrity.* The leader should be *competent* in his own technical work, so that his team mates respect him for his knowledge and skills. He should be easily *approachable,* so that the team members can reach him and seek his help and guidance for solution of their personal, technical and official problems. He should *earn respect* from his juniors and not command it by creating awe and by his blistering behaviour. The doctor, as a leader of the health team should continue to be *a good clinician,* because in him, the community see the image of a healer, who relieves their pain and suffering. He should be able to diagnose and manage common health problems of the community. The doctor leader of the health team, who overloads himself with too much administrative chores, soon loses his clinical competence and charisma as a healer. His team mates, the health assistants, nurses and midwives recognise lacunase in his knowledge and he loses their esteem. They do not seek his counsel for guidance and he fails as a good supervisor of his subordinates.*Ability to supervise is an essential quality of a leader*, since it helps him in recognising gaps in the knowledge and skills of the health team. It helps him to identify hinderances in their work, increase efficiency of work by removing constraints by appropriate measures such as retraining of workers, rescheduling of work and improving the logistics. The doctor leader should always appear to be *disciplined and well organised* in his thought and work. He should arrange to *disburse salaries of the staff regularly,* procure supplies in time and *exude an image of efficient manager* of affairs. This can be achieved only if he keeps himself free from routine chores of work and willingly *delegates responsibility for* carrying out simpler tasks to his subordinates, who if properly chosen and instructed may do the job nearly as well. Thus a leader of the health team should be *competent in his clinical skills, efficient and well organised in management techniques, sympathetic and humane towards his staff and community and willing to delegate responsibility and authority to his subordinates.*

8.3 Delegation of Authority

Essence of good management is accomplishment. A good leader gets the work done efficaciously within the allotted time, with the minimum expense and maximum output to the satisfaction of all concerned *i.e.,* workers and the consumers. The focus should be on getting the job done and not on who does the job. A manager may himself be highly qualified and skilled in certain tasks. It is not necessary for him to do all the task himself, because he must have time to think, plan and coordinate the work of his team-mates. He should not overburden himself with routine chores, as this will reduce his work output and efficiency. Some of the jobs normally done by the leader may be done nearly as well by his lesser educated and trained colleagues, if the latter are specially instructed to perform that role. The leader should personally perform those jobs which require critical judgement and assign simpler tasks requiring lesser degree of precision of his colleagues provided that such persons are reliable and can be trained to do the work efficiently. When a responsibility is assigned to a person, adequate authority should also be given to help him perform his duty well.

Delegation of responsibility and authority by the doctor to the health team is equally important in the primary-health-care setting. The efficiency of the health-care system improves because it saves time of the leader particularly, if the span of his work extends over a large geographic area. Several common illnesses in the community, which cause considerable incapacitation and mortality can be managed adequately by lesser-trained-paramedical worker. For an example, diarrheal disease is a major cause of ill health and death in young children. Deaths due to diarrhea can be dramatically reduced by oral hydration, a procedure which cab be carried out by mothers in their own homes with minimal or no medical supervision. At times, a subordinate colleague to whom responsibility for work is assigned may make some mistakes in the discharge of his duties. This calculated risk has to be taken. However, care should be taken that the authority is *not delegated to an incompetent or unreliable* person since his wrong decisions or actions may hamper the work of the entire health team or organisation. It is best to delegate the authority to a reliable person with adequate intellect, capacity and background. It is helpful to *define the extent of responsibility and authority* in clear, unambiguous terms. After the authority is delegated, the manager of the team *should not interfere too much or too frequently,* unless his specific advice or guidance is sought. The leader should be willing to give technical advice and support to his team. He should continuously supervise and monitor the work of his subordinates to minimise shortcomings in the program.

8.4 Supervision of the Health Team

The health team is expected to provide essential medical care to the people and promote their health. Since the team works collectively, functions of different members of the team need to be coordinated for achieving the desired results. If a member of the team is lazy and does not function properly, the output of the entire team is reduced. Thus health team can be likened to a chain. One weak link in the chain breaks the entire chain. A good leader or manager tries to identify the weak links in the chain and tries to reinforce them. The doctor, incharge of the health team should therefore supervise the work of members of the health team at regular intervals. He should discern gaps in their knowledge and skills and rectify these by appropriate measures such as technical guidance, administrative support and corrective retraining. Regular supervisory control helps the leader to discover other constraints such as non-availability or delay in supplies of much needed stores.

As the leader of the health team assigns responsibility to various members of his team, he should *prescribe the proper standards of norms of performance* and define the *time-scale* during which the specific job should be completed. The workers should be made fully aware of what is expected of them. The supervisor should then review their work by analysis of tasks completed in the given time in relation to the expected quality of work and standards of performance.

Good supervision is essential for efficient functioning of the team. A leader who cannot or does not supervise his team creates a chaos. The individuals then work in a haphazard, uncoordinated manner. The output is markedly reduced. The workers become frustrated and consumers are dissatisfied. Lack of supervision leads to *anarchy* in the organisation. Depending on his temperament, a manager may be *autocratic or democratic*. The *style of supervision should not be related to his temperament* but on the specific needs of the team. Authoritative or autocratic and democratic or consultative styles of supervision have a distinct place and role in taking management decisions.

The *authoritative* style of supervision is more suitable, when the end results proposed to be accomplished are consistent and uniform and need to be achieved quickly, such as in situations caused by epidemics and natural disasters or when strict policies and targets are enforced by the government. It is pragmatic to be authoritative, when dealing with large number of workes, who may be unreliable, with lesser knowledge and skills, have little aptitude and motivation for work and who do not understand goals of the organisation.

On the other hand, it is desirable to adopt a *democratic style of supervision,* when the colleagues in the team are well educated, competent, reliable and experienced. The leader should consult the workers, listen to them and consider their views carefully before taking final decisions. In a consultative style of supervision, the workers shoulder greater responsibility and give their best to the organisation. Consultative style to particularly useful when creative output is desired, such as in education and research. A consultative democratic style of supervision produces durable results and if properly executed does not lead to indecisions and vacillations.

8.5 Span of Control of Supervisor

There is a limit to the human ingenuity. Even the most skilled people can perform a task well to certain extent and beyond that their efficiency wanes. No individual howsoever skilled can exercise direct supervision very effectively over more than 6 to 10 persons. For the best results the span of direct control of a supervisor should be restricted to about than number. However, a good manager may be able to extend his supervisory control in a larger organisation indirectly by delegating to appropriate persons in the team, the supervisory responsibility over workers lower in the line of command. The leader should periodically get the feed back from them.

8.6 Coordination

The individual workers in the health team should cooperate with each other and coordinate their activities to accomplish the desired tasks. Coordination is possible only if the workers are aware of what is expected of each of them. Therefore the first essential for a supervisor is to communicate to the workers in unambiguous terms, what is to *be done, by whom, where, how and when?*

If the number of people in the health team, whose work needs to be coordinated, is large, it is useful to *convene a meeting* of all concerned at a convenient time acceptable to a majority of them. In this meeting, difficulties and doubts of the workers should be expressed and sorted out by the team leader. Agreed decisions should be taken and announced to all members. Such meetings should be convened for a specific purpose. The leader should prevent introduction of extraneous issues in the agenda. Before the larger meeting of all workers is actually convened it is expedient to call a meeting of 3 or 4 immediate colleagues for exchange of ideas or of a little larger group of 6 to 8 people for sharing their experiences, so that the discussions in the larger group are properly channelised. In such meetings, a few aggressively vocal people take the floor for most of the time. A good leader should restrain them diplomatically and encourage those who might have good ideas but are shy to speak to express their views. This ensures a balanced discussion. It is inevitable that there will be some disagreements in the presentation of views, but the leader should under no circumstance allow the members to become rude, intemperate or disagreeable to other members. It is always useful for the convener to *patiently listen to all the* viewpoints expressed, analyse these in his own mind, carefully weigh the pros and cons and announce his decision at the end of the meeting. A vague indecisive statement by the convener disconcerts the members.

They begin to feel that the meeting was a waste of their time and they had little useful role in it. It is also equally annoying if the convener announces his own decisions at the start of the meeting and then seeks comments if any of the members. In such setting, very few members express their views frankly and fearlessly.

As outlined earlier, non-health sector can play a significant role in primary health care. It is therefore necessary to establish close linkages with persons working in sectors outside the jurisdiction of the Department of Health. In such situations, coordination becomes even more vital. Such coordination of activities of different sectors cannot be accomplished by autocratic style of functioning of the leader of the health team. because to seek active cooperation and help of other workers, their genuine fears and anxieties should be assumed.

9. Monitoring of the Progress of Work

The leader is expected to set targets for different member of the health team. He should define the tasks to be accomplished within an agreed schedule of time. The efficiency of different workers may vary and certain essential inputs for optimal functioning may not be available at the appropriate time. To achieve the best results, the manager should periodically review the progress of all work at specified intervals. He should judge the pace of the work by relating it to the earlier agreed job schedules, reports of their achievements and site visits for personal observations and discussion with the staff. These site visits should be well planned and should not be too hurried. The supervisor should spend sufficient time with the workers, listen to then problems and try to find solutions for their difficulties. A flying visit disconcerts the worker who feels that supervisor had little actual interest in the quality of work and that he came only to see, if the worker was present on site.

Table 12.1

Records which should be inspected by the doctor while visiting sub-centres.

1. Maternity register for

   (a) new ante-natal cases (b) women due for delivery in the next month (c) high risk antenatal patients, not yet seen by the doctor (d) births and deaths register.

2. Eligible couples register for (a) family planning couples (b) new acceptors of family planning methods.

3. High risk children, who are not maintaining good growth and those, who are referred to the doctor for management of complex health problems.

4. Records of sick patients seen by the doctor during his last visit.

5. New cases referred to the doctor.

6. Problem cases, such as those who refuse to cooperate, those for immunisation, nutrition and family planning *etc.*

7. Laboratory reports of patients seen during the last visit.

Table 12.2

During supervisory visits, the primary health center doctor should specially look at the following aspects.

1. Cleanliness of the clinic and sub-center.
2. Arrangements made by the staff for confinement of the expectant mothers.
3. Any new pregnancies detected in the interval, since the last visit.
4. Complication of pregnancy such as bleeding and toxemia in the registered pregnant mothers.
5. Any malnourished children as detected from surveillance of growth cards.
6. Health worker's understanding of standing orders and instructions for the management of minor illnesses.
7. Number of patients attending the clinic.
8. Discussion of health matters with the village elders.
9. Visit to a few homes along with the health workers.

Monitoring of the weak periodically, helps in recognising obstacles or unforeseen difficulties in accomplishing the desired objectives. The constraints may be removed or targets revised. Monitoring is useful in good management but it should be *minimal, flexible and timely*. Too frequent monitoring upsets the schedules, creates tensions and infact may at times actually hamper the progress of the work. During monitoring control, the workers doing good work should be suitably rewarded by appreciative letters and recommendations for promotion. Inefficient workers may be trained further, transferred or even sacked.

Primary Health Care in India

In India, primary-health care is provided through community development blocks. In each community development block, there is one primary health center and 6 to 8 sub-centers at present. There were 5532 primary health centers and 5,1184 sub-centers as on 31.3.1981. An average primary health center in a community development block, covers a geographic area of 400 to 500 sq km with a population of about 100,000 to 120,000 persons living in about 100 to 125 villages. In each health center there is one medical officer for curative and preventive work and one lady medical officer for family planning work. Besides the doctors, the health team consists of (i) a dispenser (ii) a male health assistant (sanitory inspector) (iii) 2 public health nurses or lady health visitors (iv) 14 male multipurpose basic health workers including those for basic services and malaria surveillance (v) 10 female multipurpose health workers including 6 for family planning work (vi) a laboratory technician (vii) an extension educator (viii) a record keeper (ix) a store keeper (x) a driver (xi) 2 ancillary staff and (xii) about 8 female attendants. There are some variations in the staff in different states, depending on the availability of staff and budgetary allocation. The number of staff appointed in primary health centers are not optimum for the anticipated jobs. It has been envisaged that a female (multipurpose) health worker will provide maternal, child health and family planning services to women and children among a population of about 4000 living in villages within a radius of 5 km from their place of residence *(intensive area)* by making regular cyclic home visits. She will provide these services on request only to women and children in a population of about 6000 people living beyond 5 km (twilight area) from the place of residence of multipurpose worker. It is proposed to increase the number of female health workers progressively, to extend the maternal and child health coverage to the entire population in an intensive manner. One female and two male health workers generally work together in a sub-center. Two female health workers work at the primary health center to provide for nursing care to out patients and admitted patients and another for MCH and family planning work. Each male health worker looks after a population of 5000.

CENTRAL GOVERNMENT

Central Council of Health	Ministry of Health	DGHS
Policy	Administration	Appraisal
Legislation	Finance	National programs
Coordination	Manpower Research	Vital statistics Drugs
Grants	Occupational diseases	Food
	Medical Institutes	Med. Educ.

Fig. 12. 6: Areas of responsibility of Central Council of Health. Ministry of Health and Directorate General of Health Services.

Revised Minimum Needs Program

In accordance with the comprehensive National Health Policy and the need to create a model of health care service, with the objective of providing Health for All by 2000 A.D. a Working Group of the Ministry of Health of the Government of India recommended integration of the promotive, preventive and curative aspects at all levels of primary health care, Keeping in view the local topography, density of population, transport systems *etc.*, the following model of health services structure was recommended. Each State Union Territory was expected to undertake careful exercises to review the available structure and to adopt the recommended model with local variations as required, to adequately meet the local requirements.

For each District

District Health Centre with specialised curative services and public health experts.

For each Sub-Division/approximately 5 lakh population

A sub-Divisional Health Center with epidemiological wing attached to it.

For each Block/one lakh population

A Community Health Center with specialised medical care services in Gynacology, Pediatrics, Surgery and Medicine (out of the 4 non-specialised doctors, one may be drawn from any of the locally accepted traditional systems of medicine and one should be a public-health man).

For 30,000 population (or 15,000-20,000 in the case of hilly, tribal, sparsely populated or desert areas)

A Primary Health Centre (PHC) fully equipped to render preventive, promotive and curative services.

For 5,000 population (or 2,500 population in the case of hilly, tribal, sparsely populated or desert areas).

One sub-Center having one MPW (F), MPW (M) and one part-time attendant.

For each village 1000 population (or 500 population in the case of hilly and tribal areas or sparsely populated or desert areas)

One Health Volunteer preferably female, ex-serviceman, school teacher, village *vaidya* or village *dai,* etc.

A decentralised, participatory approach involving the community intimately in the planning implementation and maintenance of the health services was recommended.

13

The Health Centre

Definition. The word 'health centre' means different things to different people. When used here it is *a unit which provides a family with all the health services it requires, other than those which can only be provided in a hospital.* Fundamental to the nature of a health centre is that it takes its services and exerts its influence outside its own precincts right in the very homes of the people themselves. Once it fails to do this, and its staff stop visiting the surrounding villages, it is no longer a health centre. Its functions are promotive in that it promotes healthy living conditions, 'preventive' in that it seeks to prevent disease in the population by immunization, better environmental sanitation, better child feeding practices and early diagnosis; and curative in that minor ailments are treated in the centre and do not need to be referred to hospital.

When well developed a health centre provides general outpatient services and limited domiciliary care of the sick; it provides clinics for antenatal and postnatal mothers, school children and the 'under-fives', while, in addition to these there is usually a midwifery unit within the centre itself. It also provides environmental health services and gives advice and guidance on home living conditions, water supplies and sanitation. Simple dental care is also provided; at present this is mostly confined to tooth extraction, the relief of pain and the recognition of more serious oral pathology. Above all, and at every possible opportunity, a health centre educates the individual, the family and through them the community it serves it strives also to obtain the active participation of the community in its health promoting activities community directed health action.

Because the health centre is *the* important unit of rural medical health in its area, all other health activities must be channelled through it. It is not to be regarded as an embryo district hospital, but as an entirely separate entity with different and complementary functions. Health centres are complementary because they enable hospitals to be fewer, larger and more efficient and so make the building of multiple little hospitals unnecessary.

Health centres do not exist in isolation, their staff co-operate with other workers, especially agricultural extension officers, community development workers and schoolmasters. Co-operation must be mutual. This means for instance, that the medical assistant in charge

HEALTH CENTRE AREAS

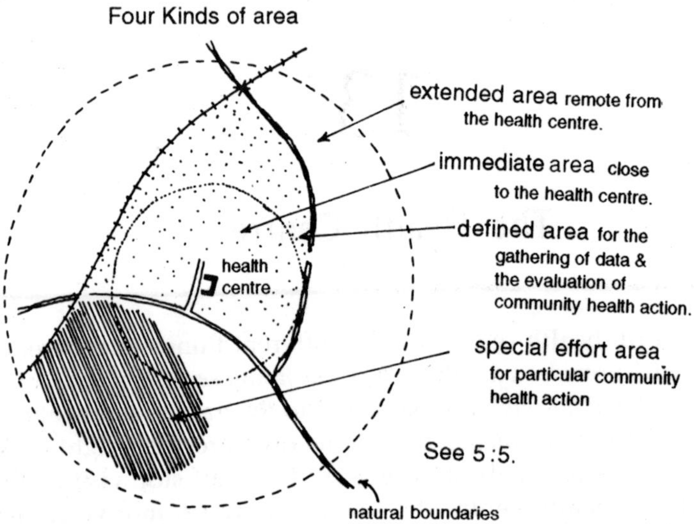

Fig. 13.1

of a centre must try to enlist the help of the local schoolmasters in the health education of their pupils. It also means that, if veterinary officers want the co-operation of the health centres in spreading information about such things as cattle diseases, then the health assistant should do his best to help them as he goes round the villages.

Health Centres Areas. In Kenya, from whence this accounts is derived, and where more than 150 health centres have been built in recent years, the ultimate objective is to have a health centre for every 10,000 persons. This is a somewhat arbitrary target but if it can be achieved it permits a very satisfactory level of health centre services to be attained. In the more densely populated regions these centres need only serve an area with a radius of about five miles, but in other areas this has to be extended. Because of a lack of sufficient capital and trained auxiliaries, 1:10,000 is not a practical immediate objective, so, for the time being at any rate, the target is to try to achieve a health centre for every 20,000 persons serving an area which may have to be ten miles and more in radius. The need for a health centre to serve a larger area than is ideal makes two developments necessary in its practice.

The first is to divide the whole area for which it is responsible into two parts, an 'immediate area' within about five miles of the centre where full services can be provided, and an 'extended area' beyond it where services are of necessity limited and have to be provided by mobile teams. These have been drawn in Figure 13.1 which also shows the 'defined area' and the 'special effort area' where the health centre team conduct a particular drive on some important health problem.

The second is to build or upgrade any dispensaries in the area into health 'sub-centres'. These play the same role as a health centre and are merely smaller and not so fully staffed.

The structure of the health centre. Two health centres are drawn in Figure 13.2, a simpler one from Embu and the standard one now being put up by the Kenya Government, the so called 'improved SIMOHNN pattern'. These plans are not hard and fast and their various rooms can be adapted to suit local requirements. For instance, the SIMOHNN type of centre can be built one wing at a time as funds permit, and the kitchen wings of both of them are optional and can be added later. In some versions of this centre the female ward is used for health education, and the male ward as the health office. On the whole, a separate health education room has not been found generally successful, and health education is

TWO HEALTH CENTRE PLANS

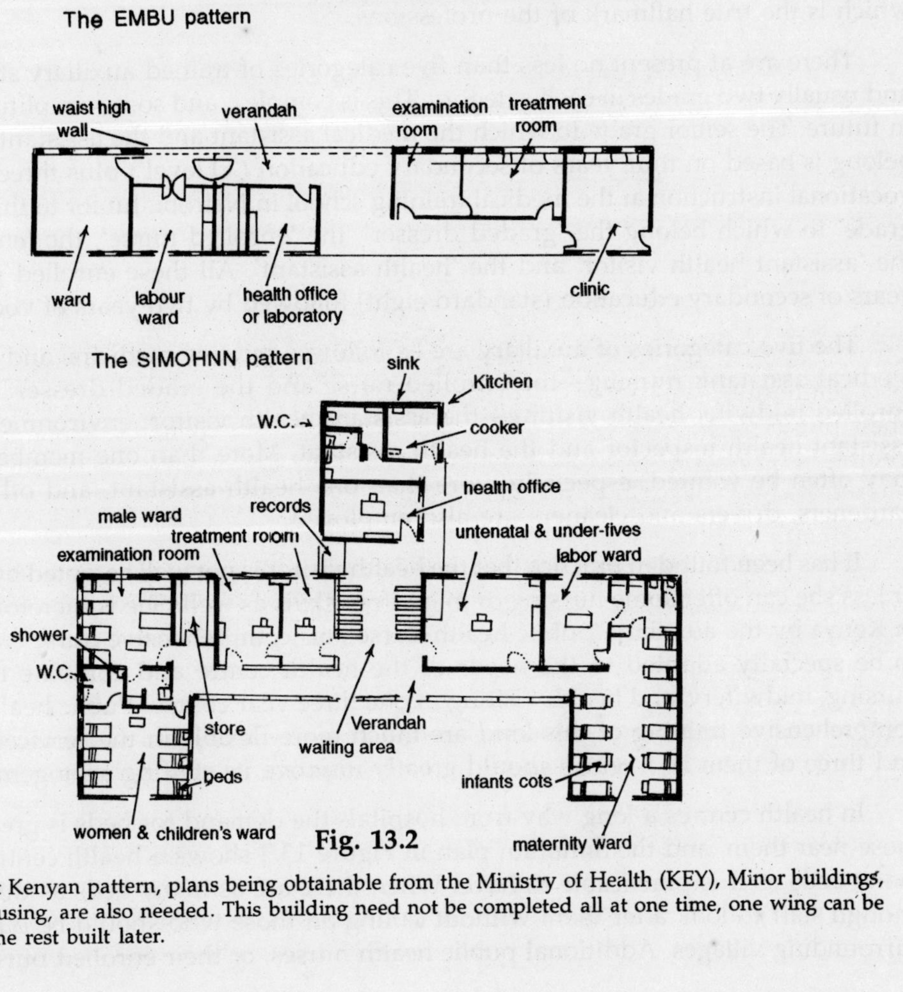

Fig. 13.2

This is the latest Kenyan pattern, plans being obtainable from the Ministry of Health (KEY), Minor buildings, such as staff housing, are also needed. This building need not be completed all at one time, one wing can be built first and the rest built later.

more conveniently undertaken in the clinics themselves, or in the waiting space where a blank wall is provided for the projection of slides and films after dark.

One point is quite clear: it is that no dispensary should every be put up except with the intention of converting it later into a health centre. This means that there must be a rudimentary 'master development plan' like that for a hospital.

STAFF

The value of auxiliary staff. In most developing countries professional staff, especially doctors, are so scarce that health centres have to be staffed by auxiliaries, and preferably by auxiliaries indigenous to the region. But this no disadvantage, for they are at the same time more economical and are generally more closely in touch with the local inhabitants than are doctors, and, very important indeed, they are also much more content to remain in the rural areas. In Kenya auxiliaries have proved to be effective substitutes for fully qualified professional people, be these doctors, midwives or health inspectors, and, when carefully selected and adequately trained, they develop that real sense of vocation and responsibility which is the true hallmark of the professions.

There are at present no less than five categories of trained auxiliary staff at the centres and usually two grades in each category. This is complex, and some simplification is planned in future. The senior grade to which the medical assistant and the assistant health inspector belong is based on four years of secondary education ('O level') plus three or four years of vocational instruction at the medical training school in Nairobi, Junior to this is the 'enrolled grade' to which belong the 'graded dresser', the 'enrolled nurse', the 'enrolled midwife', the 'assistant health visitor' and the 'health assistant'. All these enrolled grades have two years of secondary education (standard eight) followed by two years of vocational training.

The five categories of auxiliary are as follows: curative medicine and paediatrics—the medical assistant: nursing—the enrolled nurse and the graded dresser: midwifery—the enrolled midwife: health visiting—the assistant health visitor: environmental health—the assistant health inspector and the health assistant. More than one member of each group may often be wanted, especially more than one health assistant, and other staff such as gardeners, drivers and cleaners are also employed.

It has been found in practice that the health visitor is not well accepted by the community unless she can offer some nursing or midwifery skills as well. She is therefore to be replaced in Kenya by the auxiliary 'public health nurse', or 'comprehensive nurse' whose training is to be specially adapted to the needs of the health centre and combine the essentials of nursing, midwifery, and health visiting in one three year course. Public health nurses with a comprehensive training of this kind are much more flexible in the services they can offer, and three of them in a centre should greatly improve its staffing arrangements.

In health centres a long way from hospitals the demand for beds is greater than it is in those near them, and the Simohnn plan in Figure 13.2 shows a health centre with about as many beds as it is practicable to have. When there are as many beds as this there must be enough staff to look after them without calling on those who should be out visiting in the surrounding villages. Additional public health nurses, or their enrolled nurse, midwife and health visitor components, are thus required whenever the beds exceed a certain minimum number. Looking after the patients in the wards does not occupy much of a medical assistant's time, and of course none at all of that of the health inspector and his assistants, so the demand for these grades of staff is largely independent of the number of beds in the centre.

All members of the staff, particularly ambulance drivers, are instructed in first aid and emergency medical treatment, for the failure of any member to cope with a crisis may discredit the whole team.

At a health sub-centre there are only two or three staff members, all of the junior grade, a health assistant, an enrolled midwife and a male enrolled nurse.

Careful staff training in a central school, and continued supervision are the key to a good system of health centres. Because the staff will have to learn to work with one another as a team, and, as a good team spirit is vital, it is desirable to let the staff select their own teams and to train these teams together. this training and retraining of health centre staff both auxiliary and professional, for the district medical officer needs instruction too, is one of the main functions of the National Reference Health Centre.

If standards and morale are to be maintained, centres must be regularly visited and supervised, both by the district medical officers who are in direct command, and by other professional personnel, especially by the tutors responsible for training health centre staff.

The medical assistant. A medical assistant is in administrative charge of each centre; he diagnoses and treats the sick and visits patients in their homes—he is in fact the general practitioner of the area. He gives health education talks and sees that the other members of the staff do so too. Health centres provide valuable opportunities for health education, for this starts with the premise that the sick are much more susceptible to advice about preventive action than are the healthy. Medical assistants also give health education talks to the elders and chiefs, they co-opt members of other departments to help in this field and they co-ordinate their work with community activities as a whole, including community development workers and homecraft centres.

The medical assistant organizes the work of the centre and tries to see that the health assistants correlate their work to take account of the diseases shown to be prevalent by the outpatient clinics. He also conducts regular staff discussions that do much to maintain the interest and morale of the team. One half day each week is reserved for such meetings when all the staff of the centre can discuss cases and exchange information. The medical assistant is also responsible for record keeping and sends in returns to the district medical officer, whose duty it is to supervise a group of centres.

The health staff. In Kenya the assistant health inspector is of similar status to the medical or hospital assistant, and the health assistant is the equivalent of the dresser. Thus the assistant health inspector at each centre has several assistants to help him, one posted to each large village or location, and preferably centred on a dispensary or health sub-centre. They are responsible for providing safe water by digging wells and protecting springs, and often have a mason to help them in these task. These health assistants also provide latrines and see that these are used, they advise on improvements in indigenous housing, they assist in measures against diseases such as malaria, and they help to trace the contacts of infectious cases. They inspect meat and supervise markets. Like other members of the staff, assistant health inspectors and health assistants go into the patients' homes where their work is particularly valuable in times of epidemic, because it is then that the villager is most susceptible to advice and instruction.

All the health staff are taught to be active workers with their *hands* as well as their heads, and are encouraged not to be afraid of getting their hands dirty.

Graded dressers and enrolled nurses. Dressers and enrolled nurses apply all dressings, and give all the treatments and injections ordered, but, though they may give antibiotics, they are not allowed to prescribe them. In Kenya they act as a filter to the medical assistant, for they are capable of dealing with most minor complaints and need only refer the more seriously ill patients for his opinion. Dressers and nurses do not normally leave the centre and may even take temporary charge of it when the medical assistant is out in the district. If patients come up meanwhile, these dressers treat what patients they can and either save any perplexing ones until the medical assistant returns, or else send them on to hospital.

The enrolled midwife and enrolled health visitor. Enrolled midwives are able to handle normal deliveries and recognize complications which they refer to hospital. They hold antenatal and postnatal clinics at the centre and in the villages, they deliver mothers in the centre and in their homes, and they assist the health visitor with under-fives clinics. A midwife pays one postnatal visit to each case during the postnatal period, after which the health visitor takes over the care of that family.

Kenya cannot afford institutional delivery for all mothers, so, in order to encourage confinement at home, mothers are charged a fee for hospital delivery, and half fees for health centre delivery, while domiciliary delivery is free. The policy is to send abnormal cases to hospital, and to restrict health centre delivery to 'primips' and cases where the home conditions are particularly bad.

Kenya has a high birth rate, so the midwives are busy, most of them managing to deliver about 20 babies a month, half of these at home. Antenatal clinics are popular, and once mothers are assured that their pregnancy is normal, most of them are content to have their babies at home, even if it is not possible for them to be attended by a midwife. The most important aspect of this work is, however, the opportunity it gives these midwives to instruct mothers in domestic and personal hygiene.

The enrolled health visitor holds under-fives clinics in the centre and in selected villages, she visits as many families as she can in their homes, she helps the midwife and she undertakes health education and schools visits. In future her tasks will be taken over by the auxiliary public health nurse or comprehensive nurse.

THE WORK OF THE HEALTH CENTRE

The service of the health centre classified. The activities of a health centre can be summarized like this:

Personal services

General curative outpatients services
Maternity care (19:1)
The care of the under-fives—immunization.
The care of school children.
Consultative clinics.
Clinics for special diseases. e.g. tuberculosis and malnutrition.
Dental care.
Mental care.
Home visiting.
Case work.
Limited inpatient care.

Community services

Health education.
The improvement of water supplies.
The improvement of excreta disposal.
The supervision of housing conditions.
The regulation of food shops and markets.
Campaigns against communicable diseases.
The collection of statistics.

This list does not claim to be complete, nor is it always mutually exclusive, but one thing in particular is missing from it. No mention has been made of family planning which should become one of the more important health centre services in many developing countries in the years ahead. At the time of going to press there are reports that this is causing considerable concern in Kenya.

These services are provided both within the health centre itself, its 'internal services', and outside it, particularly in the extended area, its 'external services'.

Internal services. Large numbers of general outpatients are seen in the centre itself. Inpatient facilities are limited, but they are not so greatly needed, for many acute illnesses when treated early respond to two days or so of modern treatment, and require only a short admission followed by outpatient treatment if necessary. Accidents, particularly head injuries, often need observation for a day or two, so these few beds are very useful.

General outpatient clinics are held at the centre daily, but emergencies are seen at any time. Clinics for particular categories of persons, such as antenatal mothers or the under-fives are held on appointed days when there is usually more time to see and deal adequately with each person. These clinics are often finished in the morning which leaves the staff time to visit villages nearby in the afternoons. Care is taken to hold under-fives clinics on the same day as antenatal clinics, thus saving mothers a second visit. These clinics have not, however, reached the peak of development described in previons chapter, selected children only being encouraged to attend according the their need.

Though clinics for particular disease are sometimes held, special records are more important for they make it unnecessary for members of the same family to come up on separate occasions. Thus, if a tuberculous father brings up his child with a cut knee, father and son are both attended to at the same time, and the general policy is to treat such diseases as tuberculosis and leprosy along with the general outpatients. Consultative clinics by visiting doctors are routine, and the equivalent of such consultations by visiting experts in environmental sanitation, public health nursing or health education are *just as important as the strictly clinical ones* in maintaining the standards of the centres. *The real purpose of such consultations is to teach the staff who must be present whenever these visiting consultants are at work.* This is just one example of the teaching opportunities of clinical consultations. In planning these clinics efforts are made to hold the general ones at the times most convenient to the patients and the consultative ones at times that suit the consultants.

Health centres are also expected to co-operate with 'traditional practitioners', whether these be 'witch doctors' whose assistance may be useful in treating the mentally disturbed, or indigenous midwives among whom the health centre can play a very useful educational role. If it starts by supplying these women with cotton wool, umbilical tape, and razor blades to cut the umbilical cord, goodwill is rapidly established and a spirit of co-operation is soon built up.

External services. Because the staff only hold full clinics at the centre once a week they are able to hold a regular programme of clinics in the villages nearby on the four other days. A very real attempt is thus made to take the services to the people—even within the immediate area—and to make the 'care gradient' as fair as possible. Multipurpose clinics are held after the pattern described, and are staffed by two or more auxiliaries working together, usually the medical assistant and an enrolled midwife.

In the immediate area auxiliaries are able to visit the sick at home, deliver mothers at home, find cases, trace contacts, and keep a close watch on environmental sanitation—in other words to provide complete health centre care. The immediate area is mostly served by individuals working on foot, bicycle or scooter, though when occasion demands two or more members may visit together in a motor vehicle.

The extended area is visited by teams consisting of the medical assistant and the assistant health inspector, or one of his assistants, who are often assisted by a midwife or a health visitor. By working together, they gain a better understanding of each other's work and are able to look at the community as a whole. This team holds multipurpose clinics in the villages all over the extended area in a regular fortnightly rotation. While they are away, a nurse or dresser remains at the center to cope with the daily flow of sick. The schedule is arranged by the medical assistant in consultation with his team and the local authority councils, and is adhered to until sufficient progress has been made to warrant their moving to a fresh series of villages. Thus, although the team cannot visit every village in the extended area every fortnight, they are in turn able to extend their influence over the whole territory assigned to their centre.

On arriving at a village in the extended area the team select a spot to hold their clinic. It may be held in a building loaned for the purpose, in a specially built mud-and-wattle hut or 'station', or even number a tree. Clinics are preceded by a health talk in simple language given by the medical assistant or the assistant health inspector. A subject of topical interest is chosen, such as typhoid fever for example; the villagers are told what it is, how is spreads and the measures that the community should take to avoid it. At the end of the talk questions are invited. Clinics are then held, while the assistant health inspector tours the village inspecting and giving assistant and advice on general sanitation, water supplies, latrines, building standards and the food shops. He also investigates any special problems that the elders bring to his notice. The staff confer on the results and each member of the team talks for five minutes on a subject that needs particular attention by the community. The four members are able to over the subject fairly well between them. For example, if malaria is found to be prevalent the talk would cover its cause and treatment, the harm it does to children, why it is afflicting the villagers and what steps they should take to protect themselves.

Local elders and headmen are co-opted to see that the preventive measures are put into effect and to be certain of their support.

Progress is checked when the team next visit the village. If there are any local health personnel in the village, they are automatically made part of the health-centre team and carry on with its work until its next visit.

One of the most valuable results of teamwork is, that when there are outbreaks of infectious disease, the whole team can go into action together in an all-out community effort.

Attention has to be paid to the special needs of certain groups of people, and to places of particular need; schools for example, should be visited regularly. As an example of the value of school work, the prevalence of scabies in certain schools in one district was as high as 70 per cent, but, by repeated visits it was reduced to almost nothing. Veterinary and agricultural workers should be called upon for assistance in areas where malnutrition is rife.

These teams are very popular in the districts, they enable the centres to attack disease and ignorance and promote a better standard of living.

Mobility. Mobility is of critical importance, so health centres are equipped with bicycles, motor-cycles and a motor vehicle which also functions as an ambulance. While the team is their vehicle emergency cases arriving at the centre are transported in an ambulance from the district hospital, in a hired vehicle, or by public transport.

The cost of motor transport is discussed where the principle of using the cheapest vehicle capable of doing the job is emphasized. This is particularly true of mobility in the extended area, where an expensive four wheel drive Land Rover is not always required and can often be replaced by a cheaper vehicle.

There is a tendency to save on transport now that many health centres in Kenya are run by the local authorities who find it difficult to raise sufficient money for them. This is a pity because it means that the influence of the health centre team is diminished, particularly in the extended area. Transport costs form a significant fraction of the health centre budget, and detailed studies of the economics of health centre mobility are much needed.

There are areas where water-borne units are practical, the Nile and Lake Victoria, for example.

In nomadic areas with vast distances of inhospitable terrain the mobile health unit has to be much more self-contained, and undertakes sorties lasting ten days or more. In such areas a forward timetable is essential if faith is to be kept with the people. The movements of nomadic tribesmen must therefore be studied, and efforts made to meet them on specified dates at such points as their cattle watering places.

Drugs and equipment. A standard list of drugs is issued to all health centres. All centres are given drugs for the routine treatment of the more important diseases such as tuberculosis, leprosy and syphilis, for which standard treatment programmes are laid down. Sulphonamides, penicillin and chloramphenicol are issued routinely, a little morphia is also supplied, as are drugs for such conditions as trypanosomiasis, kala-azar and onchocerciasis, where these diseases are prevalent in the area. The general policy is in effect to be liberal, and to supply what is needed under the discretion of the district medical officer. Carefully constructed circulars on management routines for the more important illnesses are sent round to the health centres, both to simplify procedures and to economize in the use of drugs.

One of the present weaknesses of the health centres is the difficulty their staff have in making a definite actiological diagnosis, that is, in actually confirming the presence of malaria parasites, tubercle bacilli or schistosome ova, etc. Their staff need further elementary laboratory training, a carefully selected outfit of laboratory apparatus.

The National Reference Health Centre. Careful training and *retraining* of the several grades of auxiliaries is the key to a good system of health centres. In Kenya this is undertaken at the Medical Training School in Nairobi, but something is required to support the health centres in addition to the traditional type of school.

This supporting unit is the 'National Reference Health Centre' which has the following functions.

1. It acts as a model working health centre serving a population living in a typical rural African setting and is thus an example on which other centres can be built.
2. It serves as a unit for training and retraining all categories of staff who have anything to do with health centres, whether they be as senior as provincial medical officers or as junior as enrolled nurses. Whenever possible training is *team* training.
3. It serves as a 'community health laboratory' for detailed investigations into community health, and as a centre of operational or methodological research into health centre practice. On the outcome of this research can be based plans to be carried out on a national scale in other centres.

The World Health Organisation advise the establishment of a series of Primary Reference Health Centre. one for each province, supported by a National Reference Health Centre (47). Because this is not possible in Kenya at the present time, a single reference centre has been started at Karuri near Nairobi to combine both the functions of a Primary and a National Reference Health Centre.

A 'community health laboratory' is also discussed in connection with these centres and is apt to be considered as something distinct from them; it is not, and is inherent in the third or research function of both types of reference centre, and indeed of any health centre where a community diagnosis is made followed by carefully planned and evaluated health.

Health centre economics. These are not easy to calculate exactly, but an approximation is that a centre costing £8,000 ($22,000) to build and £4,000 ($11.000) to run each year can provide about 50,000 outpatient attendances annually. This makes each attendance cost about Shs. 1/60 ($0.23) but takes no account of the fact that the staff spend about half their time Rendering services of other kinds. Reckoning that an illness at a health centre involves 2-3 attendances, each illness costs about Shs. 4/- ($0.56).

Serving a population of 20,000 such a centre might provide an average of 2.5 outpatient attendances per person per year, which is the same as the somewhat arbitrary figure used as a basis for calculation.

There are about ten staff employed at a health centre, so each job requires a capital outlay of about £800, a figure which closely 'resembles that for the district hospital. These costs are based on standard methods of construction, and what has been said about cheap hospital buildings applies equally to cheap ones for health centres.

If the annual running cost of £4,000 is spread over the 20,000 people that a typical health centre is intended to serve, then the average cost per person per year also works out at Shs. 4/-. It is instructive to compare this figure with two others.

This first is with the amount spent on health services by developing countries. Here it will be seen that mans developing countries spend about Shs. 7/- ($1) per head per year medical services. Four shillings amounts to about half of this sum and might seem a just proportion to spend on health centre services. In practice, however, hospital services are incomparably more expensive, and in Kenya, where health centres have a very high priority, the amount spent directly on health centres in 1961 was only about £600,000 ($1,170,000), or about 13 per cent of the £4.7 million ($13 million) health budget that year. The demands for hospital medicine are so strong that in practice it is difficult to allocate health centre services a larger fraction of the health budget.

The second revealing comparison is that of the cost of health centre services with the GNP per head per year. For a typical developing country this is of the order of £25 ($70). The annual cost of health centre services (4/-, $0.56) amounts to less than 1 per cent, of this. Admittedly, this figure only covers the running costs of the centres and it is difficult to estimate how much more should be added to cover training, supervision and administration, nor is it easy to take account of the capital costs of the centres themselves, but if simple building methods are followed this should not be excessive. Even if the proportion of 1 per cent of the GNP is doubled to account for these other costs, the sum is still only half the figure of 4 per cent which is approximately the fraction of the GNP which the United Kingdom and the USA spend on health services. This can for convenience be considered as being not more than the just fraction of its GNP that a country should spend on health services. In practice, Kenya only spent 2.1 per cent of its GNP on health in 1961, and even this figure was twice what it had been only five years previously.

Looked at in this way, as a percentage of the GNP, health centre services manned by auxiliaries are cheap. They represent a substantial return in human welfare for comparatively little expenditure of money and skill. If this is granted they must be a high priority in a health service budget and money must somehow be raised for them, either by taxation or direct charges.

So convincing are the economic arguments, that a very strong case indeed can be made out of restricting further hospital expansion in a country until efficient health centre services have been built up.

14

The Cross-Cultural Outlook in Medicine

'Culture'. Though it is all around us the most important parts of our 'culture' remain invisible to us. As we slowly reach our full thoughtfulness and maturity inside it we inevitably absorb it unawares; whether we like it or not we are the product of it. Only when we have reached high level of education, and obtained something of the insight of the comparative sociologist or social anthropologist, can we see our own culture for what it is, and understand where it differs from those of other communities.

But what is this abstraction 'culture'? It is the sum total of the customs, beliefs, attitudes, values, goals, laws, traditions and moral code of a people. It includes their language and their art as well as everything they make, be it a stone axe or a spacecraft. It includes their corporate view of the universe and also their attitudes to health and disease. In all these dimensions does the culture of a people like the pygmies of the Ituri forest differ from the culture of the commuters of New York city. The reader will say that this is obvious, and in a limited sense so it is. The American doctor practising among the pygmies will immediately see that in such things as language, dress and education his patients differ from those he looked after in North America. But these are only the obvious and visible parts of a culture. Its values, attitudes, traditions and chorals are invisible and not nearly so obvious.

The almost inevitable human tendency is to accept the visible part of a strange culture, and unconsciously graft on to them invisible element from the observer's own culture, albeit in a very incomplete and has hazard way. A real understanding of the invisible elements of another culture, and even more so of one's own, requires training, effort and great openness of mind. Unless he is watchful the doctor will tend to assume that this tropical patients know about the spread of infectious diseases and put the same value on the possession of money or cows as he does. He may know that witchcraft exists, but disregard it, because it plays such a small part in his own culture. This compounded view of a strange culture—'the visibles of the strange culture plus some of the invisible elements of the observer's own culture'—is the common view of the educated but sociologically untrained person contemplating a culture new to him.

The value of a 'cross-cultural' outlook. Few doctors, even in developed countries, practise among patients who are culturally similar to themselves and this is even more so in developing ones which typically contain so many varied tribes. If this cultural difference between a doctor and his patients is granted, how necessary is it that he understands their culture, and obtains what might be called 'a cross-cultural outlook'?It may be argued that penicillin works similarly whatever the culture of the patient, that a post-partum haemorrhage requires the same treatment anywhere in the world, and that the signs of mitral stenosis depend only on disordered physiology. This is true, and it must be admitted that many doctors have practised with some success, and even achieved academic eminence with hardly the faintest understanding of the way their patients look at the world. But their success is partial and perhaps their eminence is undeserved. If medicine is to be more than just the application of technique, and indeed even if it is to be merely the efficient application of technique, then the patient's culture must be understood as it relates to their health, and in practice it is found to relate at a great many points. Why will they not give their blood for transfusion? Why, when their children are malnourished, will they not use the protein sources that seem readily available? Why are they so loath to accept family planning? Why is it so difficult to persuade them that tuberculosis is infectious? Why is gonorrhoea so prevalent in the area? All these questions and a great many others may only be explicable in their cultural setting.

Obtaining a 'cross-cultural' outlook. If it is granted that a cross-cultural outlook is necessary, how can it be obtained? How can a doctor, as it were, get inside his patient's culture and see the world as they see it?

The first step is to realize that the cross-cultural problem exists, and that active measures are needed to discover and understand a strange culture.

The next is to observe the culture closely. Why does a child patient wear such a peculiar necklace of skin and bits of hair? Has it been supplied by the traditional healer, and if so, what is the system of beliefs on which it depends? What are those peculiar herbs the patient's relatives are cooking so busily in that pot? Why do the women wear dresses which bear such a remarkable resemblance to those fashionable in Europe in 1890? Why is this adult literacy class composed mostly to women? Is it because by learning to read these women seek to gain influence over their illiterate husbands? Why are the words 'Sea never dry' written on the tailboard of that 'Mammy wagon'? These are just some of the visible starting points from which the invisible aspects of a culture can be built up by careful question and enquiry. Some of them have no obvious relation to health, yet they are well worth following because an overall view of the culture is necessary if those parts of it which are relevant to health are to be seen in their true context.

Those about to practise in a strange culture should make a point of reading whatever published work is available on the local community. Thus, Southall and Gutkind's book *Townsmen in the Making* /124/. is a classical and easily readable study of the sociology of urban Uganda and *Igbo-ora, a Town in Transition*, is a more recent account of a some-what similar kind from Nigeria /19/. Oscar Lewis's book *Children of Sanchez* /93a/. will provide vivid insight into the culture of the common man in Mexico. Though they have wider application, these are only local studies and a textbook of medical anthropology for developing countries is greatly needed. In its absence the popular works of Margaret Mead will provide some background knowledge /96/. In a few developing countries, the local novelists and playwrights provide useful insight into the culture. This is especially true of Nigeria where the works of Chinua Achebe and Wole Soyinka will be found very instructive.

Thanks to endeavours of anthropologists, many of the world's cultures have now been fairly adequately studies, and if a particular tribe has not been examined, there is likely to be an account available of a closely similar one. Hitherto, the readership of works in this field has been small and some accounts may be hard to obtain, but if local studies can be found they may well make interesting reading.

Similarly, if there are anthropologists working in the area they may have much to tell doctors working with the same tribes. Once they have learnt the local language and been accepted by the people, they are likely to be a good source of information on customs relevant to health. They are likely to have the information available in a very accessible form but should not be too difficult to elicit from them.

Educated members of the community, particularly the hospital staff, are another source of information on the local culture and here again careful questioning will be needed. Care must be taken to account for the bias of the informant, who may try to cover up what he feels ashamed of, be ignorant of what actually happens, or be incapable of conveying the true state of affairs, even if he knows it.

Lastly, but most important of all, there are the patients themselves. Besides observing them carefully, the critically important step is to learn their language, but time is short, languages are diverse, postings from one part of the country to another are often frequent, and few doctors acquire new languages with sufficient facility to enable effective two-way communication to take place. Sometimes there is a language like the Nigerian 'Pidgin' which makes communication at a certain level very easy, but interpreters have usually to be used. But working through an interpreter is time-consuming, and it is convenient to know a few clinical questions in the vernacular to which the expected answer is 'yes' or 'no', such as 'Have you got a cough?' or 'Is there blood in your sputum?' Even more useful are what might be called the clinical imperatives, such as 'Take a deep breath' or, 'Say aaah'. A few dozen phrases of this kind, and especially the local greetings, must be considered the minimum knowledge of the local language for clinical efficiency. On being posted to a place where the language is strange it is well worth making a list of the phrases and learning them. The reader could hardly do better than translate into his local vernacular the phrases compiled by Strover and Mazorodze in their *Shona Phrase Book* which is published as a supplement to the December 1965 issue (Vol. 11, No. 12) of the *Central African Journal of Medicine* '. Here at least is the basis for a planned interview and a foundation upon which a working knowledge of a language can be built.

Even so, there will be many occasions when interpreters will have to be used, and sometimes, if the the language is a very unusual one, two of them will be needed working together, one interpreting to the other. Try to make sure that the interpreter himself understands the question and that he does his best to make sure that the patient does so too. Get in the habit of insisting on being given the answer to the question asked and not the answer to a different one. Once the answer to a different question is accepted further logical interrogation becomes impossible.

But this has been a digression. The important point, as far as this chapter is concerned is, that when histories are being taken, some questions should be asked which relate to the patient's general culture. This will enable a clear picture of their society to be built up steadily over the years. In every community the doctor is in a uniquely favourable position to study his fellow men, because, with due care, he can ask almost any question he likes in the name of medicine.

Some early steps in the study of a culture. Even the simplest human society is enormously complex and the novice can be pardoned for not knowing where to begin. Large numbers of individuals play many different roles, they interact with one another, with their physical environment and with other societies in intricate and ever changing ways. The following list contains just a few of the things that have to be known in the description of every human community. They are the sort of questions to begin by asking and form some of the more obvious dimensions of a culture. Further lists are recorded in connection with health education and malnutrition.

Method: A start in the study of a strange culture

The Family, What are the common patterns of family composition? What is the age of marriage and how stable is it? What are the strongest emotional ties within it? What are the obligations towards the extended family of uncles, aunts, and cousins? What is the status of women?

After the family, what other important associations are there? Political parties? Guilds? Agricultural co-operatives?

Initiation groups? Religious communities?

Who are the influential members of the community? Chiefs? Party officials? School teachers? Ministers? Hospital assistants?

What accords status in the community? Cattle? Wives? Children? Land? Money? Education?

What are the values of a community? Leisure? Conformity? Happiness? Fulfilment of the personality?

What are the customs of the community over the use and ownership of land and money? How is the land inherited? What is the income of the average family? Is money the common property of the family? Is there available in the community for medical expenses?

What are the attitudes and practices of the community in matters of health and disease? What is the traditional system of medicine? Do people consult their healers first, or only after scientific medicine has failed? What are the concepts of causation of the common diseases? Does the indigenous system of medicine include the idea of prevention? What are the local names for the common diseases?

The practices of the community on matters of health can be divided into three groups, those which are beneficial to health, those which have no effect and those which are positively harmful. It is their effect on health that matters, not their strangeness to the observer nor their remoteness to his own culture. Some practices may seem very odd indeed and yet be either harmless or even actually helpful. Thus, the habit that mothers in some cultures have to prechewing their infant's food and giving him the masticated material straight from their own mouths is not to be discouraged; it is likely to be harmless and may even be beneficial. Mother and child share the same bacterial flora anyway, and part of the child's digesting will already have been done for him.

Some useful sociological concepts. This is no place to go deeply into the structure of human communities, but here are certain ideas that are well worth bearing in mind.

A culture is a logically integrated dynamic whole and is not merely an accidental collection of customs. Looked at overall it makes sense, and, unless great changes are taking place, most cultures are fairly harmonious. But, because a cultural is in equilibrium, a major change in one part of it is likely to cause multiple changes elsewhere, for the old balance will now be changed. For example, the assumption of professional or middle class standards of life is at variance with the traditional idea that many cultures have of the obligations to an extended family. The desire for a higher standard of living may lead to the limitation of family obligations, and this in turn may produce further changes, such as less security in sickness and old age, and lessened responsibility for the education of nephews and cousins.

A culture makes it possible for the members of a society to interact with one another in a more or less automatic manner. As they grow up its members learn the behaviour expected of them in the innumerable roles they will have to play in life, whether as sons, fathers, employees, lovers, buyers, students or professors, etc. This stereotyped activity of a stable culture is a great convenience, for it makes interaction between one individual and another so very much simpler. In an unstable or changing culture these roles will be changing too, and its members will be without the security of knowing the exact behaviour that is expected of them in each social situation.

All culture is learned by one member from another. For many individuals the learning process is complete once childhood is past, and it is only the minority of adults who are likely to learn new forms of behaviour. But this minority is of great importance, because, if we can only identify the few people who are susceptible to being taught and teach them, then the society can in time be introduced to new patterns of behaviour.

In most communities there are a few individuals to whom the rest look up. These are often, but not always, the natural leaders of the group such as chiefs, priests, schoolmasters and doctors. If these can be identified, and it may be more difficult to identify the women leaders in communities where their status is relatively low, they are the people who are most likely to be effective in spreading a change in behaviour through the group.

Every society has a few individual members who are inventors or discoverers and their activities are one of the reasons for the fact that no culture is ever quite static. But the main reason for cultural change is not a community's own inventors, but its power of absorbing the inventions of other cultures. Thus the scientific industrial culture of developed countries has in the past absorbed an immense wealth of invention from the civilizations which preceded it, coinage and the wheel to mention only two. It in its turn is now being absorbed by the traditional cultures of the pre-industrial countries at a very rapid rate. This meeting of the two cultures, the scientific and the traditional, is so extensive, and they are so profoundly opposed on so many issues, that the stress resulting can best be described as 'cross-cultural conflict'.

In this cross-cultural conflict, in which the indigenous doctor is likely to be involved quite as much as any of his patients, it is natural that the health aspects of the clash should be uppermost in his mind. Nevertheless, a doctor is well placed to observe the whole process of social change, mid though there may be little any individual can do to modify it, a doctor has a uniquely influential position in the local community.

It is suggested that he be guided by the following principles which determine whether a change in the culture is to be encouraged or discouraged. inevitably, any attitude in this matter is deeply influenced by the observer's own values. Too often, the individual is powerless and principles often conflict, but despite this some guidance may be useful.

Other things being equal, any social change is likely to be beneficial which does the following:

(a) Promotes harmonious social interaction and cohesion of any lawful kind between individuals; that is, anything which promotes 'togetherness' or 'community. Thus, unless there are compelling reasons against them, clans and societies, rites and rituals, etc. are all to be fostered.

(b) Enables the individual to realize his innate potentialities; this includes any kind of education.

(c) Preserves or enhances the uniqueness and creativity of the group. Thus, art, in any form, folk tales, local languages and customs are to be preserved as valuable components of the total achievement of our species.

When two cultures meet it is unusual for one to displace the other completely, a more common result is for elements of the two to fuse in some way, the process being given the name of 'syneetism'. For example, in societies where scarification or tadtooing is done with non-medical intent, it is possible for the populace to interpret the scientific process of vaccination merely as an addition to their present beliefs and not as an entirely different concept. Should such a process of integrating scientific medicine with the local beliefs be encouraged or discouraged? Opinions differ, but most workers would probably agree that it is better to get a desirable practice adopted by this means than not to get it adopted at all.

Summary. Before summing up there is one final message to leave with the reader. This is the importance of learning from the culture being studies. One thing that compels admiration in so many tropical societies is their intense sense of community. This is surely *the* critical ingredient in human happiness, and how far removed from, and how infinitely preferable it is to the loneliness and social fragmentation of the industrial suburbs of Europe and America. The incorporation of deep and vigorous community life in a technological society is widely held to be one of the major problems of our age.

Method: Obtaining a 'cross-cultural outlook' in medicine

Observe the society closely. Use what is visible to lead to what is invisible in terms of attitudes, values and goals etc.

Read some anthropology.

Read what novels and plays may be relevant.

See if there have been any specific studies of the tribes in the area and read them.

Make the acquaintance of any anthropologist working in the vicinity.

Obtain an insight into the local culture by carefully questioning some of the more educated members of the local community.

Follow this by obtaining more information in routine case histories taken from the patients.

Take at least some steps to learn a local language, even if it is only the greetings and the necessary clinical questions and imperatives.

Lastly, all the old's cultures are equally fit for study, be they those of affluent technology or pygmy aborigines. Anthropology is the study of man in all his variety and is in no sense limited merely to the study of remote and barbarous tribes. It has been rightly said that anthropology is not merely barbardology.

15

Administration of the Indigenous System of Medicine

A. Genesis and Need

Genesis

Before the advent of the Western system of medicine in the world, some indigenous systems were prevalent in every country which provided medical care to the people. These systems were developed independent of one another. Each system developed its own rationale of treatment. Even today, this traditional system is being practised all over the world. The prestige of the traditional system of medicine has gone down over the years because of its neglect and absence of pursuit of proper researches to keep the system in tune with the changing conditions. Modern medicine has been accepted all over the world as a reliable system to provide health care to the people. The basic problem in the developing world is to provide medical care to all the people with their meagre resources. Is it possible to open costly hospitals and dispensaries based on the Western system of medicine to provide health care to all? The answer is plain and simple, i.e., 'NO' because of the huge investments involved in establishing and maintaining modern clinics and hospitals. Only the few rich or influential people can afford this system. Millions of people living in rural areas have no access to the system of modern medicine. How can we provide the health care to the neglected 80 per cent of the world population? They must be provided health care to ensure social justice within the country and among the countries in the world. It has also been found that the indigenous system of medicine can provide care to a number of diseases for which there is no treatment in allopathic system. The Secretary of the Ministry of Health and Family Welfare (Govt. of India) stated:

> "We do recognise that there are quite a few diseases where the modern system of medicine has not been able to give an answer but where the practitioners of Indian systems of medicine have got an answer. They claim that they can treat such diseases with effectiveness. . . For instance, we have not been able to find a cure for diabetes so far as modern systems of medicine is concerned. We have medicines to treat it. But Ayurveda claims that they can cure it."

Dr. Mahler, Director General of the WHO has rightly said that:

> "The age-old arts of the herbalists too must be tapped. Many of the plants familiar to the `wise-woman' or the `witch doctor' really do have the healing powers that tradition attaches to them; the pharmacopoeia of modern medicine would be poorer if one removed from it all the preparations, chemicals and components whose origins lie in herbs, funguses, flowers, fruits and roots."[1]

Integrated Approach

Eighty per cent of the people who are not getting access to modern medicine still use the traditional system. Thus, there is a need to refine those systems, to prevent them using such practices that might pose possible risks for their patients. The practitioners of these systems can be given training to exploit them for providing health care. The Estimates Committee has also stressed that :

> "While every effort should be made to appropriate the best in knowledge of the West and make modern medicine and science available in India, the high cost of Western system of treatment makes it difficult for universal application and it is therefore necessary to develop an alternative strategy of medical care combining the good features of both the Western and indigenous systems."[2]

It was further indicated that, "It is evident that indigenous medicine which has served the country for ages, can be used effectively after a scientific evaluation of its effects. The committee would therefore stress on the need for making concerted efforts to develop an appropriate integrated relationship between modern and indigenous systems of medicine."[3]

The Western system of medicine and traditional systems should not run parallel to each other but must supplement each other's efforts. Some experiments are being conducted on the use of medicine used in the traditional systems. Dr Mahler has beautifully said,

> "For far too long, traditional systems of medicine and `modern' medicine have gone their separate ways in mutual antipathy. Yet are not their goals identical—to improve the health of mankind and thereby the quality of life ? Only the blinkered would assume that each has nothing to learn from the other."[4]

A recent International Conference on Asiatic Medicine was held at Canberra, with 300 participants from 29 nations. The conference presented no confrontation between Eastern and Western practitioners. On the contrary the Western doctors paid close attention so that they overcome their inculcated blindness towards the patient.[5]

Comparative Merits of Traditional Systems of Medicinevis-a-vis Western System of Medicine

In our efforts to provide community health care to all, we must exploit all the systems of medicine available to us. The advantage of using traditional systems are that they are cheaper as they do not require costly and sophisticated equipment and are also effective in dealing with chronic ailments. We must make use of the available material, financial and manpower resources that are rooted in traditional medical practices. These systems use cheap medicines based on local preparations and these medicines are devoid of side-effects. The Western system of medicine uses drugs which can produce harmful effects. The people have become drug addicted. A health education programme is essential to inform people of the dangers of excessive drug usage. On the other hand, the medicines given through the indigenous system are cheap, less harmful and have in some cases nutritional value. The medicines in these systems are derived from herbal, mineral and animal origin and considered to be non-toxic.

Furthermore, the practitioners of traditional systems can devote more time to their patients and thus can develop good doctor-patient relationship. These practitioners are rooted in the community and have deep understanding of the ailments of the patients. Dr V.T.H. Gunaratne, Regional Director, WHO, SEARO, in his address to the participants of the Seminar on Traditional Medicine in South-East Asia, said :

> "The relationship between physician and the patient is particularly important for the success of health programmes. This relationship is not impersonal as between an infection and a drug. It is a relationship between two human beings—the sick on the one hand and the person endowed with the knowledge required to treat him on the other—both belonging to the same society. The physician should be close to the culture of his society and serve as a natural attorney to handle health and social problems."[6]

The practitioners of traditional systems of medicine command faith and respect from the community to which they themselves belong. The best method to provide medical care to all is to find out the best in all the systems. "No single system can thrive or be useful to all irrespective of its origin, location or merit. Anything that is good in all these systems should be made available, while false claims or ineffective practices and faulty approaches that may be currently in vogue should be eliminated through intensive and systematic research."[7]

Assessing Traditional Systems of Medicine

What we can do is to find the number of personnel engaged in traditional system of medicine. Next, we should try to judge their competence against the background of well laid-out norms and standards. If they are deficient in their art, we can provide them refresher courses. After this, these practitioners can be absorbed into the general health system to provide health care to the people.

Recent Developments

In 1976, WHO's Regional Committee for Africa had 'Traditional Medicine and its role in the Development of Health Services in Africa' as the topic for technical discussion. The Regional Committee for South-East Asia also adopted a resolution,[8] at its Twenty-ninth session in September, 1976, urging the Regional Director to initiate studies on alternative approaches to provide health care to the people by using traditional systems which have lasted through ages in conjunction with modern science. Seminars on various aspects of traditional systems were held in Colombo and Sri Lanka to implement training, service and research programmes. WHO headquarters have also been taking keen interest in promotion of the traditional systems of medicine. The Twenty-ninth World Health Assembly has requested the Director General of WHO : "to encourage the development of health teams, trained to meet the health needs of the populations, including health workers for primary health care and taking into account, where appropriate, the manpower resource constituted by these practising traditional medicine."

The thirty-first World Health Assembly held in 1978 had chosen "National policies and practices in regard to medicinal products" as the subject for technical discussion. A programme to coordinate the various activities relating to traditional medicine was prepared at the WHO headquarters with the following objectives :

— foster a realistic approach to traditional medicine so as to promote and further contribute to health care;

— to explore the merits of traditional medicine in the light of modern medicine so as to maximise useful and effective practices and discourage harmful ones;

— to promote integration of proven valuable knowledge and skill in traditional and modern medicine.[9]

B. Classification of Traditional System of Medicine

The traditional system may be classified into two categories:

(1) *Formalised systems* such as Ayurveda and Yoga, Unani-Tibbe, Siddha, Chinese system including Acupuncture, and Amchi system (Tibetan system).

(2) *Non-formalised systems* comprising herbalists, the Thood (Hindu Buddhist system), mantras and tantras, Malaysia's Bomohs.

Let us discuss in brief some of these systems. Ayurveda has a distinct place of significance. The available literature starts with *Sushruta, Samihta* and *Charaka Samhita* which were compiled during the fifth century B.C. This system influenced the medical systems of Egypt, Greece, Rome and Arabia. This is being practised in all the countries of the South-East Asia. Yogic practices are conducive to keep the body fit and promote positive physical and mental health. These practices influence some visceral and metabolic functions which help to maintain homeostatic conditions in the body. It is claimed that yogic exercises can cure chronic diseases for which modern medicine has no answer. Such exercises can bring physical and mental relaxation, economy in energy-utilisation, voluntary control over the functioning of the body, etc. There are about 200 institutions of yoga in India.

Table 1: Pattern of Training in Institutions of Traditional Medicine in the South-East Asia Region

Country	*No. of Instit-utions*	*Admission Standard*	*No. of Student Admissions*	*Duration of Course*	*Degree/ Diploma*	*Remarks*
1. Bangla Desh	4	Matric (10th Class)	200	4 years	Diploma	—
2. Burma	1	-do-	30	3 years	-do-	—
3. India	108	Intermediate (12th Class)	3000	4½ years + 1years internship	Degree	Facilities available for post-graduate course of 3 years or Ph.D. for 2 years
4. Indonesia	—	No Training Institutions				
5. Nepal	1	10th Class	30	3 years	Diploma	—
6. Sri Lanka	1	11th Class	150	5 years	Degree	—
7. Thailand	?	Literature	—	3 years Apprenti-ceship	Registered Practioner	—

Note: 10th Class: Matriculation
11th Class: Secondary
12th Class: Intermediate

Source: SEA/Trade. Med./1 Annex. 8, page 33, July, 1977.

Unani-Tibbi system of medicine is practised in Bangladesh and India to a great extent. Its origin can be traced to Greek medicine.

Sidha system is largely practised in Tamil-speaking areas of India and Sri Lanka. The Chinese system is being practised in the Democratic Republic of Korea.

Let us review, in brief, the prevalence and practice of the traditional system of medicine in some of the countries of the South-East Asia.

Table 1 summarises the existing training arrangements in the countries of South East Asia.

India

This table reveals that there are elaborate training arrangements for imparting instructions in traditional system of medicine in most of the countries of the South-East Asia region, i.e. India has 108 such training institutions/centres which are carrying out multidisciplinary research in traditional systems of medicine. The results of the research studies have proved of great value in providing better health care facilities to the people. In addition to the number of private pharmacies, almost all the State governments are maintaining their own pharmacies for the production of standard medicine. There also exist separate directorates for traditional systems of medicine in all the states. There are in all 215 hospitals and 14000 dispensaries in the country.

Nepal

Ayurveda is practised in this country. About 75 per cent of the population depend on Ayurvedic treatment. There are 200 institutionally qualified practitioners and about 1000 traditionally trained persons.

Sri Lanka

There are three traditional medicine systems in practice in Sri Lanka, viz., Ayurveda, Siddha and Unani. In all, there are 3030 institutionally trained physicians and 14590 non-institutionally trained physicians.

Bangla Desh

There are mainly two system viz., the Unani and the Ayurvedic systems. A Board regulates and registers the practitioners of these systems. At present 4350 *hakims* and *kavirajas* are registered with this Board, including 500 who have qualified for the four-year regular course.

Burma

The traditional medical practitioners, numbering 30,000 provide medical care to about 85 per cent of the country's population. There are 11277 trained practitioners and about 22000 non-institutionally trained practitioners.

C. The Indian Systems of Medicine and Homeopathy

Let us now discuss the indigenous system of medicine (Ayurveda, Siddha, Unani, Yoga and Naturopathy) in India in depth. It has been accepted as an integral part of the country's total health care services. There are 108 undergraduate teaching institutions, 2 postgraduate institutions and 18 post-graduate departments awarding post-graduate and doctoral degrees in traditional systems of medicine. A national institute of Ayurveda was established at Jaipur in 1976. There are proposals to set up a National Institute for Unani and Yoga. A General Research Institute (Yoga) has been established at New Delhi as a registered society. There are 14000 dispensaries and 215 hospitals which provide medical care through the traditional systems of medicine. Separate directorates for traditional systems of medicine exist in all the States of the Indian Union.

(i) Central Council of Medicine

It was established by the Government of India in 1971 by an Act of Parliament mainly to develop uniform standards of education in these systems of medicine and to maintain a central Register for these systems. The Council has been functioning and has succeeded in finalising the uniform syllabus for under-graduate education in Ayurveda, Unani and Siddha.

The Council has finalised various other regulations and may start the operation of the central Register soon.

(ii) Pharmacoeopia and Pharmacies

The first volume of the standard Ayurvedic Formulary for 444 compound formulations has been finalised. The Unani and Siddha formularies are also being finalised.

The Indian Medicines Pharmaceutical Corporation, a joint venture of Central and UP Government, has been registered as a public sector undertaking a Ranikhet Uttar Pradesh to make available, at reasonable rates potent and genuine Ayurvedic and Unani medicines.

The Pharmacoecopial Laboratory for Indian Medicine was established in 1968 to prescribe standards developing tests for single drugs and compound preparations used in Indian system of medicine. The laboratory has developed a small museum of medicinal plants which can facilitate identification of herbs.

The Government of India provides financial assistance to State governments for development of State Pharmacies and Herb Garden upto a ceiling of Rs. 8 lakhs per pharmacy.

(iii) Central Council for Research in Indian Medicine and Homeopathy

This Council was constituted in 1969 to initiate, aid, develop and coordinate scientific research in different aspects, fundamental and applied, of Indian system of medicine including Homeopathy and Yoga. The Council has 15 full-fledged research institutions and about 115 research units for carrying out multi-disciplinary research. The Council has undertaken many other schemes—Drug Research, Literary Research, Clinical Research, Mobile Clinical Research and Survey of medicinal plants in various parts of the country. In addition, the Council has also evolved an Ayurvedic Medical Kit and published books containing simple remedies in Siddha, Unani and Homeopathy for common ailments and some more books are under publication. A research unit at Laddakh for research on 'Emchi System of Medicine' has been established. The Council has taken steps to establish a Regional Research Institute in Bihar, Madhya Pradesh and Gujarat. In pursuance of the decision to reorganise the Central Council for Research in Indian Medicine and Homeopathy, four separate research councils have been set up one each for Ayurveda and Siddha, Unani medicines, Homeopathy and Yoga and Naturopathy.

(iv) Homeopathic System of Medicine

There are 94 institutions imparting training in Homeopathy which have been recognised by various State Boards and Councils. Eight of these are government institutions. The Homoeopathic Advisory Committee advises the Central government on development of homeopathy.

(v) Central Council of Homeopathy

A Central Council of Homeopathy was constituted on 8 August, 1974, in pursuance of the Homeopathy Central Council Act 1973, for maintenance of the Central Register for Homeopathic physicians and for bringing about uniformity in standards of education in this discipline.

(vi) National Institute of Homeopathy, Calcutta

It was set up in December, 1975 as an autonomous body to provide facilities for advance training, research and patient care in Homeopathy. Short Training courses for Homeopathic teachers are being organised here since September, 1976.

(vii) Homeopathic Pharmacopoeia Laboratory, Ghaziabad

It has functioned as a subordinate office of the Ministry of Health and Family Welfare, since September, 1975. It fixes standards of raw-material and finished products of Homeopathic drugs. The laboratory maintains a museum of raw-materials as reference standards and herbarium. There is Homeopathic Pharmacopoeia Committee to lay down the standards of various medicines for inclusion in the Homeopathic Pharmacopoeia of India. Two volumes containing standards for 280 drugs have already been published.

(viii) Central Council for Research in Homeopathy

The Council which has been established as an autonomous body, conducts its research programmes through its 8 units in different places in the country and two Regional Research Institutes at New Delhi and Kottayam and one Central Institute at Calcutta. Encouraging results have been obtained in the treatment of amoebic dysentry, tonsillitis, allergic dermatitis and bronchial asthama. Research programmes were also undertaken (a) to evaluate the efficacies of homeopathic drugs with those of modern drugs at the All India Institute of Medical Sciences, and (b) to evaluate anti-fertility drugs in homeopathy as a result of which three drugs have been established to possess anti-fertility effect on animals with very low side-effects.

Proposals during the Plan Period 1978-83

The plan proposals for 1978-83 are mainly aimed at:

(a) re-orienting the existing traditional practitioners in various systems and strengthening their professional knowledge;

(b) reviewing and prescribing uniform syllabi for under-graduate and post-graduate education;

(c) assisting in equipping under-graduate colleges to meet the standards laid down by Central Council of Indian Medicine and Homeopathy and to train teachers thereof;

(d) evolving and publishing pharmacopoeia;

(e) providing organisation arrangements for manufacture and testing the medicines; and

(f) encouraging intensive research in all these systems. The development of these systems of medicine should aim more towards supplementing the health care facilities in the country keeping in view the needs and the demands for these systems of medicine in different parts of the country.

D. Critical Appraisal of the Functioning of ISM Including Homeopathy in the Developing Countries with Special Reference to India

We have examined the existing potentialities and the future prospects of these systems of medicine. It has been amply demonstrated that these systems can contribute to the provision of health care to the people. What are the reasons which stand in the way of its adoption?

Dr. B. Thirumalara, FRCS, Edinburgh, DLO, London: Surgeon, King George Hospital has stated that:

> "There is a still great deal to learn from ancient systems of medicine. They have got an extensive pharmacopoeia. They have developed dietetics almost to a fine art. We may have yet to learn from the observations of the ancient physicians, their decisions, and the principles they have laid down and the methods they adopted for treatment."[10]

Dr. P.N.V. Kurup, WHO consultant, has said in his keynote address to the participants of a seminar 'Traditional medicine in South-East Asia':

> "A system which has the prime object of maintenance of health and the prevention and cure of disease certainly deserves to be investigated and introduced in the health care programme of any nation. Owing to historical reasons, these systems could not make enough progress during the last few centuries. In spite of this disadvantage, the majority of the population in the various parts of the world is still served by the traditional system which only speaks for its potentiality for further development."[11]

What has gone wrong with the application of these systems? How can we integrate these systems with modern medicine? How can we make these systems scientific and reliable? How can we imbibe the confidence of the people in these systems? We shall discuss here the solutions to all the problems posed in these questions. The facts and suggestions mentioned below are based on the study of documents, proceedings of the seminars, records of the Estimates Committee and Public Accounts Committee, Records of world Health Organisation, discussion with health experts and practitioners of Western medicine as well as indigenous system including homeopathy and the beneficiaries. Beneficiaries were contacted in different institutions of ISM on random basis to solicit their views. We shall also discuss the experiences prevalent in other countries to support our viewpoints.

Absence of Parity in the Status of the Personnel/Institutes of Traditional Systems of Medicines vis-a-vis Personnel/Institutes of Western System of Medicine

Most of the States in India have instituted separate directorates for ISM and Homeopathy. At present there is great disparity in the status and pay scales of directors and teaching staff pertaining to ISM as compared to the Western system of medicine. The scales of pay and non-practicing allowance in the case of Ayurvedic and Homeopathic physicians are lower than those admissible to allopathic doctors. The same situation was prevailing in the field of education where the teachers of Indian languages were accorded lower status and poor conditions of service. The Government has taken a wise step in removing these distinctions by granting parity in status and emoluments. The situation in the field of health can also be improved by:

(a) recognising traditional practitioners on an equal footing with those of the Western medicine;

(b) the health personnel of traditional system of medicine should be involved in the health policy formulation and implementation,

(c) the health personnel of traditional system of medicine should be provided the means to develop professionally through fellowships, research grants etc.;

(d) more recognition should be accorded to the health personnel of ISM at District and Block levels.

Lack of Cooperation and Coordination Among the various Systems of Medicine

At present, the ISM and Western Medicine are working in water-tight compartments. They are so much envious of each other that it is difficult for them to function harmoniously. Besides, a lot of propaganda is done to tarnish the image of one system of medicine against the other. The people get baffled and confused in assessing the relative merits and efficacy of each system. One of the patients remarked that, "Before a physician administers medicine, he advocates for the most of the time about the good points of his medicine and warns of the evil consequences if other systems are used." No medical system can serve the people in insolation. "They can continue to serve through collaboration and cooperation and by complimenting and supplementing each other. All the systems in their own way have their strong and weak points, but a synthesis of these may help in evolving unified medical care system devoid of disadvantages and weak points."

The experience of China in the integration of traditional and Western medicine has been quite effective. Prof. Wu-chich-Ping of Chinese Academy of Medical Sciences, while elaborating this concept said:

> "Priority is given to the work of helping the medical and health workers understand better the importance of traditional medicine, a valuable cultural heritage. We organised the private practitioners of traditional medicine to work in hospitals, with an equal social status to doctors of Western medicine. The doctors of Western medicine are encouraged to learn traditional medicine and doctors of traditional medicine, for their part, learn the strong points of Western medicine. In addition to the setting up of hospitals of traditional medicine, a department of traditional medicine is formed in most general hospitals."[12]

Their attempts at integration have evolved into what they now call the (new) traditional Chinese medicine, which can be described as the application of modern scientific principles to the traditional Chinese system.

In order to bring about effective cooperation and coordination among all the systems of medicine and to provide effective health care to all, the following points are suggested:

(a) Institute the departments of ISM in all the medical-education institutions imparting education in Western medicine.

(b) Introduction of elementary syllabus from these systems in under-graduate and post-graduate medical education.

(c) Setting up of common administrative set-up to bring about fruitful and meaningful coordination.

(d) Encourage learning from each other's system wherever useful.

(e) Specific and comparative researches may be conducted in different systems of medicine simultaneously and later on adopting the findings of that system which are economical and useful.

(f) Providing common building to all the systems. This would encourage exchange of views and information.

The Estimates Committee has also desired effective coordination. It was stressed that: The co-existence of Allopathic, Homeopathic and Ayurvedic systems of medicine provides an ideal laboratory where modern technology and ancient knowledge react on one another and can be used to bring about effective remedies for various diseases. Government should not deny full facilities to the indigenous systems of medicines so that these systems are fully utilised for bringing relief to the beneficiaries who wish to avail of them." [13]

Poor Financial Allocations to the Traditional System

There is a lot of disparity prevalent at present in the allocation of financial resources to modern medicine and traditional medicine. For example, In India, an allocation of Rs. 60 crores has been made for ISM and Homeopathy for the plan period 1978-83. This has been reduced from 5.6 per cent during the 5th plan period to 4.6 for the current plan. During 1978-79 only 445 lakhs have been provided for ISM out of a total budget of Rs. 2,67,47.44 lakhs for health. How can we expect good results from the traditional systems without providing facilities? We have to put them to life after a neglect of long period. The activity which is to be revitalised needs more resources. We have on the other hand given step-motherly treatment to these systems of medicine. It is, therefore suggested that:

(a) More financial allocations be made to tone up the traditional systems of medicine.

(b) Financial allocations may be stepped up slowly to cope with the present and future activities.

(c) Expenditure on Western medicine may be decreased and those national institutes which are not relevant may be wound up. This 'sunset approach' may be applied to prune the unwanted growth and the resources may be diverted to other productive fields.

(d) While allocating the money to these systems care may be taken not to creat unwieldy and unmanageable institutes resulting in wastage of resources.

Unsatisfactory Utilisation of Health Manpower Available in these Systems

At present we do not posses the information regarding the availability of health manpower in these systems in terms of their educational background, training, experience, and academic background etc. Thus, there is a need to collect data about the availability of health manpower in these systems. These health personnel who are mostly half-baked are administering health care to the people. Most of the experts remarked:

> "Such health personnel treat the patients without much knowledge or background. These cases later on become complicated and chronic and become either incurable or need long hospitalisation". what can be done to ward off such dangers? It is suggested that:

(a) Different types of training courses may be arranged for these health personnel so that they may function scientifically. This would also increase their morale and develop self-confidence in them.

(b) Those who have no background should be asked to wind up through a strict legislation so that they may not play with the lives of the patients. One expert remarked: "Everybody is a physician in India". So we must weed out those who have no knowledge at all about these systems.

Lack of Proper Standards of Medical Education in Traditional Systems

The standards of medical education in these systems are not upto the mark. There is a dearth of standard texts to enable the students to have through knowledge. Because of the paucity of funds, many medical educational institutions cannot employ the highly qualified teachers, and provide facilities to the students. Just as the Western medical education system should adopt from these systems some elements of traditional systems of medicine, similarly the traditional systems of medicine must incorporate the good points of Western medicine. This cross-breeding would benefit all the systems of medicine. The following suggestions are given to improve the image of medical education in these systems.

(a) There is an urgent need for systematic research into the various aspects of these systems to make them scientific and relevant.

(b) Liberal financial assistance may be provided to the institutions imparting education in traditional medicine to effect modernization in their programmes.

(c) Financial Assistance may be provided only if Central Council of Indian Medicine and Central Council of Homeopathy approve the functioning of their respective institutes.

(d) Basic conditions must be laid down before giving approval to a new institution.

(e) The syllabi must be examined thoroughly so that the medical education in these systems can be improved.

(f) More post-graduate departments and institutions must be set up to set standards for under-graduate education.

Absence of Researches and Case Studies to Develop and Modernize the Traditional Systems

Modern medicine has progressed because of researches in the medical sciences. They have evolved standard terminology which is applicable throughout the world. Traditional systems of medicine have not so far developed standards which can be uniformly applied. All these standards differ from person to person. It is very difficult to get the same treatment from different persons of the same system. Researches can revolutionize the medical sciences. It is, therefore, suggested that the traditional systems of medicine should encourage research through the National Institutes and the postgraduate institutions to evolve generalisation based on case studies. It was remarked by a patient that

"Everybody would boast of curing the disease in his own way."

What is lacking is the need to develop common pool of knowledge which can be administered to benefit the people. Xavier Lozoya, Coordinator of the Mexican Institute for the study of medicinal plants in Mexico City in his article "Balance between Man and Nature" tells the uses of plants as medicines. He suggests researches to find the hidden treasures. He remarks, "The more they are in vestigated and studied in the light of a science which once more reverts to serving the public good, the more they will contribute to the development of a system of medicine adapted to the needs, the cultural demands and the overall health of one country."[14]

Dr (Mrs) S. Kataria, Principal, Homeopathic Medical College, Chandigarh, warns the followers of the traditional system of medicine to develop the system on modern lines otherwise they would be thrown out. She further stated that Samuel Hahnemann discovered Homeopathy when allied sciences like Physiology, Bacteriology and Pathology, were in the process of being born. Her science of therapeutics at that time laid stress in symptomology, which the common man thought was a simple thing. Because there were no schools and colleges to study this method of treatment on scientific basis and teach the same, this art went into the hands of non-scientific people, and further the so-called homoeopaths started flourishing. This easy achievement on their part was a booster to their morale, and they became egoists. The result was that such a highly and thought provoking system of medicine was transferred from highly qualified scientific giants like Hahnemann, Kent, Tyler etc., into the hands of quacks, and no further research or advancement was done to the credit of Homeopathy. People got an impression that this system of medicine was harmless, but later on, because of the non-scientific basis and the poor results as well as bad effects of misguided medicines, the Government's took up the question of modernizing and regularising this system of medicine. This created a fear complex in the minds of the unqualified homeopaths and they, being in a majority, put up a lot of resistance to these proposals and science, which was losing its popularity. The result was that no qualified scientist or a high intellectual would venture to take up the research in this field of medicine. A science which closes its doors to all scientific advancements cannot progress. While other systems of medicines, particularly Allopathy, have engulfed scientists from various fields of science like Physics, Chemistry, Biology etc., Homeopathy even today when governments are trying hard to rejuvenate it, is being obstructed by the so-called homeopaths, and,therefore, unless the authorities make a firm and determined effort to transfer this system of medicine into the hands of scientists and people of high intellect, this science will become obsolete in due course of time as has happened in other parts of the world.[15]

We may mention here the recommendations of a recent seminar on Traditional Medicine in South-East Asia held at Colombo (1-5 April, 1977) which need examination and adoption by the member states to improve their health systems.

(1) Governments should make a policy declaration at the top national level to recognize, promote and rehabilitate the traditional systems of medicine prevalent in their respective countries and to maximise their utilisation in health teams, particularly in providing primary health care to the rural population.

(2) Governments should conduct national surveys to collect information about the number of traditional medical practitioners (including traditional birth attendants their methods of treatment, the nature of their training and such other information as may be necessary for their utilisation in extending health care to a large number of people.

(3) Based on the information collected, steps should be taken to identify the most appropriate manner of participation by traditional medical practitioners in the health team with a view to promoting their activities in the provision of basic health care, particularly to the vulnerable sections of the rural population.

After identification of the manner of their participation at various levels of the nation's health care system, orientation/training programmes should be organized for these traditional practitioners in community surroundings in keeping with the needs of the people.

(4) Governments should design and supply standard medical kits to trained health workers which should contain traditional medicines for common ailments wherever these are not available, the kit may also include certain specific allopathic drugs for the delivery of primary health care.

(5) Governments should intensify their efforts at:

(a) inter-disciplinary research into the practice of traditional medicine;

(b) the proper training of personnel;

(c) documentation, and

(d) the conservation and cultivation of medicinal plants.

(6) Governments should make freely available to other governments and relevant agencies information regarding traditional medicine practices, research findings on flora, fauna and minerals used in the preparation of traditional medicines.

(7) Governments should include in the curriculum of all health workers (medical and paramedical) an orientation course in the principles and practice of traditional/ indigenous systems of medicine.

(8) WHO should: (a) Collaborate in the implementation of the above recommendations; (b) Assist member-countries in organising group educational and research activities and award fellowships for training in research techniques, studies of health care systems and other technological procedures related to the traditional/indigenous systems of medicine.[16]

Conclusion

We must encourage the growth of all the systems to provide total health care to all the people. The good points of all these systems must be integrated to alleviate human sufferings.

We may conclude with the observations made by Sir William Osler:

> "unless we develop the spirit of tolerance between the practitioners of different systems of medicine originating from different countries there cannot be any progress."[17]

References

1. Dr H.Mahler "The Staff Aesculapius". in *World Health,* Nov., 1977, p. 3.
2. Lok Sabha Secretariat: Estimates Committee, *Hundred and Second Report* (Fifth Lok Sabha), April, 1976, p. 100.
3. *Ibid.*
4. Dr H. Mahler, op. cit., p. 3.
5. The *Tribune,* Chandigarh, 12 September 1979.
6. SEA/Trad. Med/I, p. 23, Annex. 4.
7. P.N.V. Kurup, Advisor to the Govt. of India for indigenous system of medicine, "The Science of Life" in *World Health,* November, 1977, p. 15.
8. SEA/RC 29/RII; Fifth Meeting, 17th September, 1976, SEA/RC/29/Min. 5.
9. Dr H. Bannerman, "WHO's programmes," in *World Health,* November, 1977 p. 16.
10. Quoted in SEA/Trad, Med./I, pp. 15-16, Annex. 3.
11. SEA/Trad. Med./I, p. 27, Annex, 6.
12. WHO, *World Health,* july, 1976, p. 33.
13. Lok Sabha Secretariat: Estimates Committee, *57th Report* (5th Lok Sabha) April, 1974, p. 113.
14. WHO, *World Health,*November, 1977, P. 11.
15. Based on Personal Interview with the Principal. She was kind enough to give her views in writing to the author.
16. WHO, SEARO: SEA/Trad. Med./I,pp. 8-9.
17. Quoted in SEA/Trad. Med. I, p.31, Annex. 6.

16

Voluntary Health Agencies and Health Care Administration

A. Nature and Functions

Genesis

Voluntary agencies have a long history of active involvement in the promotion of human welfare and well-being. Lord Beveridge called them "a private enterprise for social progress". Voluntary agencies came into existence spontaneously, voluntarily and without any compulsion or control to fulfil the particular needs of some groups of people. These agencies are flexible and possess the virtues of human service with dedication. Voluntary action is the soul of democracy as this medium secures the active involvement of the people from policy-making to implementation of social services. It is the life and blood of democracy. Their programme covers a diverse range of functions embracing human welfare in the field of health. The programmes of voluntary organisations include the strictly professional, specialised and technical organisations; broadly-based associations of persons or groups organized for a particular purpose, e.g., information and service activities, educational institutions and associations, social welfare organisations, religious groups, women's organisations, youth groups, childrens' councils, trade unions, family planning associations. Many voluntary organisations at national level are linked with international federations or associations. There are many which though not directly involved in health care administration, indirectly influence the promotion of the programmes of health administration as human development cannot be fragmented. Social and economic sectors are closely allied and interdependent, e.g. it is useless to promote a health insurance scheme if employment opportunities are so limited that participation is beyond the reach of many. Provision of a source of clean water to a community will have impact on water-borne diseases only in so far as the community is educated in its use and management. Thus, the work of other voluntary organisations influence the functioning of total health care administration in a country. The programme of other voluntary organisations which is of great and direct relevance to health care administration includes projects to improve nutrition, food production, housing, provide potable water, promote literacy, provide educational and instructional material, enhance community development, improve environmental sanitation, child and woman welfare, etc. Thus they are helping to create conditions to the protection, promotion and maintenance of health, and the prevention of illness.

Meaning and Definition of Voluntary Health Agencies

A voluntary health agency may be defined as: "An organisation that is administered by an autonomous board which holds meetings, collects funds for its support, chiefly from private sources, and expends money, whether with or without paid workers, in conducting a programme directed primarily to furthering the public health by providing health services or health education or by advancing research or legislation for health, or by a combination of these activities."

Voluntary health agencies are functioning in almost all the countries of the world. In some countries, voluntary health services have played an important role in stimulating and initiating the development of social services while in other countries they have given leadership in promoting the establishment and progressive extension of Government responsibilities. In some countries these agencies carry the major responsibilities and may provide the only social services available to the people. For example, the voluntary health services in India have played a significant role as the problems are so large that it is not possible for the Government alone to tackle it. The main object of planned development is to mobilise the total, known as well as hidden material and human resources in such a way as to improve the socio-economic living conditions of the people to the maximum at a given time. They have been supplementing the efforts of the government from ancient times to this date. Thus, we find that "such agencies and the services they provide differ widely in terms of auspices and objectives, types of services, methods of operation, extent of coverage, standards maintained, source of financing and relationship to Government and to other non-governmental agencies."[1]

Functions of Voluntary Health Agencies

(a) *Participation of beneficiaries*. Voluntary organisations are nearer to the people and get better response from them in the implementation of programmes than official agencies and thus they are in a better position to render effective service. By and large, they have a better knack of communicating with the beneficiaries than members of official agencies. This of course, is a natural manifestation of the ancient civilisation of India, which has attached the greatest importance to the participation of the people in decision-making. The mobilisation of the energies and resources of the beneficiaries themselves is the key factor in increasing their welfare and self-reliance. People's participation through voluntary agencies in the promotion of health care means involvement of the people in the process of health care voluntarily and willingly. Such participation cannot be forced. People's involvement can be assured through the participation of the beneficiaries in the decision-making, implementation, monitoring and evaluation of health programmes carried out by the voluntary agencies. This will lay the solid foundation in the prevention and promotion of health care services and the people would become self-reliant rather than depend on the help from the Government. According to Dharma Vira: "Work of voluntary organisations and citizen participation are two sides of the same coin. Citizens work in organisations but on their work depends the quality of the service the organisations render. Voluntary Organisations provide a frame for citizen participation. Without effective citizen participation, the organisation would only be empty forms."[2]

(b) Creating a sense of responsibility through direct involvement. Programme results are more successful and meaningful if the potential beneficiaries take part in their design and implementation through the forum of voluntary organisations. For example, if uncollected garbage draws flies, or drains become clogged and overflow or if dirt pathways become ankle-deep mud sloughs in the rainy season, they will like to do something to remedy the situation-from complaining to the Health Department to dredging canals and filling in muddy pathways themselves.

(c) Rectification of planner's misconception. The planning now is without involving and understanding the needs of common people. It is very difficult for people to let their views be known individually. And planners find it difficult to appreciate their needs. People's participation through voluntary agencies can rectify planning errors by making it possible for clients to point out to planners, policy-makers and administrators what will work and what will not. For example, if the rural people participate through various voluntary health agencies in the process of planning, the disparity between the urban and rural health care can be removed. If things are left only to the specialists, they would ignore the demands of the masses. The higher status experts thus set the framework of discussion and carry it through in categories meaningful to themselves but often incomprehensible to the ordinary, poor and lowly educated laymen.

(d) Greater understanding and positive attitudes among the beneficiaries (formation of public opinion). The involvement of the beneficiaries in the socio-economic development or national reconstruction is dependent to a great extent upon their enlightenment. This can take place when voluntary health agencies interpret and explain the issues and problems of health care administration to the public e.g. Family Planning Association of India with its branches in all the States has been quite active in the population education programme of the public. The voluntary agencies are also trying to help by creating in the people an urge, an attitude to adopt new methods of health care, by arranging for the people services and opportunities to acquire new knowledge and techniques and by acting as a mediator between the people and the official machinery to interpret the problems and needs of the one to the other in order to develop better appreciation of each other.

(e) Effective policy formation through interpretation of public opinion. The voluntary health agencies can present the real needs of the health care of the people to the various decision-making bodies. They can also interpret health care plans based on their contacts with bilateral and multilateral agencies. Information is the policy makers' raw material, forming the basis for his diagnosis, strengthening his projections and permitting him to evaluate the programmes which have been planned. The degree to which a health planner will be able to plan in terms of health needs will depend on the degree to which he is able to obtain information about them which is valid and reliable. The information supplied by voluntary health agencies can be reliable as it is based on the outcome of their intimate contracts with the population.

(f) Flexibility and experimentation. The voluntary agencies are autonomous in their functioning. They are not bound by well-defined laws and regulations which are difficult to change. This gives the voluntary agencies an opportunity to experiment with a given programme and adjust it according to the environmental conditions. The programme must develop environmental linkages in order to be of lasting value and benefit to the people. The autonomous character of the voluntary agencies provide them flexibility to adopt their programme according to the needs and aspirations of the people. We know that the best structure can come up only in a congenial soil. The health problems of the people differ from area to area and hence, it is difficult to solve the problems for all the areas with the same solution. The voluntary organisations can experiment with different models in different areas and adopt and develop the best for the area for a given time dimension as the models of development are bound to change with the time dimension.

(g) Initiative and leadership. Voluntary agencies involve the people in the policy formulation and implementation of the programmes. This encourages the local potential leaders to develop as agents of socio-economic change. The people are not dependent on the initiative of the Government. They take the initiative and believe in self-help rather than help from outside.

(h) Channelise human resources. It is very difficult to provide all the social services to the people through the Government as it is very costly and rigid. The voluntary agency can exploit the unused energies of the people for the development of the country. Energy of the people, if unused, cannot be preserved. This unused energy "like the unused vast water resources flowing down the Himalayas is not only wasted like those rivers, but also, like the river waters that take with them the top soil of the Himalayan region causing permanent loses in soil erosion, cause permanent damage to the human spirit and will in a community through dependence and frustration born out of ever increasing level of abject poverty over the generations."[3]

We can explain this in the context of the provision of Primary Health Care Services. Voluntary health agencies can train the educated and willing workers in the art of elementary health care and health education. Such trained and motivated people in turn would be cheaper and efficient as can be seen from the Chinese experience.

(i) Advancing health legislation. In a welfare state, public health laws are as essential as security laws. These come under the purview of social legislation. It is the tool with which the health administrator is able to help the community from health hazards and promote the cause of health. The health legislation needs radical changes to cover all the people under health care, e.g., there is a need to make a law for the severe punishment for adulteration which is slow poisoning. Voluntary agencies can mobilise public opinion in support of such legislation. These agencies can prepare the people to act as a pressure group to compel the Government to enact legislations for the welfare of the masses. A political system remains in equilibrium only if it channelises the demands of the people into policies and decisions beneficial to the people.

(f) Supplement the efforts of government. The problems of development are so vast and stupendous that it is difficult to solve these problems with the efforts of the Government machinery alone. There is a need to share this responsibility and the voluntary sector which possess immense potential can take up this burden. During the last three decades the

government have been trying to bring about socio-economic revolution but the progress has been halted because of the non-availability of needed resources. Thus, there is a need of a voluntary sector to supplement the efforts of the Government. The working group appointed by the Planning Commission remarked that the country's social and economic problems are so vast and multi-farious that the Government's administrative machinery alone cannot tackle them. The establishment of a self-reliant society implies progressive curtailment of people's dependence on the Government. From time immemorial voluntary agencies in our country have played a significant part in promoting people's welfare.[4]

(k) Help in efficient programme implementation. Voluntary agencies can help in the programme implementation, collaboration and coordination of primary health care activities. They can contribute to primary health care in many ways through programme implementation. They can.[5]

"(1) Provide assistance to develop and/or strengthen local NGO capabilities and activities with particular attention to local community development groups.

(2) Conduct reviews and assessment of existing health and development programmes and assist communities in the exercise of their own role in such reviews. A greater emphasis on evaluative techniques will render all new programmes more accountable to real community needs.

(3) Develop innovative programmes placing primary health care in the context of comprehensive human development.

(4) Ensure that their existing programmes and new initiatives promote full participation by individuals and communities in the planning, implementation, and control of these programmes.

(5) Expand their training efforts to respond to the need of primary health care programmes, e.g. training of health workers, supervisors, administrators, planners and various agricultural and development workers. Included would be training schemes which build on the skills of traditional healers and midwives.

(6) Extend their efforts to develop locally sustainable and appropriate health technologies and use of resources, with particular attention to energy, water, agriculture, sanitation and medical care.

(7) Contribute to the creation of new and effective methods of health education which enable both individuals and communities to assume greater responsibility for their own health.

(8) Recognise the essential role of women in health promotion and in the full range of community development concerns.

(9) Further extend their capacity to work with poor, disadvantaged, and remote populations, enabling them to break the cycle of deprivation, and in this way contribute to the search for greater social justice."

B. Voluntary Health Agencies in India

In India, voluntary action by individuals, communities and organisations has existed from ancient days. India developed a unique tradition of social work through the in-built mechanism of providing security to members through the joint family system, kinship and other supporting social structure. The role of the state has varied in the past from indifference to benevolent interest depending upon the interest of individual rulers. For instance, Emperor Asoka organised a group of volunteers called 'Gopas' for social welfare work. During the Gupta period, the state had established workshops for the amelioration and training of handicapped persons. During the Mughal period, the state had separate departments to supervise charity and endowment to the poor. Community support rather than the state benevolence was the mainstay of voluntary agencies throughout the centuries preceding independence. Whether the case was an individual in distress or an emergency caused by a famine or flood, the voluntary agencies were the first to initiate social services. The voluntary system has been influenced by the economic structure of 'Jajmane' and Zamadari systems and by the religious values of *karma* and *dharma*. During the British period, some eminent political and social leaders set up a network of voluntary agencies mostly geared towards removing the social disabilities and barrier to development. These agencies became more active during the Gandhian era.

In the post-independence period, Government became committed to promote social welfare. The measures to achieve objectives of a welfare state have been enshrined in several articles of the Constitution. "The Directive Principles of State Policy", which *inter alia* states that

> "The State shall strive to promote the welfare of the people by securing and protecting, as effectively as it may, a social order in which justice, social, economic and political shall inform all the institutions of national life."

Articles 39(e), 41, 42 and 47 are of direct relevance to the promotion of health.

> "That the health and strength of workers, men and women, and the tender age of children are not forced by economic necessity to enter avocations unsuited to their age and strength."
>
> 39(e)

> "The State shall, within the limits of its economic capacity and development make effective provisions for securing the right to work, to education and to public assistance in cases of unemployment, old age, sickness and disablement, and in other cases of underserved want."
>
> (41)

> "The State shall make provisions for securing just and humane conditions of work and for maternity relief."
>
> (42)

> "The State shall regard the raising of nutrition and the standard of living of its people and the improvement of public health as amongst its primary duties."
>
> (47)

Article 24 of the Constitution (relating to Fundamental Rights) provides that no child below the age of fourteen years shall be employed to work in any factory or mine or engage in any other hazardous employment.

Planning was adopted as the mechanism to exploit the socio-economic resources. In such a scheme of planning, it is the people who have to organise themselves to safeguard their own interest. Voluntary agencies represent the organised expression of such public opinion and social action. Our five-year plans have been giving special incentives to the voluntary agencies. In the field of health, they are playing a significant role in the promotion of health, creation of awareness among people about the various measures to prevent sickness and the provision of welfare measures for the victims of different types of diseases.

India is a big country where governmental effort alone may not be able to meet the health needs of its large population and hence involvement of voluntary organisation is not only welcome but essential and desirable. Let us mention some of the important voluntary agencies engaged in the field of health care administration.

The Indian Red Cross Society

It was established in 1920 and works in close cooperation with national and international agencies. It plays an important role both in war and peace. It trains members of the community in health care procedures as well as focuses attention on certain health problems. The Indian Red Cross Society with its headquarters in New Delhi and branches in the States and Union Territories has been in the forefront of many projects to help people by voluntary effort.

Tuberculosis Association of India

It was formed in 1939, and has branches in all the states in India. It offers expert advice and serves as a coordinating agency in standardising methods, promoting consultations and conferences, starts model institutions, trains tuberculosis workers, etc. It administers the following institutions: The New Delhi Tuberculosis Centre. The Lady Linlithgow Sanatorium at Kasauli, the King Edward VII Sanatorium at Dharampur and the Tuberculosis Hospital at Mehrauli.

The Hind Kust Nivaran Sangh

It was founded in 1950. It renders financial assistance to various leprosy homes and clinics, training of medical workers, conducting research and field investigations. It organises All India Leprosy Workers Conference. It publishes *Leprosy in India*, a quarterly journal.It provides health education through publications and posters.

Indian Council for Child Welfare

It was established in 1952 with its branches in all the States. It is affiliated to International Union for Child Welfare. It is devoted to secure for children those opportunities and facilities which will help them "to develop physically, mentally, morally, spiritually and socially in a healthy and normal manner and in conditions of freedom and dignity."

The All-India Blind Relief Society

It was established in 1946 to coordinate the different activities of different organisations for the blind. It organises eye relief camps.

Family Planning Association of India

It was established in 1949, with its branches in the States. It provides support to the Family Welfare Planning Programme of the Government of India. We would examine the functioning of the Family Planning Association of India (Haryana branch) in detail.

Professional Bodies

Besides the above, there are some other voluntary professional organisations of various categories, e.g., Indian Medical Association, the Indian Public Health Association. The Trained Nurses Association of India, All-India Dental Association, etc., which are also making substantial contribution to the health programmes in the country. These bodies hold annual conferences, arrange discussions and lectures on important health problems, foster research and set up standards of Professional Education.

International Agencies

These include the Rockefeller Foundation, Ford Foundation and Care.

Semi-Official Organisations

These include the Medical Council of India, the Indian Nursing Council, Dental Council of India and the Central Social Welfare Board, etc.

C. A Case Study of the Family Planning Association of India (Haryana branch)[6]

The affairs of the association are looked after by an Executive Committee with a President, two Vice-Presidents, Honorary General Secretary and an Honorary Treasurer. Then, there are 12 more members of the Committee. Local committees have been constituted in those areas where there is more than one project. Five such committees were functioning at Ambala, Yamuna Nagar, Karnal, Sirsa and Kurukshetra. The day-to-day administration is carried out by the organising secretary of the association.

The Family Planning Association of India (FPAI), Haryana branch set up on 24 July 1972, since its re-organisation is a voluntary organisation engaged in promoting acceptance of family planning as a way of life. It is a body of socio-medical experts, both social workers and professionals, committed to the concept of planned parenthood. The branch is affiliated to the Family Planning Association of India with headquarters at Bombay, which is further affiliated to the International Planned Parenthood Federation, London.

Activities

Let us discuss the activities in brief (for details see Tables 1 and 2).

The branch is managing 17 projects, both in the clinical and educational fields. Besides rendering clinical services efforts are made to create a good will about the plans and programmes being implemented by the State government. Major emphasis is these projects is laid on establishing rapport with the community through educational and motivational efforts. During the year 1977, more than 74,000 people were contacted through personal counselling, group discussion, etc. There were more than 1,600 group discussions followed by 223 general meetings, 20 mass meetings, film shows and exhibitions.

Table No. 1: Family Planning Association of India, Haryana Branch `Statistical Tables'

Combined performance since inception (Period: January-December)

Particulars	*Period*						*Total since* inception
	1977	*1976*	*1975*	*1974*	*1973*	*1972*	
Clinical Service							
Sterilisation done	253	1,910	634	472	241	167	3,677
Sterilisation referred	66	2,404	304	136	396	75	3,381
Total Cases	319	4,314	938	608	637	242	7,058
IUD	189	1,029	683	703	84	56	2,744
Conventional Contraceptives (Number of pieces distributed)	1,30,124	2,25,960	2,33,471	1,82,221	82,718	3,450	8,57,944
Extension Service							
Personal Counselling	23,748	42,289	75,992	31,225	9,314	4,442	1,86,810
Repeat Contacts	10,420	1,24,397	88,656	39,051	18,893	7,641	2,89,058
Group Discussions	1,624	2,494	4,801	1,953	1,304	354	12,530
General Meetings	223	1,375	149	160	166	86	2,159
Mass Meetings	7	13	11	11	3	7	52
Film	20	15	22	36	25	—	118
Others	1	5	5	5	4	7	27
Population Education							
Continuing Lesson Series	378	355	230	330	—	—	1,293
Talks	630	340	176	67	—	—	1,213
Stories	500	417	358	306	—	—	1,581
Discussions	108	242	210	143	—	—	703
Debates	14	20	14	1	—	—	49
Exhibitions	12	6	2	12	—	—	32
Film Shows	15	20	44	77	—	—	156
Others	140	9	32	1	—	—	182

Table No. 2: Extension Service and Population Education (Number of Persons Contacted)

Particulars	*1977*	*1976*	*1975*	*1974*	*1973*	*1972*	*Total*
Extension Service							
Personal Counselling	23,748	42,289	75,992	31,225	9,314	4,542	1,87,110
Repeat Contacts	10,420	1,24,397	88,650	39,051	18,893	7,641	2,89,052
Group Discussions	19,280	16,498	33,967	12,077	8,335	2,636	92,793
Mass Meetings	1,470	6,345	10,805	3,008	4,500	10,400	36,528
General Meetings	13,869	18,124	12,915	16,435	10,266	2,300	73,909
Films	5,600	3,500	31,550	17,250	12,500	3,030	73,430
Exhibitions	200	2,000	2,890	15,000	26,808	17,000	63,898
	74,587	2,13,153	2,56,769	1,34,046	90,616	47,549	8,16,720
Education							
Continuing Lesson Series	15,432	12,446	7,861	19,630	—	—	55,169
Talks	24,053	11,047	8,846	8,110	—	—	52,056
Stories	16,165	22,477	10,810	14,922	—	—	62,374
Discussions	4,348	12,665	7,121	12,133	—	—	36,267
Debates	3,074	4,218	1,640	650	—	—	9,582
Exhibitions	321	2,462	300	4,826	—	—	7,909
Films	1,870	1,505	10,500	11,651	—	—	25,526
Others	3,58	2,005	1,270	15	—	—	6,929
	68,652	68,875	41,348	71,937	—	—	2,55,812

Teachers and social workers are also oriented in the new and innovative techniques of imparting population education to children. Let us now review the functioning of important projects.

Surgical Centre, Panipat

The Centre is one of the most important projects started by the branch. It aims at monitoring fertility through target-oriented and time-bound family planning services integrated with pre-and post-natal activities encompassing a wide range of medical, clinical and surgical services. It is a 10-bed clinic providing all sorts of family planning services under one roof and a single group of personnel. The MTP & MR services are made available to the patients with proper follow-up and motivation. The Centre has an additional facility in the form of creche for the children of mothers who come to receive family planning services. The Centre, since its inception in 1971, has been doing commendable work in promoting both the temporary and permanent methods of birth control which include sterilisation, orals, IUD and conventional contraceptives. The team of medical and extension staff, which goes around the operational area with Mobile Education Service Unit (MESU) attached to the Centre, motivates cases for family planning. Motivational work is also done at the Centre through its out-patient department.

Urban Family Welfare Planning Centre, Ambala Cantt.

The project came into existence on 1 May 1975, when the State government transferred an Urban Family Welfare Planning Centre covering 25,000 population, to the branch. The Centre was upgraded by adding an additional population of 25,000 in 1976. The entire finances to cover personnel costs and contingency are provided by the State government. The Centre has further been developed by starting MCH and Mobile Education and Services Unit.

Urban Family Welfare Centre, Jagadhri

This project was installed in early 1975, when the State government started providing finances for maintaining an urban family welfare centre covering more than 50,000 population, in the twin cities of Yamuna Nagar and Jagadhri. The project is managed by the branch through a local committee.

Mobile Clinics

The branch is running three mobile clinics at Ambala, Panipat and Kalka. These units aim at extending family planning services in the outlying rural areas by intensifying educational network and providing on-the-spot clinical services to the rural and semi-urban community which is not well served. These units also cater to the needs of rural and semi-urban people by providing efficient family planning clinical and educational services and help in strengthening the work being done at static clinics.

Mtp, Mr and Tubectomy Centre, Jagadhri

The branch, during the year 1977-78 was able to start a new project for providing facilities for MTP and MR services. The Centre is attached to an MCH care unit which serves as a basis for increasing the acceptability of MTP and sterilisation. The project is expected to cover more than 50,000 people which is largely urban, semi-urban and falls within the backward pockets of the cities of Yamuna Nagar and Jagadhri. The project is expected to cope with the rising demand of MTP and MR services in view of improved social acceptability and statutory liberation of early abortion as a means of family welfare and of preserving the health of the mother.

Population Education

The population education programme has been launched with the objective of creating awareness, interest and rational decision-making abilities among the younger group of people about population phenomenon and make them understand the significance of the population characteristics for the present and further quality of life including socio-economic development and attainment of the higher level of basic needs and amenities of life.

The programme, in its wider fold, covers four major components, i.e., population dynamics, population awareness, family life education and the basic value orientation. Based on the above programme, the following five projects have been developed and maintained by the association. These are:

1. Population Education Project, Kalka-Naraingarh Complex.
2. Population Education Club, Kurukshetra University.
3. PEN Form.
4. Population Education Project, Sirsa.
5. Research and Evaluation Cell.

The first four help the students and teachers to understand the dynamics of population education. Through direct teaching the students are made familiar with the population situation, small family norm, family life education etc. The elements of demography, population trend, implications of growing population and population equilibrium are the major components of population dynamics.

Pen Forum

The project started during the World Population Year 1974, and the Silver Jubilee of the FPAI, completed four years in 1978. It aims at generating population awareness amongst the youth through creative writing. It also provides the school, college, and university students a forum for exchange of ideas and experiences about population education, sex, family-life education and environmental issues.

A monthly publication entitled *Population Education News* is being brought out regularly. The publication intends to serve as a medium for exchange of information and experiences about population education. It is circulated amongst all the colleges, community centres, primary health centres and public libraries in Haryana. Besides, it is sent to all the branches of the FPAI all over the country. The Department of Education, Government of Haryana, has approved the publications for all the libraries and schools in the State. Likewise, the Kurukshetra University, has approved it for all its affiliated colleges and institutions. Three special numbers have so far been brought out. It has drawn the attention of a number of national and international research institutions, libraries and study centres engaged in population education work. UNESCO, IPPF and NCERT have included the publication in the standard bibliographies on Population Education. The writer has also contributed a number of articles to PEN.[7] Some of the ideas contained in these articles have been adopted by the association for experimentation.

Finance and Accounts

The total grant received from various sources during 1978-79 amounted to Rs. 4,85,685 out of which the headquarters alone provided Rs. 2,90,700 and the balance was made available by the State government. The major amount of the grant was spent on the maintenance of Surgical Centre, Panipat, Mobile Education and Service Units, MCH care and providing incentive to the acceptors.

Critical Appraisal

This association has been doing useful work in both clinical and educational fields relating to family welfare as is evident from the Tables 1 and 2. For example, personal counselling has increased from 9,542 persons (1972) to 23,7 8 (1977). We can find similar achievements in other fields. The dedicated leadership of its Organising Secretary has been responsible to a great extent for this effective performance. The quantitative performance is satisfactory but there are qualitative weaknesses. On close examination, we find that its activities are concentrated in cities and places nearer Chandigarh. We have to awaken 80% of the rural population and weaker sections of the community. It is suggested that its activities should penetrate in the interior of Haryana and cover far-flung areas. A perusal of the list of Executive Members reveal that there is no representation of rural people on this Committee resulting in the poor participation of the unprivileged and needy people. It is also suggested that this association may develop active linkages with the multipurpose workers and community health workers to provide educational services rather than set up its own costly institutions. It should plan for more coverage rather than multiplying institutions in the areas already having such institutions. Besides it must work in coordination with the allied agencies to make the best use of resources. Most of the functions of the association were held either at Panchkula, a place about 7 km from Chandigarh or Sirsa, the constituency of the ex-Chief Minister of Haryana. It clearly indicates that the functions are not being organised for the benefit of the beneficiaries but to suit the convenience of the organisers and to please political masters. Thus, there is a need to re-orient its machinery to serve the cause of Family Welfare and ultimately its clients, i.e. people. The association should design a cheap administrative set-up to motivate the people to adopt family planning as their way of life. This requires a missionary zeal on the part of the executive members and other functionaries of the association.

D. Critical Appraisal of the Functioning of the Voluntary Health Agencies

The critical examination is based on the writer's discussions with the officials, non-officials and beneficiaries of the voluntary organisations. The writer got the opportunity to examine the functioning of some of the organisations in depth. Some of the observations and comments in this analysis are born out of this study.

Lack of Effective Collaboration among the Voluntary Agencies Themselves

Coordination implies the prevention of both duplication and overlapping so as to avoid administrative wastes of efforts, manpower and resources and pool resources and experiences in dealing with problems and in achieving common objectives. Coordination—a means to an end and not an end itself—must be considered in relation to its practical purpose which is to facilitate better performance and greater administrative efficiency in the system. To ensure efficient and economical functioning of an organisation, coordination is not only desirable but even essential. For the same reason, inter-organisation coordination is advisable, especially when the activities of the various organisations concerned are of a complementary nature.

Apart from the continuing need to avoid overlapping and inconsistencies, coordination is more and more conceived in a positive and dynamic sense aimed at providing an agreed direction and a framework for action and at ensuring not only that activities dovetail into one another but there is also full measure of forethought and harmony in carrying out our responsibilities.

Coordination is distinct from the hierarchical process of authority, command and control. It requires collection of information about other organisations whose operations have identical objectives.

Coordination may lead to one organisation performing services or attacking a problem on behalf of all organisations in the system. It may also lead to one or more parties on the basis of information and consultation, to refrain entirely from the participation in a given activity so as to avoid duplication of efforts. Coordination under such circumstances is accomplished by a decision to work in concert. According to H.K.D. Tandon,

> "The experience of social work and social welfare institutions in different countries has revealed that the resources of voluntary agencies can be utilised more fruitfully and voluntary efforts could be mobilised more effectively if there is proper coordination between the voluntary agencies."[8]

There is no coordination among the voluntary agencies. Uncoordinated activities can be wasteful and may even have a damaging effect on the beneficiaries. It was mentioned by a non-official in one of the voluntary health agencies; "It does seem to me that one of the defects that should be remedied in the work of the voluntary health agencies that concern more than one agency is the absence of a greater degree of collaboration in many matters. So far as I am aware, there is not at the present moment sufficient machinery to deal with this problem. I think steps might be considered for greater collaboration and consultation on problems that are common to more than one agency, which would make the work much more useful."

According to M.R. Malkhani, "The need for coordination and cooperation among voluntary organisations and the state agencies is very urgent but remains unfulfilled."[9]

It was also mentioned as one of the handicaps of voluntary effort in the National Plan of Action for women. It was stated that,

> "Most of the voluntary organisations have been operating independently of each other. They have, therefore, not been able to fully benefit the community. The role

of existing organisations should be determined and measures should be initiated to coordinate the efforts of various organisations at each district level."[10]

It is suggested that the following steps may be taken to improve inter-agency relationships:

(i) representation at each other's meetings on all appropriate occasions;

(ii) early consultation when one organisation felt that the other might be interested,or involved in an activity;

(iii) creation of standing or *ad hoc* joint committees whenever circumstances warrant;

(iv) full and continuous personal contacts among the officials of allied voluntary agencies;

(v) housing all the offices at various levels in the same building; and

(vi) exchanging information on a regular basis.

Governmental Interference

Governments provide financial assistance and technical guidance. In some places, financial assistance may be provided in the form of grant-in-aid which help in establishments, extension or improvement of services by the voluntary agencies. Voluntary agencies have to fulfil certain criteria to be eligible for grants-in-aid. As stated in a UN publication, 'The objective of such controls should be to facilitate the provision of social services in keeping with national social policy and plans; to safeguard the interest of all the people, to ensure at least minimum standards of services and efficiency, to avoid duplication of effort and to ensure the most effective use of available resources."

This necessitates the cordial relations between the Government and the voluntary agencies. The Government has a right to supervise the functioning of the voluntary sector to ensure its efficient functioning and to help it improve the standards of service. The officials of the voluntary agencies, however, complain of excessive control by their respective departments and bureaucratic machinery of the Government. Their autonomy is thus vitiated resulting in inefficiency and poor standards of service. They are subordinated like the other departments of the Government and their functioning plagued by interference. There is a need to find out the methods which can help in the synthesis of control and autonomy. In a document, presenting a draft resolution on social policy for the consideration of the governments, the Council of Social Development has described the relationship between Government and voluntary organisations as:

"The nature of relationship between the government and voluntary organisations reflects the nexus between the state and the society, representing two approaches, namely, the legal and the non-legal to the tacking of social problems and meeting of social needs. A co-partnership between governmental and non-governmental organisations and sharing responsibilities for the information and execution of social policies between them is in keeping with the spirit of true democracy and genuine welfare-state".

Lack of Competence to Develop Integrated Area Plans

Who should be responsible for the socio-economic planning in a particular sector and area—say Block level—in India? The present situation of voluntary organisations is that there is no clear-cut demarcation of objectives, functions, and activities between this sector and the Government on the one hand and among the voluntary agencies themselves. In such a situation, we cannot entrust the task of planning in a particular sector or area to any one of the voluntary agencies howsoever competent it may be. Besides, most of the voluntary agencies lack planning competence. However, the Government must seek the active cooperation, guidance and advice of the voluntary agencies while planning in a sector in which these agencies have developed competence and expertise. The working group appointed by the Planning Commission to initiate Block level planning recommended:

> "The responsibility for preparing an integrated area planning cannot be handed over to a voluntary agency, however competent. This responsibility must be squarely borne by the government. The planning team at the district level should consult and actively seek the assistance of the voluntary agencies in their area while preparing the plan and selectively entrust to them the implementation of some sectoral plans in which they may have requisite expertise and experience. It can even be joint venture but the ultimate responsibility will be that of the Planning team."[11]

Lack of Identity with the Programmes among the Personnel of the Voluntary Agencies

Most of the persons working in various capacities in the voluntary agencies are not committed to the ideals and philosophy of these agencies. They have not developed identity and faith with the task environment. Mrs Gresst pointed out in an interview to the *World Health* the secret of success of the eradication of the small-pox from the world. This secret must be adopted by all personnel concerned with the execution of a programme. She says:

> "A good programme needs only a few highly experienced and qualified people at the top level. We had these; out of the hundreds recruited by WHO, many had no past experience in small-pox eradication when they first arrived. The qualities they needed rather than past experience, were faith in their work, courage, perseverance, adaptability to any situation, imagination, efficiency, capacity to take on responsibility yet flexibility to work easily as part of a team, but not least, willingness to work hard."[12]

She equates good people with a good programme. It is better to have a post vacant than have it filled with a wrong person. The ideal solution is worthless if it cannot be implemented. Efficiency is every aspect is more important than hypothesis or long reports. Workers at all levels must spend more time working in the fields has in the offices. Besides, the effective supervision from the highest to the lowest level is essential for getting the job done.

The personnel engaged in these voluntary organisations must be ready to accept hardships. Because of centuries of neglect, the people have become apathetic to taking a hand in matters beyond their immediate family domain. Voluntary workers must keep in mind this apathy of the people generated after years of powerlessness and neglect. Their ambition and enthusiasm should not be dampened by local conditions which may not provide them with the necessary facilities. This should, rather, motivate them to exert more and find innovative ways to bring them out of this morass. Unfortunately, the sense of dedication has been the greatest casualty of the prevailing atmosphere of cynicism bred by increasing propensity towards expediency. We should try to train the workers of these agencies so that they can develop identity with the programme and have faith in them. *Faith is as contagious as any infectious disease and is perhaps the most important factor for the successful implementation of the objective of these agencies.*

Ornamental Membership of the Non-officials in the Governing Bodies

The governing bodies of the voluntary agencies formulate policies and supervise their implementation. Policy making is an art and depends upon the sound knowledge of social work in the country. The nomination of the members of these governing bodies is made on the basis of the status and not on the basis of skill, interest, aptitude and competence. On critical examination, we find that the wives or relatives of high-ups in the Government are appointed and this becomes a status symbol for them. In other words, the governing bodies can be called as the clubs of the vested interests in the government. It is strange as to how this vested interest group can be motivated to help the down-trodden and needy people suffering from poverty, disease, hunger, etc. The governing bodies meet at the State or district levels, that is, in an environment completely divorced from the reality of the situation. It is suggested that the chairman and the members of these bodies should be appointed on the basis of the interest and not on the basis of status.

Poor Linkages with the Beneficiaries

The present relationship between the beneficiaries and the voluntary agencies is not cordial and harmonious. The success of the voluntary agencies depends on their response to the social milieu and to the ideas, beliefs, expectations and values of the people. These agencies must try to solve the problems without disrupting people's customs or straining their emotional susceptibilities to the point of social recoil or disintegration. This clearly means that the objectives of these agencies must be understood and accepted by the people. They must render the services through the personal human touch and sympathy rather than through an impersonal bureaucratic machinery. The programmes of these agencies can be effectively implemented only through a favourable environment for cooperation between various cooperative agencies, governmental and non-governmental, and the community. These agencies must be given freedom to administer, to execute, to change and adapt, to find their own solutions for the problems which may arise from day-to-day within each community. It is suggested that women may be involved actively in the work of social welfare as many of them have spare time which is wasted in idle pursuits. Today, developing countries are not utilising more than 15 per cent of the potential capacity of human beings.[13] This calls for an active participation of women on a bigger scale in the task of development, national reconstruction and social change. As Helvi Sipila, a Finish lawyer, UN Deputy Secretary General for Social Development asserted: "We cannot hope to solve the increasing international problems of economic and social development and improve the quality of human life while leaving aside half the resources of humanity."

We can involve the women in this stupendous task through the institutions of mothers' club. This experiment has been a great success in the Democratic Republic of Korea. On the suggestion of the author, the Family Planning Association of India (Haryana Branch) is experimenting with this idea at three places. The details of the mothers' club were published by *PEN*, an issue of FPAI (Haryana Branch) in their issue of May, 1977. The important ideas about the club are reproduced below.[14]

The basic requirement of such clubs is that the voluntary agencies and the Government must plan in advance as to what information is necessary to enlighten the people which is a prerequisite for their involvement in socio-economic development. This information in a coordinated fashion must reach the members of the mother's club who would diffuse such information to the beneficiaries. Once the beneficiaries get functional literacy, political consciousness and the understanding of their responsibility for socio-economic development, the process of national development would be accelerated.

A mothers' club implies a group of 25-40 women depending upon the size and population of the village or city. Those who have skills to spare, and those who have the will to do something for others by using their time and energy, can be provided with an organisational framework whereby their contribution could be made more meaningful and satisfying to themselves. The problem lies in providing the organisational framework. These women must be married and sufficiently influential. The other women of the village or city must have confidence in them. It is the task of sociologists to locate such women from all the mohallas/wards through sociometry etc. It would be better if the women from all the mohallas/wards are represented on it. As the work progresses, more mothers can join the club if the village or city is vast; then two or more mothers' clubs can be constituted. So we must find out women who possess the following qualities to carry out the challenging task of social change and modernisation—missionary zeal, the capacity to communicate with others, the ability to get along with colleagues and the people, cultural adaptability, the capacity to organise and manage, the capacity to instill confidence in others, patience and dignity. Besides, they must have faith in the ideals of the programme. They should be willing to accept hardships and be prepared to work in the spirit of service.

The mothers' club, to start with, may have limited objectives, e.g. the promotion of the Family Planning, the programme for Child Nutrition, the Education programme (especially functional literacy), programme against disease and dirt, or even prohibition. As the work progresses, these clubs can extend their activities to the whole cultural, social and economic (small-scale industries) aspects of the village/city life. This would also have the positive effect of utilising their energy for constructive purposes. Most of the women interviewed by the author revealed that "half of their working time is spent for uncalled and uninteresting problems, which are born because the women are idle".

Voluntary Agencies Not Action-Oriented

The appraisal of the performance of most of the agencies reveal that there is something wrong with the implementation of the objectives. On personal discussion with the beneficiaries, it was revealed that "the existence or absence of such agencies is immaterial to them. These agencies are existing for their own sake. The benefits of these agencies are usurped by the well-to-do sections of the society. It is only accidentally that some benefits may percolate to the deserving people."

The objectives for which these agencies exist are laudable—the Family Planning Association of India and its branches are exerting themselves to help the Government in population control, but without concrete results Words, spoken or written, are of no use unless they lead to action. Thought—the essential basis of human endeavour—is translated into words but words should be spoken or written only if they make others think and act. More time should be given to the thought and action, and words should be cut down to a minimum.[15] Voluntary agencies lay more emphasis on seminars. How can we improve upon it? The answer is to introduce managerial planning to control the output. In implementation scheme may be designed to develop certain amount of details for its effective performance. Management must work to ensure that all tasks are accomplished according to the implementation schedule. We should fix in advance of the implementation process the indices of expected input and output. This will help us in effective monitoring and evaluation of the programme.

Absence of Controlled and Regulated Growth

There is a haphazard growth of the voluntary agencies. Even the social welfare department is not aware of the number of such agencies operating in a State. Such agencies are set up on *ad hoc* basis to deal with a particular and pressing problem but such agencies continue even though their functioning have become obsolete. It is high time that we must scrutinise the existence of all the voluntary agencies. We must examine their utility in terms of their objectives and performance. We would find that 75 per cent of such agencies are only a drain on the resources of the State and the people. A new technique called 'sunset' has been devised to weed out the bogus and paper agencies. It means that we should apply this and other techniques to make the operation of these agencies worthwhile. This would strengthen the agencies which are already doing useful work. The State should patronise only those agencies which are really contributing to socio-economic development of the country.

Thus, in order to develop a good image of these agencies, the Government must appoint a committee to go into the performance of these agencies and recommend the winding-up of such agencies which are out-dated, worthless, bogus and not serving the objectives for which these were set up and extend help to such agencies which are doing useful work.

Not Properly Equipped and Staffed

It is perhaps not unfair to say that voluntary organisations by and large are not properly equipped and are understaffed. Competent and qualified persons do not usually remain with these agencies for long due to the uncertain circumstances of voluntary organisations. A recent study carried out by the Central Institute of Research and Training in Public Cooperation identified some important gaps in the field of voluntary action. It mentioned that voluntary work has been on the decline since independence. Voluntary workers now tend to feel that the State should assume greater responsibility for various welfare programmes.Voluntary agencies are also in need of workers who are committed and remain with these agencies for longer assignments. Voluntary workers, often, have been unable to fulfil their commitments to the agencies due to rising transportation cost and lack of long-term incentives. This study recommended that a bureau be set up to enlist the services of workers and to place them appropriately with the agencies. Voluntary workers will have to be trained for short period so that they can better appreciate the requirements and expectation of the beneficiaries as well as those of the agencies. This training would be broadly in the areas of organisation of services, administration and account keeping and developmental services with an emphasis on the rural reconstruction. Since most of the agencies surveyed did not have adequate financial and organisational support to undertake such programmes, the study recommends that this could be done through the existing schools of social work and other professional organisations. The universities can play a great role in this direction. The rapport between the voluntary workers and the agencies would depend to a large extent on the mutual perceptions of their problems and common causes.[16]

Absence of Systems Mechanism to Coordinate the Functioning of Allied Agencies in a Geographical/ Functional Area

Human development cannot be fragmented. We find that in the same area many voluntary agencies are working without any coordinating mechanism, e.g. in the field of child welfare there were more than 558 voluntary agencies rendering welfare services for children. Of these 152 organisations provided education for children, 98 offered nutrition services, 95 rendered welfare services for socially handicapped children, 89 provided recreational and cultural programmes, 76 promoted medical and health facilities, 23 organised maternity and child welfare services, 29 undertook research work and another 10 provided facilities for psychological services. It is suggested that in a particular area, e.g. State headquarters or at the district level, some organisations may be entrusted to function as a coordinating agency as has been done in the UN system. United Nations Development Programme has been designated by the UN system to serve as the coordinating agency at the national level on behalf of all the agencies of the UN system. In the same way, we may entrust this function to the central social welfare board and its branches in the State to serve as coordinating agency for the welfare services provided in every State.

Lack of Interest among the Intellectual Elite

The universities and colleges as in the German Democratic Republic can really serve as the bridges between government and community. At the moment, intellectual elite in India—teachers in the universities, colleges, schools and training institutions have not much perception of their responsibility to the community. The intellectual elite can help these agencies in improving their functioning with their innovative ideas based on basic and applied researches. It is suggested that these voluntary agencies must involve the teachers from these institutions to help them grow and live up to the expectations of the beneficiaries.

Misappropriation and Improper Utilization of Funds

There is a general feeling among the beneficiaries that the funds of these voluntary organizations are utilised only for the chosen few. On behalf of these voluntary organisations, few individuals get the privilege to travel abroad or in India to attend the conferences, or seminars. These organisations provide lip-service to those who are in need. A report of the Study Team on Social Welfare on "Economy and Efficient Utilisation of Resources" has stated that there is a "chaotic situation in which the grants are given in an haphazard manner without any well-deyined criteria to go by and there are no means of ensuring that they contribute to a proper and balanced growth of the institutions."

Besides, there is a lot of pilferage and embezzlement of funds. The funds are spent in arranging activities in the urban areas. In this way, the real purpose of these organisations is defeated. It is suggested that an efficiency audit may be conducted of the operations of these organisations by a committee of the people or legislators belonging both to the ruling and the opposition parties. These efficiency audit reports may be published in the daily newspapers for the enlightenment of the people.

Absence of Sound Administrative Set-up to deal with Social Work

Administration is the vehicle through which the objectives of voluntary agencies can reach the beneficiaries. The administrative structure, processes and procedures of these agencies are not conducive to the functioning of such agencies.The ability to assume new tasks, to cope with complexity, to solve novel problems, to mobilise resources, depends upon the administrative capacity based on increased professionalisation and administrative talent. According to Tara Ali Baig, "What is increasingly clear, however, is that the improved management principles, geared to the worker potential of the country could greatly increase the positive contribution to progress that we seek in community activity and more efficient techniques in social welfare services."[17]

We have to examine the existing structure and process of these agencies so that they can be fit instruments to cope with the existing functions and future development. One of the officials in these agencies mentioned that: "Administration of these agencies is bureaucratic and is more legalistic than result-oriented."

The administrative culture of these agencies is unsuitable for the tasks imposed on them. The administrative system cannot function properly and administrators lack the necessary skills and environment for adequate performance. To achieve pre-conceived plans over a period of time, these two agencies should develop common working rules, right policy-formulation, proper inspection and review of work, high quality decision-making, decentralised operations, monitoring of information, managerial planning, cost accounting, immediate error correction mechanism, committed workers professionalisation, improved administrative techniques and administrative adaptability including organisational research and the built-in administrative mechanism to gain the confidence, loyalty and participation of the beneficiaries.

B. Chatterjee[18] has mentioned some of the areas in which voluntary agencies have to give greater attention in the last quarter of the present century. These are as follows :

(a) Voluntary organisations need to develop a reasonable personnel policy to attract qualified and stable personnel to implement their programmes.

(b) They need to evaluate their programmes and performance so as to improve the quality of services.

(c) They need to develop a sound accounting system which not only meets their demands but also the demands of the government and the community.

(d) Voluntary agencies should play an increasing supportive role to Government programmes and complement the Government's efforts.

(e) Voluntary organisations at present are too much programme-oriented , they should develop a broader perspective of the field in which they are working and enlarge the scope of their activity to meet the problems faced by the majority of the population.

(f) There is a need for them to work in the area of social action and thereby facilitate social change.

(g) The majority of voluntary agencies are concentrated in urban areas and there is an urgent need to expand their work in rural areas where the majority of India's population lives."

References

1. UN, *Report on the Organisation and Administration of Social Services*, New York, 1962, p. 19, ST/50A/44/E/CN5/360/Rev. I.
2. Dharma Vira, "Citizen Participation" in *Encyclopaedia of Social Work*, Vol. I, p. 102.
3. Malhotra, R.C., op. cit., p. 11.
4. GOI, Planning Commission, *Report of the Working Group on Block Level Planning*, 1978, pp. 139-140.
5. World Federation of Public Health Association, op. cit., pp. 45-46.
6. Data obtained from the official records of the Family Planning Association of India (Haryana Branch).
7. (1) Development Demands Managerial Improvement, Dec. 1975, (2) Role of communication in Family Planning, setting up of mothers' club May, 1977, (3) Shaping Tomorrows, Destiny, April, 1978, (4) Education for Family Health, June, 1978, (5) Challenges of Health and Family Welfare Administration, March, 1979.
8. Tandon, H.K.D., "Public Cooperation" in *Encyclopaedia of Social Work in India*, Vol. 2, p. 132.
9. Malkani, M.R., "Voluntary Agencies and Social Welfare" in *Encyclopaedia of Social Work*, Vol. II, p. 409.
10. GOI, Department of Social Welfare, *Blueprint of Action and National Plan of Action for Women*, New Delhi, 1977, p. 23.
11. GOI, Planning Commission, *Report of the Working Group on Block Level Planning*, 1978, p. 140.
12. WHO, *World Health*, Nov. 1975.
13. UNDP, 12th session of the UNDP Governing Council, 7-23 June, 1971, pp. 112-114.
14. For details refer to *PEN*, an issue of Family Planning Association of India, Haryana branch, May, 1977.
15. WHO, *World Health*, Nov. 1975, p. 36.
16. National Institute of Public Cooperation and Child Development : (NIPCO): *Study of the Young Child India: Case Study*, New Delhi, 1976, pp 64-65.
17. Tara Ali Baig, "Social Administration in Voluntary Social Welfare Agencies" in *Encyclopaedia of Social Work in India*. Vol. II, p. 245.
18. B. Chatterjee, "Voluntary Agencies for Social Welfare" in *Social Development*, Edited by B.N. Ganguli, Sterling Publishers Pvt. Ltd., New Delhi, 1977, pp. 258-259.

17

Modernising Health Administration

A. Need and Nature of Management Improvement

People of advanced countries get their health services as much for granted as the essential utility services like water, electricity, public transport, etc. Despite the magic bullets of the modern medicine, the health services in the developing countries are far from satisfactory. The people living in the developing world, and especially 80 per cent of them living in rural areas, have little or no access to modern medical and health care resulting in high rates of morbidity and mortality from diseases which are preventible. If we want to reach the objective of providing health care to all by the year A.D. 2000 we will have to introduce innovations in technical and administrative fields. It has been recognised by health experts in all the countries that the difficulties in meeting the health needs of the community are largely dependent upon the capabilities to design and manage the health care delivery system. The management of health care system can help in the greater achievement of goals through the optimum utilisation of resources available—men, money and material. To quote Dr. Chi-Yuen Wu of UNDP:

> "To create administrative capabilities, commensurate with requirements, developing countries must be able among other things, to use modern management techniques more effectively than in the case of the industrially advanced countries."

Unfortunately, present health management systems are not functioning well as these are managed by untrained personnel. This is the common management challenge faced by those in charge of the health services. To quote from a recently published book:[1]

> "In the field of health, we rarely have consciously trained executives...We have expected a vast army of professional care givers to fill individual human needs, mainly on a *laissez faire* basis, mostly without planning, without coordination, without sufficient concern for (those) who either do not look for care, cannot afford it or cannot get to it."

> "With little or no formal training, administrators...have arisen from our midst willy-nilly, too few through natural ability, too many by virtue of their staying-power on particular job, lack of available competition, or the administrator's uncritical need for power and control..."
>
> "In health administration, there are few theoreticians, few training centres, few books, and an almost absolute dearth of strict scientific investigations."

Thus there is a great need to improve the functioning of health care management with the help of modern management techniques. A modern management system is one which is designed to make the existing health care delivery process effective and efficient. Modern management methods and techniques are in reality, only techniques for improving this process by making it more accurate and reliable, by making the process respond faster, or by giving the health-manager the ability and capability to manage better.

Health administration in a country is a part of the total administration and thus influences and is influenced by this general administrative culture. Let us have a look at the general administrative apparatus prevailing in developing countries. In India, for instance, the administrative machinery has not been adequate to handle the tasks of economic and social development. The administrative inadequacies in a national government has a retarding influence on economic and social development. This lack of efficiency in administration equally holds good for the health organisations as well. The widespread feeling of inefficiency of the administrative machinery was rightly sensed and expressed by Mrs Gandhi in a broadcast to the nation shortly after assuming the high office of the Prime Minister. She said:

> "In economic development as in other fields of national activity, there is a disconcerting gap between intention and action. To bridge this gap, we should boldly adopt whatever far-reaching changes in administration may be found necessary. We must introduce new organizational patterns and modern tools and techniques of management and administration. We shall instill into the government machinery greater efficiency and sense of urgency and make it more responsive to the needs of the people."[2]

In the health sector, it was emphasised that "better management of health services is essential if higher standards of health care are to be achieved...that progress... today is to a higher extent dependent on education and development of the management, than it is on medical research and increase of material resources."[3]

The development of public administration remains an essential prerequisite for successful economic development of the country. Therefore, far-reaching improvements in public administration are required if the objectives of planned socio-economic development are to be realised.

Before we analyse the meaning, nature, scope and application of management techniques for administrative improvements and reforms, let us be clear about the concept of administrative improvement first.

Administrative improvement means the act or the process of improving the administration. As stated in a United Nations Report:

> "Management improvement comprised the planning, implementation and evaluating of various measures conducive to the increase of organisational effectiveness and efficiency."[4]

Administrative reform is still widely regarded as a special type of improvement activity, even when it is often closely connected with other activities. The concept of the "administrative reform", as it is applied in practice, also has its weakness. In a report by the Secretariat of the United Nations Programme in Public Administration for the period from 1950 to 1966, it is stated that:

> "Efforts at administrative reform too often stop with the preparation of reports of promulgation of law."[5]

In a number of countries the word 'reform' has also a close relationship to political concepts and attitudes, which makes it less suited for general use than the broader concept of 'improvement' or 'effectiveness'.

Public administration in any country cannot remain static over a period of time. There are always scientific, economic, political, social, cultural and other changes taking place in a country. Health organisations like other organisations, must adjust themselves to these changes in order to be effective and responsive to the needs of the people. Peter Drucker, an expert in the field of management has said: "Social awareness is organisational self-interest. The needs of the society, if left unfilled, turn into social diseases. No institution whether business or hospital or University or Government agency is likely to survive in a diseased society."

The design of an administrative system is a basic aid to the achievement of its primary objectives; if the design is unsound, the achievement of objectives is likely to fall short of expectations. Therefore, there is a great need to improve the structure and functioning of the administrative organisations.

Most of the economic and social progress in the developing countries is halted because the administrative apparatus in these countries is not upto the mark. Therefore, there is an urgent need of administrative improvement in these countries. H. Paul Appleby has rightly remarked that the full success of the plan, therefore, turns rather exclusively on administrative reform to make the Government as an organism equal to its identified goals.

The administrative capability of a Government and the manner in which the development programmes are likely to be carried out are intimately related. On the other hand, administrative inadequacies in a national Government have a retarding influence on economic and social development. These deficiencies prevent the vast flood of money, talent and material from achieving their objectives. As early as 1950, the Secretary General of the United Nations pointed out that, "Any systematic effort towards economic development must be preceded by or coupled with efforts to make more effective the functioning of Governmental machinery."[6]

During the last few decades, phenomenal changes are taking place at a fast rate in the field of science and technology as well as in external environment. These changes have their impact on public administration also, which today, has to shoulder multifarious tasks designed to fulfil the rising aspirations of the people. In the words of Prof Waldo, Public Administration is, "a part of the cultural complex, and it not only is acted upon, it acts." It is a great creative force. There is an urgent need to re-orient (improve) the system of public administration to cope with changes in technology and social behaviour and maximise opportunities for raising productivity, and thus the standard of living of the people.

According to Sir Isaiah Berlin, "It is certainly a reasonable hypothesis that one of the principal causes of confusion, misery and fear is blind adherence to outworn notions, pathological suspicion of any form of critical examination, frantic efforts to prevent any degree of rational analysis of what we believe, we live by and for."

Thus public administration including health administration must be recreated, renewed and revitalised to produce the predesigned changes and output in the modernization of societies. This necessitates a different trend and magnitude of administrative culture and capability.

Scope of Management Improvement

If the need for change and effectiveness is to be fulfilled, management improvement must be considered to be an organisation-wide continuous activity. The important function must embrace the total needs based on the objectives and goals of the public administration and the resources available. The improvement effort must be regarded as a whole involving a spectrum of different types and levels of activity. There is, in principle, no reason why 'administrative reform' and 'organisations and methods' should be set up as separate and isolated activities. These and other new activities should rather be merged and coordinated into a total, carefully planned and organised "management improvement programme" involving the whole organisation. The needs require centrally planned improvement programme, and for coordination purposes decentralized programmes in different ministries and institutions. Each agency or institution of importance should be responsible for its own programme, planned in cooperation with the central authorities.

As the implementation of significant changes in organisational structure and behaviour is complex and time consuming task and is closely related to the long-term development planning of the country, improvement programme must be planned on long-term (from ten to fifteen years), medium-term (from four to five years) and short-term (yearly) basis.

Strategies and Policies in Administrative Improvement

As stated in a UN publication[7], the following strategies and policies are necessary to bring about administrative improvement:

(a) Improvement work must be a systematically planned organised activity with specific work programmes, a continuous activity, and it should be based on long-term planning and development.

(b) Classification of objectives and goals is necessary to be able to measure or evaluate the effectiveness and manage the improvement work.

(c) Improvement work must be recognised as a responsibility of the management; and in planning and organising improvement projects, participation and involvement of management in the organisations affected by possible changes are of great importance.

(d) Special resources must be allocated to the improvement projects including the support of professional staff of high quality with special qualifications in the management fields.

(e) Improvement work must be based on the concept or the organisation as a socio-technical system where human and social factors are of primary importance.

(f) Training and development of the members of organisations—both management and staff, usually constitute one of the most important parts of improvement work.

(g) Improvement projects should from the beginning, be oriented towards implementation and change, step by step, and not only towards writing reports and giving recommendations. Such projects should include specific implementation plants.

(h) As a rule, there is need for both centralised and decentralised (though coordinated) improvement programmes. It is advisable first to build up a strong, central activity.

(i) An improvement work programme should be formalised as an obligation for the public administration, institutions and tied with long-term development plans, and budgeting and accounting control procedures.

(j) The improvement project organisation should be flexible. A task force, under a responsible project leader and a Steering Committee, is often a useful type of organisation.

(k) In larger projects, pilot studies of the implementation of new organisational structures in a limited part of the administration are often necessary and useful to demonstrate effects and results.

(l) Improvement projects must be planned in terms of activities, time and resources. The setting of deadlines or time-limits in the work programmes has frequently proved most helpful in the effort to obtain a high level activity and results.

After explaining the concept of administrative improvements and administrative reforms, let us discuss the need, types and utility of management techniques as an instrument of administrative improvements and reforms.

B. Need for Management Techniques

In a developing country, such as ours, there is a great haste to achieve maximum growth and progress in the shortest time possible. It is felt that the scope of experimentation is a costly and slow process. As such, we need to learn from the experience of others and use their results to help achieve our goals. A word of caution at this point is in order. Nothing succeeds like success. So too is the case of the glamorous instances of technology and management techniques and their tall claims of progress and development. Such a philosophy has done more harm than good. A few years before, modern management techniques were thought to be a panacea for all problems. Some problems did get solved while a host of others took birth as a results; many of the overpopular techniques have found their graveyards whilst a lot of organisations which should have gone to the graveyards for not putting into use the 'overpopular' techniques, have passed the test of time and resistance. In this context, Ernest Dale and L.C. Michelon observes that:

> "Today's manager lives in a world of rapid change, and yet the rate of change is likely to increase in the years ahead. Unless, he can keep up with this change, he is likely to find himself obsolete—perhaps unpromotable or even unemployable."[8]

Thus, there is a great need to enhance the administrative capability of health administrators so that they can use these techniques profitably. Administrative capability is an important means of converting or processing programme inputs into outputs such as goods and services. It has been mentioned by Gabriel that, "What makes the leadership variable so crucial in implementation process, is its dynamic, not passive quality, i.e., its capability to act and react on these critical inputs. It is this manipulative and transferring quality of leadership that could significantly determine the administrative capability of implementing organisation."[9]

Administrative capability is "the capacity to obtain intended results through organisations."[10]

Katz says:

> "Administrative capability for development involves the ability to mobilize, allocate and combine the actions that are technically needed to achieve development objectives."[11]

Organisations are not simply structures but action-oriented system and the success and failure of the organisations are to be measured in terms of this action system. Action system is a structured device in which resources are mobilised and transformed by use of certain skill and technology to produce predesigned output all taking place by the influence of administrative capability within an environmental context.

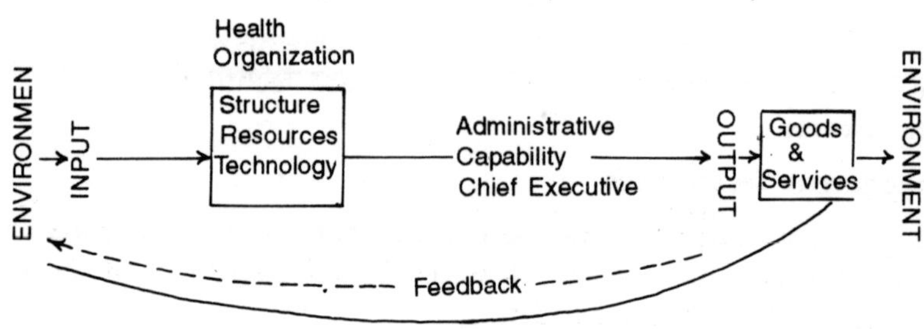

Fig. 17.1

Health administrators should facilitate the accomplishment of desired objectives with the least friction and the most satisfaction to those for whom the task is done and those engaged in the enterprise, as has been shown in the chart below:

Thus, there is a need to understand and portray the management techniques in all its various facets.

Management techniques are of added significance for the health sector as this sector deals with preventive, promotive, and curative and rehabilitative aspects of health care activities and uses the services of Government, private and voluntary agencies. Most of the practitioners, academicians and political elite are not happy with the performance of this sector as the majority of people in the developing world do not have access even to rudimentary health care. After personal discussions with some of the health experts and top management of health personnel at Chandigarh, it was revealed that the present administration was in a bad state and needed radical reforms. It was confirmed by personal visits to some of the health institutions and their field establishments, as also by the health and medical personnel at District and Block levels. This is resulting in huge wastage of resources. There have been a large number of administrative problems which account for the unsatisfactory working of the health administration. These problems have already been examined in the earlier chapters. Some of the specific problems which need immediate solution can be mentioned as:

(a) Absence of effective health policy to meet the need of the people.

(b) Absence of coordination between the health and socio-economic sector; between Western and indigenous system of medicine and among Government, Private and Voluntary administration.

(c) Lack of effective planning, monitoring, implementation and evaluation machinery.

(d) Lack of an effective manpower planning resulting in the concentration of health services in the urban sectors.

(e) Absence of people's participation in the health care delivery system.

(f) Absence of decentralisation resulting in inefficiency of operations.

(g) Disproportionate investments for secondary and tertiary health care.

(h) Top heavy administrative set up.

(i) Defective organisations and procedure—an obstacle in the way of efficient services.

(j) Lack of interest to improve administrative structure and procedure i.e. absence of innovative leadership.

In reviewing the management of health services, the delegates who came to attend the 25th Regional Committee meeting of the South-East Asia Region of WHO, noted the following considerations and constraints:[12]

(a) lack of a clear development policy and clear objectives for health services in relation to socio-economic development;

(b) inadequate understanding of health problems and the problem of tackling it from the viewpoint of consumers and providers of health care;

(c) poor utilisation of existing resources and inadequate harnessing of potential resources, human and other for health;

(d) inadequate coordination and integration between different authorities and organisations providing health services in the same geographical areas;

(e) inadequate or no integration of preventive, curative and family planning services;

(f) the increasing cost of health services and their inequitable distribution, with the result that the basic health needs of all the people were not being met;

(g) the participation of communities in the promoting of their own health and in contributing to health services policy, financing and decision-making;

(h) the need to find ways of developing new types of health man-power, including local multi-purpose health workers, and of employing them on a wider scale;

(i) the need to develop an organisations in the countries of the region for improved delivery of health services within the existing constraints—both financial and manpower—for the masses in rural areas, which along constitutes about 80% of the population, and

(j) meagre allocation of funds (3% to 5%) for health in the overall socio-economic development plans in most countries of the Region.

C. Nature and Classification of Management Techniques

Nature

In order to understand the meaning of 'management techniques' we must be clear about the two concepts namely, 'management' and 'technique'. In words, management is the handling of tools and techniques to achieve desered goal. In other words management simple infers planning, organising and controlling of human and other resources to achieve the specified goal. A technique is a set of procedural steps which may be loosely or rigorously stated, which embody a multiple idea content and which are concerned with doing work to achieve an objective.

In other words, we can say that management technique is a set of procedural steps which may be loosely stated, embodying a multiple-idea content and which are either concerned with decision-making in general or with decisions relating to planning, organising or controlling of human and/or other resources with a view to achieving the specified objectives. Management techniques make positive efforts to analyse the situation in a systematic and scientific manner and provide a rational basis for decisions. Adoption of these techniques would encourage greater professionalism in administrative activities. If a new administrative culture is also developed side by side, it would be possible to make optimum use of available and potential resources. According to one of the ILO publications, management techniques are systematic procedures of investigating, planning, controlling and supervising which can be applied to management problems.[13] Thus modern management techniques in actuality, are the techniques for improving the management process by making it more accurate, by making the process respond faster, or by giving the manager greater control. From the above discussion, we can say that management techniques have the following features:

1. Thy are a set of procedural or formal steps. This is basic for any management technique. Procedural or formal steps lead to 'systematic' approach which has been the highlight of any scientific method, the root of all sound modern management theory. They take us from the known facts to the unknown parts of the problem.
2. They have a multiple-idea content. They do not have a single idea, but a number of them through related ones.
3. They help in decision-making in general or with decisions relating either to planning, oganising or controlling or to any combination of these three processes of planning, organising and controlling of human and/or other resources with a view of achieving certain specified objectives.
4. They give the idea of efficiency which, according to Clay, can further be broken into five components:
   a) economy of efforts in terms of money and other resources;
   b) speed;
   c) quality;
   d) stability; and
   e) aesthetic or rhythmical approach.
5. They are consistent in their results.

Functional Classification of Management Techniques

Management techniques can be classified in different ways. For example, they can be grouped according to the outlet and the department in which they are applied as, for example, preventive techniques, promotive techniques and curative techniques. This does not, however, cover all techniques. For example, where would we place the techniques of brain-storming or critical examination? An alternative can be classification according to parent discipline. But it is more an historical approach than a current use, because many of the techniques are developed in one field but later on used in a number of fields. Clay gives a classification which is based on the objective of the technique, i.e., what does the technique hope to achieve? He mentions the following eight objectives which various management techniques attempt to achieve.[14]

1. *Detection*. (To find out or discover something e.g., what is happening or what is wrong?): We can include such techniques here as input-output Analysis, Attitude Survey, Production Study, Activity Sampling, Critical Examination, Break-even Analysis.
2. *Evaluation*. (To measure or estimate the value of an item): We can include such techniques here as Job Evaluation, Work Measurement, Work Estimation, Performance Appraisal, Cost-Benefit Analysis.

3. *Improvement*. (To improve performance): We can include such techniques here as Management by Objectives, Method Study, Value Analysis etc.
4. *Optimisation*. (To optimise performance): We can include such techniques here as Linear Programming, Ergonomics, Operations Research, etc.
5. *Specification*. (To specify a desired value or situation or action): Here we can include such techniques as Layout Planning for Offices and Plants etc.
6. *Control*. Here we can include such techniques as Cost Control, Credit Control, Labour Control, Inventory Control, Production Control, Budget Control etc.
7. *Communication*. (To communicate information): Here we can include such techniques as Visual Aids, Suggestion Schemes, Report Writing, Communication Theory, Information Theory, Management information etc.
8. *Demonstration*. (To demonstrate something): Here we can include such techniques as Programmed Learning, Job Instruction, Management Development and Training, etc.

This achievement criteria tells us that these techniques can help us in discovering or finding something in evaluating the performance, in improving the performance, in optimising the performance, in specifying a desired value or a situation, in controlling a variable, in communication or in demonstration.

S.No.	*Source*	*Management Techniques*
1.	Human Resources	1. Organisational analysis
		2. Job Evaluation
		3. Training
		4. Incentive Schemes
		5. Suggestion Schemes
		6. Method Study
		7. Work Measurement
2.	Material	1. Inventory Centrol
		2. Value Analysis
		3. Material Handling
		4. Standarisation
		5. ABC/VED
3.	Machinery and Equipment	1. Method Study
		2. Value Analysis
4.	Space and Building	1. Layout Planning
		2. Method Study
5.	Money	1. Cost Benefit Analysis
		2. Budgetary Control
		3. Performance Budgeting
		4. Management Accounting
6.	Time	1. Method Study
		2. Work Measurement
		3. Network Analysis (PERT/CPM)

The management techniques can also be classified in terms of various resources employed in an organisation, viz., human material, machinery and equipment, money and time. As such, some of the techniques which can be applied to bring about increased managerial capability, efficiency, effectiveness and productivity can be categorised as tabulated on p. 191.

Before we proceed to discuss the systematic applicability of management techniques according to the level of activities of management, let us discuss in brief the meaning and utility of some of the important techniques.

Organisational Analysis

It helps in critical examination of an organisation with a view to evolving a systematic and harmonious arrangement of work with reference to its objectives. This technique can be applied to assess the effectiveness of hospital services especially the teaching-cum-research institutions.

Work Study

It is a generic term for those techniques particularly Method Study and Work Measurement which are used in the examination of human work in all its contexts, and which lead systematically to the investigation of all the factors which affect the efficiency and economy of the situation being reviewed in order to effect improvement.

O&M

It is generally used to describe the activities of groups of people in Government or other public bodies or in private firms who are asked to advise administrators or managers on the question of Organisation and Method so as to increase the efficiency of work for which they are responsible, either by providing a better service, or a cheaper one or both.

Personnel Administration

Participative Management and Organisational Development (OD): The health of an organisation is measured in terms of its capability to adjust with internal and external environmental challenges. We find now-a-days that in big health organisations like hospitals, three is a lot of friction amongst the experts and other staff generating an atmosphere of frustration and low morale, resulting in the overall inefficiency. We can introduce the technique of OD in such large hospitals to maintain the healthy atmosphere of work. A comprehensive definition of OD has been given by Backhard. According to him:

> "Organisational Development is an effort (1) Planned; (2) Organisational wide; (3) Managed from the top to (4) increase organisation effectiveness and health through (5) Planned interventions in the organisations' `Process' using behavioural science knowledge."[15]

OD depends upon the purely internal initiative of the employees of an organisation. The present emphasis in health administration is only on structural changes but structural changes without personnel dedication and capabilities would be of no avail. It is high time that we introduce OD in all our big institutions to ward off the bureaucratic attitudes which result in low output and stagnation. We have also the other techniques to achieve this objective, e.g. Management by Objectives, Participative Management. We must try to integrate all these techniques for optimising the efficiency of personnel is an organisation.

The most important task of Personnel Department must be to give abundant evidence of its belief that personnel in an organisation are key to development. This requires proper motivation of the employees. Motivation is of utmost importance as it constitutes the base for the management functions of planning and organising. It has been noticed that the performance of the personnel either as individuals or members of a group is less as compared to their capabilities in terms of skills, abilities, and capacities. Finer, for example, states that demonstrated performance generally never exceeds more than fifty per cent of the individual's ability to perform.[16] Most individuals tend to balance their efforts around an assessment of relative costs (time and energy) and benefits.[17] A climate of creativity must be developed and maintained by management Maier and Hayes say that "the optimal climate for creativity...in whatever human conditions is optimal for individual freedom and self-expression in social setting."[18]

It is the duty of the officers of such units to make the employees feel that their work and their association with a given organisation represent a vehicle which will accelerate the achievement of personal goals as well as the achievement of goals of the organisation. This would require the active participation of the employees in the decision-making process of the organisation.

> "Participation is...an individual's mental and emotional involvement in a group situation that encourages him to contribute to group goals and to share responsibility for them."[19]

The concept of participative management views the employees as:

1. *A unit of energy* that seems to spend itself and, in the process, both processes and exercises the choice of how to spend this energy; that is to say, whether to conserve it, waste, it, or use it productively.
2. *An organism possessing the dynamic ability to grow and adjust and select quantitatively*. In other words, man has the power to extract from his environment the nourishment he needs to build himself more both physically and mentally. Because the environment. . . can be conditioned, growth may be accelerated or slowed down.
3. *Purposeful*.. therefore that induces him to expand his energy to become more perfectly what he wants to become. This drive may be conscious or unconscious...
4. *Unique*... Each human being has his own personality and each has the capacity to direct his energies. Thus capacity... magnifies the effect of experience upon his ultimate development... Each...is...always in the process of becoming more and more different from his fellows.[20]

It is, therefore, important that management always views the employee—either as an individual, or as a member of group or both.

Management Information System

The significance of information for administration can be compared to what Napoleon said about the army: "an army marches on its stomach," - any administration marches on information. As the universe is saturated with information, health administration must select pertinent information for their programmes otherwise it is difficult to make any rational policy or decision. This technique is tailored to provide such information to the decision-makers which is most relevant, accurate, complete, concise, timely, economic, reliable and efficient. A good information system provides data for monitoring and evaluating the programmes and gives the requisite feedback to the administrators and planners at all levels.[21]

The development of a suitable technique for a health information system would improve the capacity of health administrators to make appropriate policy-decisions. The information system may not serve the purpose if the health administrators are not committed to use the information constructively. The health administrators should use the available information sensibly and logically rather than construct complex information system which may not be used. We can show with the help of the diagram the functions of information for policy formulation.

ABC Analysis

It is a technique which would enable a busy executive to chase those activities ardently which would quicken the wheels of administrative machinery. By arranging his work into an order of priorities, he can decide on which items to concentrate first, which others to deal later, and yet which others to delegate to his assistants. When done more systematically and in quantiative terms, this system of building up priorities of work is called the ABC Analysis. ABC Analysis can be of great use in dealing with materials management in hospitals. Forty to sixty per cent of the total expenditure of an organisation is generally spent on materials. The other form of ABC Analysis is VED, i.e. arranging the activities in the orders of Vital, Essential and Desirable.

Network Analysis (Pert/CPM)

Both the Critical Path Method (CPM) and Programme Evaluation and Review Techniques (PERT) emphasise efficient performance and temporal dimensions of a project. In the simplest form of PERT, a project is viewed as a total system and consists of setting up of schedule of dates for various stages and exercise of management control, mainly through project status reports, on its progress. The CPM is basically a technique to reduce the time required to implement a project. By breaking the project into activities that must be undertaken for its implementation and by determining their time sequence, it is possible to isolate the most critical activities in the project and to compute the critical path schedule for their implementation. Network planning provides the basis for both CPM and PERT.[22]

Moder and Philips enlist the following key advantages of using PERT:

1. It encourages logical discipline in planning, scheduling and control of projects.
2. It encourages more long-range and detailed project planning.

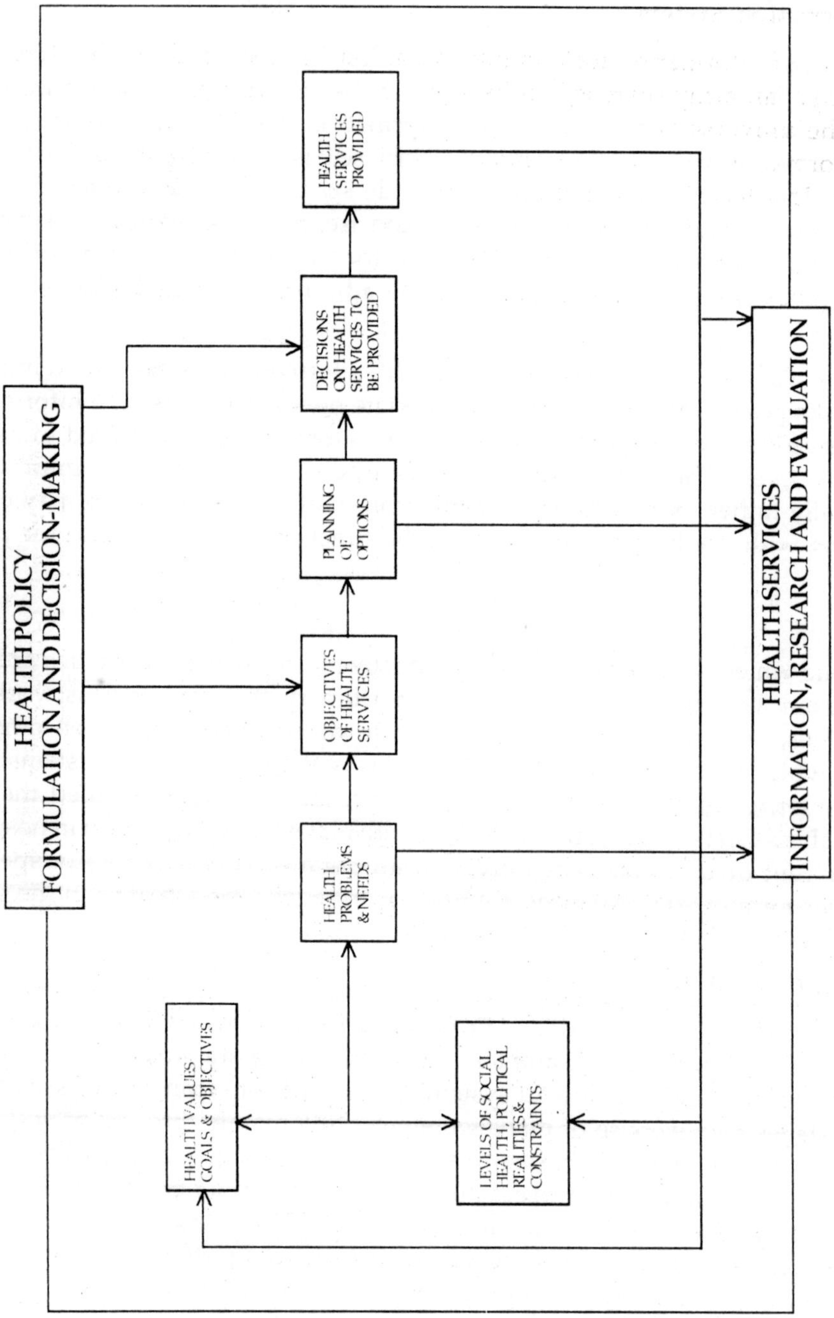
HEALTH POLICY
FORMULATION AND DECISION-MAKING
HEALTH VALUES GOALS & OBJECTIVES
LEVELS OF SOCIAL HEALTH, POLITICAL REALITIES & CONSTRAINTS
HEALTH PROBLEMS & NEEDS
OBJECTIVES OF HEALTH SERVICES
PLANNING OF OPTIONS
DECISIONS ON HEALTH SERVICES TO BE PROVIDED
HEALTH SERVICES PROVIDED
HEALTH SERVICES
INFORMATION, RESEARCH AND EVALUATION

Fig. 17.2

3. It provides a standard method of documenting and communicating Project Plans, Schedules and Time and Cost Performance.
4. It identifies the most critical elements in the Plan, thus focussing management attention on the 10-20 per cent of the project that is most constraining on the schedule.
5. It illustrates the effects of technical and procedural changes on overall schedules.[23]

The application of PERT\CPM can be profitably utilised in the Programmes and Projects of Health, e.g., construction of Hospitals, Eradication of Communicable Diseases, Family Planning Programmes. Administration of Environmental Programmes etc. Care should be taken that the cost of the PERT\CPM should not take away large resources of the Project.

Cost-Benefit Analysis

This technique is designed to consider the social costs and benefits attributable to the project. The benefits are expressed in monetary terms to determine whether a given programme is economically sound, and to select the best out of several programmes. Its advantage lies not in making decision-making simpler, but in its possibilities for systematic examination of each part of a problem in hand, for putting diverse decisions at a par and following logical sequence.[24]

Cost-Benefit Analysis is an aid to systematic thought and helps the planners to decide as to what should be done—on the relative merits of different programmes. How far, for example, should resources be devoted to health education or maternal and child health services or immunisation against particular disease? Any given budget for health may be distributed between programmes by including, first, those with the highest ratio of benefits to cost, then those with the next largest and so on, until the budget is fully allocated. The limitation of this method in the field of health administration is that it is difficult to express the benefits in monetary terms. We must encounter this limitation by making our tools of research methodology perfect.

Cost-Effective Analysis

Cost effectiveness methods are those that search for the least costly way of achieving a defined result. Cost effectiveness analysis are easier to make as the aim is clear. It helps the health administrator in managing his health resources at the local level. The problem is to find the way of achieving the objective at lowest cost, e.g., to find effective ways of treating patients without sending them to hospital. Linear Programming can help in this direction.

Systems Approach

A system is an integrated assembly of interacting elements, designed to carry out cooperatively a pre-determined function.[25] There are five major elements in a systems approach—selecting objectives, designing alternatives, building models, weighing cost against effectiveness and the application of suitable criterion. It can be represented with the help of a diagram.

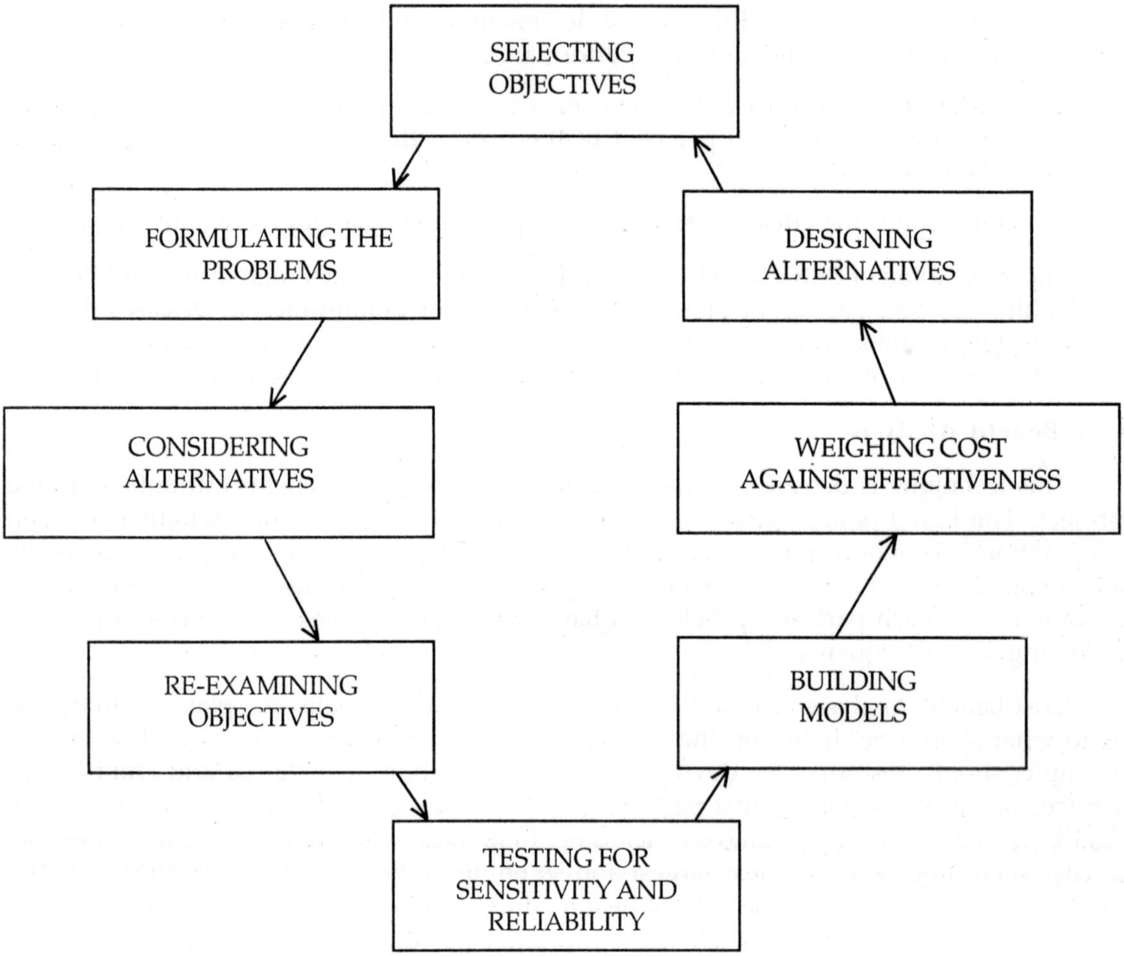

Figure 17. 3
Elements of Systems Analysis

Systems and Health Management

The application of systems analysis is useful in health management in that it provides for:[26]

1. consideration of all variables, over and above the biological and technical, that affect health intervention programmes;
2. a planning approach that relates input to output;
3. an emphasis on quantification;
4. rigour in analytical methods;
5. orientation towards health problems rather than towards categories of service;

6. communication with key governmental decision-making centres that utilised comparable methods;
7. early attention to planning and priority setting;
8. improved interdisciplinary collaboration; and
9. the use of wide range of analytical models and methods of considerable power.

Decision-Making

One of the important tasks of the health and hospital administrators is to take sound and effective decisions in the interest of the efficiency of their organisations. A health administrator who cannot take the right decision at the right time cannot aspire to be a successful executive. Decision-making is the nerve-centre of all human activity. It is an act of intelligence, will and precision. It is the process by which out of the various alternatives, one alternative is selected by health administrator to solve a particular problem. The Government in their reply to WHO felt concerned that there was no point at which there was sufficient authority to take decisions that effective coordination required. It was told that there are currently in simultaneous operation, "several levels of health care delivery, without defined authority patterns vis-a-vis each other or defined shares of operation."[27]

New problems demand new solutions and the health administrators who can come out from the routines are highly prized. This requires creativity in the decision-making. Newman has indicated the distinct stages which can help the Chief Executive in this process:

1. *Saturation*—to the familiar with the problem.
2. *Deliberation*—to consider alternative solutions and to rearrange them.
3. *Incubation*—to let the subconscious mind work on the problem.
4. *Illumination*—to get new ideas and sensing that it may work.
5. *Accommodation*—to work out the new ideas so that it is a practical solution to the problems.

Hicks[29] gives the following types of creativity in sound decision-making:

1. *Innovative*—creativity to think totally new ideas.
2. *Synthesis*—creativity to absorb, combine and use ideas from different sources and making it new.
3. *Extension*—creativity to use the old or new ideas.
4. *Duplication*—creativity to use the other's successful ideas.

No administrator can boast of perfect decision-making. His effort should be to arrive at correct decisions as far as possible.

According to L. Mehl, the structure of decision consists mainly of three zones, e.g., calculable zone, uncertain zone and axiologic zone.[30] These zones can be presented as under:

(c)	*(b)*	*(a)*
Axiologic zone	*Uncertain zone*	*Calculable zone*
CHOICE	Concept Choice v/s Reasons	Reason

In order to improve the decision-making, the administrators have to make efforts to reduce the uncertain zone to the maximum possible. This way, the calculable zone can be extended further. This would be possible if health administrator take decisions on the basis of new concepts, new methods, and new tools rather than on the basis of intuition, experience, rule-of-thumb and outdated and inadequate facts. We can make use of marginal theory, scientific theory, mathematical theory psychological theory to take correct and reliable decisions.

(c)	*(b)*	*(a)*
Axiologic zone	*Reduced uncertain zone*	*Calculable zone*

Extended
Calculable zone

Electronic Data Processing

The rationale in using this technique is to reduce the manpower required, the time taken for a given process and to reduce the possibility of error.[31]

Performance Budgeting

Performance Budgeting not only correlates physical and financial aspects of every programme or activity but also aims at improving budget formulation, review and decision-making at the levels of management.[32]

We shall discuss the other Management Techniques applicable to health administration in the relevant chapters.

Application of Management Techniques for Administrative Improvement and Administrative Reforms.

Having discussed the importance and utility of some of the important management techniques, we shall explain the application of the management techniques at different levels of management and to situations covering time horizons with the help of a chart.

The Chart reveals that one technique or the other is applied in one form or the other at all the three levels of management. Because the lowest level has to perform operational functions, management techniques like Work Study, Network Analysis, Capacity Utilisation studies are adopted. As the middle level, where the policy is executed, some more important techniques like Man Power Planning. Cost-Benefit Analysis, Statistics and Forecasting, etc. are applied to effect improvements. The top management uses more strategic techniques like Technological Forecasting, Performance Budgeting, Operational Research Studies, etc., etc.

D. Utility and Limitations

Utility

Let us explain the use of these techniques in improving the health services with some examples.

1. In a Case Study, a 750-bedded hospital (Medical Institute) was facing acute shortage of nursing personnel. The study of the utilisation of nursing personnel in this hospital revealed that 33 per cent time of the nurses was being spent on non-nursing duties. Besides, there was 25 per cent turnover of the nurses. There was a great delay in appointing the new incumbents.The study suggested that if the nurses are not given non-nursing duties, a saving of rupees three lakhs can take place. This was studied with the help of the techniques of organisational analysis.
2. A study was conducted by the writer of a university Health Centre where there was a problem of pilferage of drugs. The Chief Medical Officer of the Centre was finding it very difficult to plug this loop-hole as he himself was busy in examining the patients for all the duty time. It was suggested that the whole stock of the medicine may be classified on the cost with the help of the technique of ABC analysis. It was suggested to the Chief Medical Officer to keep 'A' category of drugs under lock and key to be issued only under his signature. He could check for other drugs once a month concentrating only on A and B categories. This helped the Centre to save about Rs.25,000 annually.
3. A Study was carried out by C.R. Prasad on the 'Application of Quantitative methods in Hospital Management'. He studied the problems of patients who were wasting

APPLICATIONS OF DIFFERENT TECHNIQUES ACCORDING TO THEIR LEVEL OF FORMALITY AND TO THE LEVEL OF ACTIVENESS OF MANAGEMENT

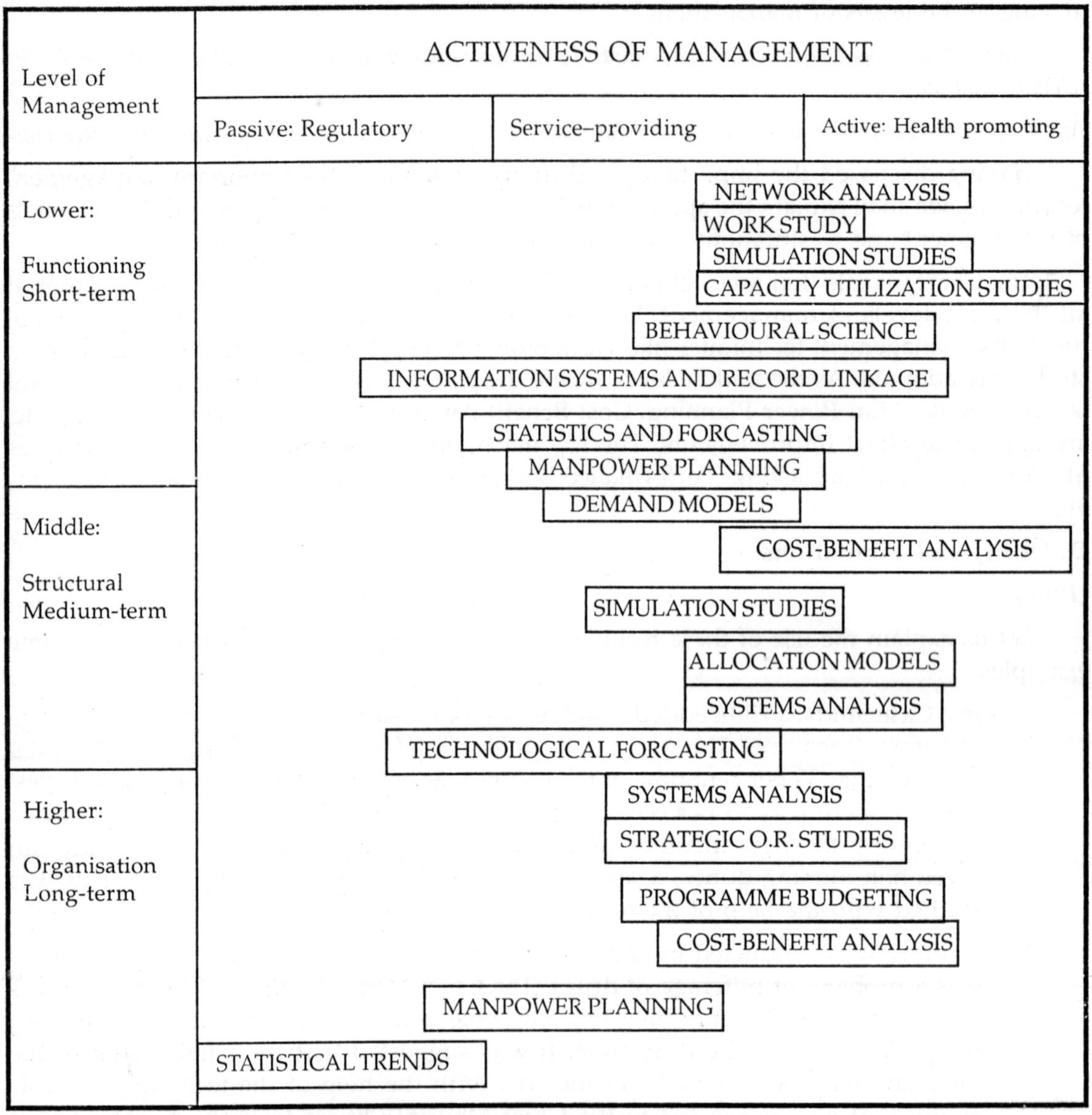

Fig. 17.4

a lot of their time to get the prescriptions, (to pay the cash and to receive the medicine). The patients had to stand in line for about 45 minutes. Prasad applied Sampling techniques and used Simulation Procedures. He was able to suggest a model by which the average time of waiting could be reduced to 16 minutes from 45 minutes.[34]

The examples of the use of other techniques would be taken up in the relevant chapters.

Thus, we find that there is an ever-increasing array of methods and techniques available to assist the management for the acceleration of national socio-economic development, with stated policies, objectives and priorities. Further, the impact of interdependence of the management techniques solely depend upon the development of improved management. But it is generally acknowledged that the availability and application of modern management skills do not meet the needs that are felt to exist.

Shortages and difficulties for the greater development and application of management skills are always encountered. Some of them are as under:

1. Shortage of experts in management techniques, and especially of those with knowledge and experience of the special problems of the health sector;
2. Difficulty in recruiting staff to specialize in health management and managerial technologies because of working conditions or lack of career prospects for personnel other than physicians;
3. Shortage of general management capability, together with lack of appreciation of 'systems thinking' and orientation to modern management on the part of doctors and health administrators;
4. Insufficient ability to identify situations in which the available consultants and other sources of expertise could best be used;
5. Lack of form of organisation that can fully utilize the available management skills;
6. Shortage of staff of various kinds (not just those with specific management skills);
7. Shortage of teachers in management for medical schools etc; and
8. Insufficient development of management methods for dealing with such difficulties, characteristic of health services as: defining objectives, public participation, coordination, motivation and supervision.

From the above, it is inferred that there is a room for improvement to make simultaneous progress on several fronts by:

(a) spreading the determination to overcome the difficulties mentioned and establishing confidence in using techniques;

(b) general management training and experience for health professionals;

(c) production of management specialists of various kinds, especially those with a broad experience in addition to their specialist skill;

(d) organisational changes necessary to utilise management skills and provide appropriate career and working conditions for their practitioners; and

(e) research and development to adapt management techniques to the health needs.[35]

No doubt, the theory of management techniques in the context of administrative improvement and administrative reforms can be learned in a classroom, from a text-book or through correspondence, but, these cannot replace the practical experience, only through which one acquires the skill of the technique.

Critical Appraisal of Management Techniques

Although the needs for modern management technology differ from country to country and from situation to situation, it is not to be expected that these differences will always be accurately interpreted, or that the most appropriate techniques will automatically be invoked. In fact, techniques like most other things, are susceptible to the influences of fashion. Their value depends on the circumstances in which they are applied. In other words, the use of management techniques, just as the exploitation of any other resources, have to be subject to continuous feedback and review.

There have been many instances when in a hurry to borrow from West, we blindly adopt the management techniques/technology in the 'as-it-is' form without even taking into consideration their limitations. John Argenti in one of his papers observes that "after all, many of the sophisticated techniques have not been employed by a great number of organisations in U.K.—we should not blindly employ the technique. We should be sure of its potentialities and also skilled in its use."[35] This means that suitable technology has to be devised to provide for decent health care to the people much more economically than the affluent and advanced countries. Thus, there is a need to evolve appropriate management techniques and technology to suit our environment.

We are in a hurry; we wish to achieve much; we cannot afford the luxury of wasting our resources for experimentation. What is, therefore, needed is a proper identification of opportunities, setting out of priority areas and accordingly, continually devising technology and techniques appropriate to our set up, our value system and to our environment. Let us strive to usher systems/techniques/technologies that are compatible. The call is, therefore, to stress on the 'know-why' rather than just on the 'know-how' of techniques and technology. This can materialise only when we bear in mind the following motto:

THE RIGHT TECHNIQUE/TECHNOLOGY

AT THE RIGHT PLACE

AT THE RIGHT TIME

AT THE RIGHT COST

BY THE RIGHT METHODS/MEANS

BY THE RIGHT PERSONNEL

References

1. Milton Greenablitt, Myron Sharaf, R. and Evelyn Stone M., Dynamics of Institutional Change, Pittsburgh, University of Pittsburgh Press, 1971, pp. 239-240.

2. All India Radio Broadcast, June 26, 1966; Selected Speeches of Mrs. Indira Gandhi, January 1966 to Aug., 1969, Publication Division, March, 1971.

3. W.H.O. Public Health Papers, 55, p. 68.
4. UN: "Inter-regional Seminar on Administration of Management Improvement Services", Vol. I, Copenhagen, Denmark, Oct. 1970, p.24.
5. UN: United Nations Programmes in Public Administration (E/4296-ST/TAO/M/38), pp. 11-12.
6. UN: Official Record of the Economic and Social Council (E/1708), Agenda Item No. 10, p.3.
7. UN: Inter-regional Seminar on Administration of Management Improvement Services.
8. Dale, Earnest and Michelon, L.C.: "Modern Management Techniques", Penguin Books, 1974, p. 9.
9. Gabriel Legisias V.: College of Public Administration, University of Philippines, "Administrative capability as a neglected dimension in the implementation of development programme and projects" Seventy General Assembly and Conference of EROPA on "Implementation, the Problem Achieving Results", 24-31 October, 1973, Vol. III, pp. 3-14.
10. Katz Saul M. : A Methodological note on appraising administrative capability for development" (UN Publication, Sales No. E-69-II. 4-2) p. 8.
11. *Ibid*, pp. 99-100.
12. World Health Organisation, Regional Office of South-East Asia, New Delhi (SEA/RC/26/pp. 31-32).
13. ILO: "Introduction to Work Study" Geneva, 1969, p. 26.
14. Clay, M.J. General Theory of Management Techniques, Part I, in Work Study and Management Services, London.
15. Bechhard R : Organisation Development : Strategies and Models, Addison-Wesley, 1969, p.9.
16. Finer, H: *Theory and Practice of Modern Govt.*, p. 106.
17. Eli Ginzberg: "Perspectives on Work Motivation" *Personnel*, Vol. 31, No. (July), 1959, pp. 48-49.
18. Maier, Norman R.F. and Hayes John, J: Creative Management (New York: John Wiley & Sons, Inc. 1962), p. 36.
19. Davis, Keith: "The Case for Participative Management", *Business Horizon*, Vol. 6, No. 3 (1963), p. 141.
20. Walters, Albert F: "Management and Motivation: Releasing Human Potential", *Personnel*, Vol. 39, No. 2 (March-April, 1962), pp. 8-16 as reprinted in Harold Koontz and Cyrill O'Donnel, *Management: A Book of Readings* (New York: McGraw-Hill Book Company, 1964) pp. 382-83.
21. For details refers: *Information Systems for Modern Management* by Murdicks Robert G. and Ross, Joel E. Prentice-Hall of India (P) Ltd., Delhi, 1977.
22. For details see: PERT & CPM — Principles and Applications by Srinath, L.S. Affiliated East-West Press, Delhi, 1975.
23. Joseph, J: Moder and Cecil Phillips R.: "Project Management with CPM and PERT, (New York: Reinhold, 1964), pp. 5-6.
24. For details see: *Cost-Benefit Analysis in Administration* by Trevor Newton, George Allen & Unwin, London. 1972, and Weisbrod, B.A. "Concepts of Costs and Benefits," in Chase, S.B. (ed.) *Problems in Public Expenditure Analysis*, Washington, D.C., Brookings, 1968, pp. 257-262; and Williams, A. "The Cost-Benefit Approach," *British Medical Bulletin*, 30, 25256 (1974).

25. Ralph, Gilson E. "The Recognition of Systems Engineering," in *Flagle*, p. 58.

26. WHO *Technical Report Series*. 596, "Application of System Analysis and Health Management" 1976, pp. 7-8.

27. *World Health*, Paper 55, op. cit. p. 61.

28. Newman, William H. *et al., The Process of Management*, (Englewood Cliffs, N.J. Prentice-Hall, 1967), pp. 338-45.

29. Hicks, Herbert, G. *The Management of Organisations*, (New York, McGraw-Hill, 1967), pp. 169-71.

30. Mehl, Lucian in his article in *Institutional d'Administration Publique*, Oct.-Dec., 1968.

31. For details refer, *Report of the Inter-Regional Seminar on Electronic Data Processing in Government*, UN, Vol. I & II (ST/TAC/M/63) 1971.

32. For details refer, *Reading on Performance Budgeting* (Ed.) by M.J.K. Thavaraj and K.B. Iyer, IIPA, Delhi.

33. WHO, *Public Health*, Paper 55—"Modern Management" Methods and the Organisation of Health Services, Geneva," 1974, pp. 15/16.

34. Prasad, C.R., Application of Quantitative Methods in Hospital Management in *Management in Govt.*, Vol. IV—No. 3, Oct.-Dec. 1972 pp. 238-248.

35. WHO *Public Health*, Paper 55, pp. 70-71.

36. Argenti John: "Whatever Happened to Management Techniques" in *Management Today*, April 1976.

APPENDIX–I

BASIC INFORMATION RELATING TO HEALTH

Sl.No.	Item		Bangladesh	Burma	India	Indonesia	Maldives	Mongolia	Nepal	Sri Lanka	Thailand
1	2		3	4	5	6	7	8	9	10	11
1.	Population (in thousands)		80.560	32.206	625.820	143.280	140	1.555	13.136	13.970	44.160
2.	Urban population (%)		8.8	20.0	20.6	18.2	11.3	46.0	4.0	22.4	15.9
3.	Annual rate of population growth		2.4	2.2	2.1	2.6	2.0	2.7	2.3	2.2	2.6
4.	Expectation of life at birth	M	45.8	48.6	52.6	47.0	—	64	46.0	64.2	57.6
		F	46.6	51.5	51.6	47.0	—	64	42.5	67.1	61.0
5.	Population under 15 year (%)		43.5	40.5	40.1	44.1	44.9	46.2	41.2	39.0	43.7
6.	Crude birth rate		49.5	32.9	35.2	42.9	45.3	37.1	44.7	27.6	35.0
7.	Crude death rate		28.1	11.9	15.9	16.9	11.5	9.9	19.5	8.0	9.0
8.	Infant morality rate		153.0	77.0	122.0	137.0	106.2	60.0	M 141.2 F 123.0	— 51.2	— 44 to 49
9.	Maternal mortality rate		30.0	1.0	(h)	—	11.9	—	—	1.0	2.6
10.	Number of doctors		6.508	5.700	154.000	8.977	9	3.184	378	4.427	6.000
11.	Population per doctor		12.379	5.409	3.884	15.553	15.444	488	34.751	3.156	7.160
12.	Doctors per 10,000 population		0.81	1.85	2.60	0.64	0.64	20.5	0.29	3.17	1.40
13.	Number of nurses/midwives										
	(a) professional		1.749	5.878	113.455	1.683	8	—	249	6.022	11.832
	(b) auxiliary (including midwives)		—	10.949	162.671	41.192	43	6.871	582	3.482	15.816
14.	Population per nurse/midwife										
	(a) professional		46.061	5.245	5.377	80.832	16.250	—	52.755	2.320	3.539
	(b) auxiliary		—	2.816	—	3.303	3.023	226	22.570	4.012	2.647
15.	Nurses/midwives per 10,000 population										
	(a) professional		0.22	1.91	1.86	0.12	0.62	—	0.19	4.31	2.83
	(b) auxiliary		—	3.56	—	3.03	3.31	44.19	0.44	2.49	3.78

Contd..

1	2	3	4	5	6	7	8	9	10	11
16.	Number of hospital beds	18.358	27.453	377.464	84.146	40	15.749	2.393	41.051	60.590
17.	Population per hospital bed	4.388	1.123	1.658	1.617	3.500	99	5.489	334	709
18.	Hospital beds per 10,000 population	2.28	8.90	6.03	6.19	2.86	101.28	1.82	29.90	14.10
19.	Number of health centres	RHC 150 MCW 93 SHU 24	RHC 1077 MCW 285 SHU 49 UHC 54	PHC 5.373 SC 37.931	HC 3934 Poly 6.752 MCH 3.762 Others 946	HC 21 Fld HU 1046 SANEPID 26	Phy HU 272 HP Ay Disp. Others 9	433 82	HC 25 MHC HC MCH MWY	HC 1.369 DH& 255 3.500 37 1.450
20.	Health expenditure as percent of total expenditure									
	Government	3.8	6.4	2.1	1.6	6.0	10.0	5.31	4.6	6.2
	Private	4.0	-	-	-	-	-	-	-	-
21.	Per capita health expenditure									
	Government	7.66 Takas	5.70 Kyats	9.44 Rupees	1.111 Rupiahs	7.00 Rupees	180.3 Tughriks	12.49 Rupees	29.79 Rupees	88.49 Bahts
	Private	41.00 Takas	-	-	555 Rupiahs	-	-	-	14.64 Rupees	231.39 Bahts
22.	Literacy rate (%)	24.3	60.0	29.5	60.0	60.2	100	14.92	78.5	70

Ay Disp.	Ayurvedic Dispensary
DH & MHC	District Hospitals and Medical and Health Centres
Fld. HU	Feldshers' Health Unit
HC	Health Centre
HP	Health Post
MCH	Maternal and Child Health Centre
MCW	Maternal and Child Welfare Centre
MWY	Midwifery Centre
PHC	Primary Health Centre
Phy. HU	Physician's Health Unit
Poly	Poly-clinic
RHC	Rural Health Centre
SANEPID	Sanitary and Epidemiological Station
SC	Sub-Centre
SHU	School Health Unit
UHC	Urban Health Centre
WHO	Regional Office for South-East Asia, SEA/VHS/154 Rev. 2, July 1978

Appendix II*:
Studies Regarding Economic Implications of Population Growth in India

Name of the Author and Year of Study	*Methodology*	*Period covered and main finding*
1	2	3
1. Coale and Hoover 1958	(a) Economic Model of Harrod-Domar type. Population variable incorporated in investment function. (b) Use of the model based on Cobb-Douglas Production function for long-term analysis.	(a)(1956-81) Increase in per consumer income by 38% in unchanged fertility case and by 95% in reduced fertility case. (b) (1956-2001) Income per consumer under low fertility case double that of unchanged fertility case.
2. Stephen Enke 1960	Investment model approach. Cost-benefit technique applied.	Value of preventing a birth Rs. 1500 or 100 times the return on other investments.
3. Robert Cassen 1968	Net gain in per capita income due to family planning compared with returns from other forms of investment.	(1965-75) Net gain from birth control will be 15 times the return from other investments.
4. J.L. Simon 1969	Value of preventing a birth in India estimated on the basis of Coale and Hoover's population and income projections by using discounting procedure.	(1956-81) Value of preventing in a birth in India at 15% discount rate is Rs. 750 and at 5% rate of Rs. 1160 at 1956 prices.
5. George B. Simmons 1971	Three Growth Models (I) National Income growth independent of population (II) Harrod-Domar model with population variable incorporated in investment function (III) Growth model with adjustment in model II by introducing labour force component under alternative population situation.	(1967-1991) Benefits by per capita income criterion (I) Rs. 5311 (II & III) Rs. 8290.
6. K.C. Seal 1974	Net gain due to family planning compared with returns from other forms of investment.	(1951-71) Net gain from family planning three times the returns from other investments.

Contd..

1	2	3
7. V.S. Badari 1976	Value of averting a birth calculated at 10% discount rate of using 1960-61 estimates of annual consumption per survivor in different age-groups and the productivity of 'marginal' worker.	(1961-96) Value of averting a birth in Rs. 1300.

* Quoted in by K. Srinivasan and S. Mukerji: *Dynamics of Population and Family Welfare in India*, Bombay Popular Parkashan, 1979.

Sources:

1. Ansely J. Coale and Edgar M. Hoover, *Population Growth and Economic Development in Low Income Countries: A Case Study of India's Prospects* (Princeton: Princeton University Press, 1958).
2. Stephen Enke. 'The Gains to India from Population Control: Some Money Measures and Incentive Schemes". *Review of Economic and Statistics*, 42, (May 1960, pp. 175-81).
3. Robert Cassen, 'Population Control: Aims and Policies' in Paul Streeton and Michael Lipton (Eds.), *The Crises of Indian Planning* (London: Oxford University Press, 1968), p. 258.
4. J.L. Simon, "The Value of Avoided Births to Underdeveloped Countries", *Population Studies*, Vol. XXIII, No. 1, March 1969, pp. 61-69.
5. George B. Simmons, *The Indian Investment in Family Planning*, (New York: The Population Council), 1971.
6. K.C. Seal, "On Alternative Efficiency of Family Planning Programme over other Developmental Programmes", *Studies on Population and Family Planning in India* (New Delhi: Planning and Evaluation Division, Department of Family Planning, Ministry of Health and Family Planning, Government of India, 1974), pp. 133-34.
7. V.S. Badari, "The Economic Benefits of Fertility Control: *Journal of Institute of Economic Research*, Dharwar, Vol. XI, Nos. 1 & 2 (January and July 1976), pp. 26-27.

Appendix–III

National Population Policy*

16 April, 1976

With 2.4 per cent of the world's land area, India has about 15 per cent of the world's people. It is estimated that our population as on 1 January 1976 has crossed the 600 million mark, and is now rising at the rate of well over one million per month. Since independence 250 million have been added, equivalent to the entire population of the Soviet Union with six times the land area of India. The increase every year is now equal to the entire population of Australia which is 2½ times the size of our country. If the present rate of increase continues unchecked our population at the turn of the century may well reach the staggering figure of one billion. Indisputably we are facing a population explosion of crisis dimensions which has largely diluted the fruits of the remarkable economic progress that we have made over the last two decades. If the future of the nation is to be secured, and the goal of removing poverty to be attained the population problem will have to be treated as a top national priority and commitment.

2. Our real enemy is poverty, and it is as a frontal assault on the citadels of poverty that the Fifth Five-Year Plan has included the Minimum Needs Programme. One of its five items is integrated package of health, family planning and nutrition. Far-reaching steps have been initiated to reorient the thrust of medical education so as to strengthen the community medicine and rural health aspects, and to restructure the health care delivery system on three tier basis going down to the most far-flung rural areas where the majority of our people reside and where child morality and morbidity are the highest. Similarly, ignorance, illiteracy and superstition have got to be fought and eliminated. In the ultimate analysis it is only when the underlying causes of poverty and disease are eliminated that the nation will be able to move forward to its desired ideals.

3. Nonetheless it is clear that simply to wait for education and economic development to bring about a drop in fertility is not a practical solution. The very increase in population makes economic development slow and more difficult of achievement. The time factor is so pressing, and the population growth so formidable, that we have to get out of the vicious circle through a direct assault upon this problem as a national commitment. The President in his address to the Joint Session of Parliament this year reiterated the importance of stepping up family planning efforts, and the Prime Minister has on several occasions laid stress upon the crucial role that population control has to play in the movement towards economic independence and social transformation, specially in the light of the 20-Point Economic Programme.

4. Considerable work has been done in our country in the field of family planning, but clearly only the fringe of the problem has so far been touched. In this context, after a thorough and careful consideration of all the factors involved as well as the expression of a wide spectrum of public opinion, Government have decided on a series of fundamental measures detailed below which, it is hoped, will enable us to achieve the planned target of

---

* From a statement by Dr. Karan Singh on 16 April 1976, then Minister of Health and Family Planning.

reducing the birth rate from an estimated 35 per thousand in the beginning of the Fifth Plan to 25 per thousand at the end of the Sixth. Allowing for the steady decline in the death rate that will continue due to the improvement in our medical and public health services and the living standards of our people, this is expected to bring down the growth rate of population in our country to 1.4 per cent by 1948.

5. Raising the age of marriage will not only have a demonstrable demographic impact, but will also lead to more responsible parenthood and help to safeguard the health of the mother and the child. It is well known that very early pregnancy leads to higher maternal and infant mortality. Also, if the women of our country are to play their rightful role in its economic, social and intellectual life, the practice of early marriage will have to be severely discouraged. The present law has not been effectively or uniformly enforced. It has, therefore, been decided that the minimum age of marriage should be raised to 18 for girls and 21 for boys, and suitable legislation to this effect will be passed. offences under this law will be cognizable by an officer not below the rank of a Sub-Divisional Magistrate. The question of making registration of marriages compulsory is under active consideration.

6. It has been represented by some States that while on the one hand we are urging them to limit their population, those States which do well in this field face reduction of representation in Parliament while those with weak performance in family planning tend to get increasing representation. It is obviously necessary to remedy this situation. It has, therefore, been decided that the representation in the Lok Sabha/and the State Legislatures will be frozen on the basis of the 1971 census until the year 2001. This means in effect that the census counts of 1981 and 1991 will not be considered for purposes of adjustment of Lok Sabha Legislatures seats. Necessary constitutional amendment will be brought forward during the current year. Appropriate legislation for other elective bodies will also be undertaken.

7. In a federal system, the sharing of Central resources with the States is a matter of considerable importance. In all cases where population is a factor, as in the allocation of Central assistance to State Plans, devolution of taxes and duties and grants-in-aid, the population figures of 1971 will continue to be followed till the year 2001. In the matter of Central assistance to State Plans, eight per cent will be specifically earmarked against performance in family planning. The detailed procedures in this regard will be worked out by the Planning Commission.

8. While there is a direct correlation between illiteracy and fertility, this is particularly marked in the case of girls' education. Wherever female literacy improves, it has been seen that fertility drops almost automatically. It is therefore, necessary that special measures be taken to raise the levels of female education, particularly above the middle level for girls as well as non-formal education plans for young women especially in certain backward States where the family planning performance so far has been unimpressive. The same is true with regard to child nutrition programmes, as high infant mortality and morbidity have a direct impact on fertility. The Ministry of Education is urging upon the State Government the necessity to give these matters higher priority than has been accorded so far and fully earmarking adequate outlays both for girls education upto the middle level and child nutrition.

9. My Ministry is also in close touch with the Education Ministry with regard to the introduction of population values in the educational system, and the NCERT has already made a beginning in bringing out some text books on these lines. It is essential that the younger generations should grow up with an adequate awareness of the population problem and a realization of their national responsibility in this regard. Indeed, if I may venture to say so, exhortations to plan families are more important for the younger generations than for those who have already made their contribution to our demographic profile.

10. The adoption of a small family norm is too important a matter to be considered the responsibility of only one Ministry. It is essential that all Ministries and Departments of the Government of India as well as the States should take up as an integral part of their normal programme and budgets the motivation of citizens to adopt responsible reproductive behaviour both in their own as well as the national interest. A directive to this effect is being issued by the Prime Minister to all Ministries of the Government of India, and a letter will also be addressed by her to all Chief Ministers. The performance of family planning in the States will be more carefully and intensively monitored than in the past, and the Union Cabinet will review the situation in depth at least once a year.

11. Experience over the last 20 years has shown that monetary compensation does have a significant impact upon the acceptance of family planning, particularly among the poorer sections of society. In view of the desirability of limiting the family size to two or three it has been decided that monetary compensation for sterilization (both male and female) will be raised to Rs. 150 if performed with two living children or less, Rs. 100 if performed with three living children and Rs. 70 if performed with four or more children. These amounts will include the money payable to individual acceptors as well as other charges such as drugs and dressings, etc., and will take effect from 1 May, 1976. Facilities for sterilization and MTP are being increasingly extended to cover rural areas.

12. In addition to individual compensation, Government is of the view that group incentives should now be introduced in a bold and imaginative manner so as to make family planning a mass movement with greater community involvement. It has, therefore, been decided that suitable group incentives will be introduced for the medical profession, for Zila and Panchayat Samities, for teachers at various levels, for cooperative societies and for labour in the organised sector through their respective representative national organisations. Details of these group incentives are being worked out in consultation with the concerned organisations.

13. Despite governmental efforts at Union, State and Municipal level, family planning cannot succeed unless voluntary organisations are drawn into its promotion in an increasing measure, particularly youth and women's organisations. There is already a scheme for aiding voluntary ogranisation and it has been decided that this will be expanded. Also, full rebate will be allowed in the income tax assessment for amounts given as donations for family planning purposes to Government, local bodies or any registered voluntary organisation approved for this purpose by the Union Ministry of Health.

14. Research in reproductive biology and contraception is under way in several of our scientific institutions, and there are some very promising developments which, we hope,

will lead to a major break-through before too long. This is a great challenge to our scientists, and efforts in this direction will receive special attention so that necessary research inputs are ensured on a long range and continuing basis.

15. The question of compulsory sterilization has been the subject of lively public debate over the last few months. It is clear that public opinion is now ready to accept much more stringent measures for family planning than before. However, the administrative and medical infrastructure in many parts of the country is still not adequate to cope with the vast implications of nationwide compulsory sterilization. We do not, therefore, intend to bring in Central legislation for this purpose, at least for the time being. Some States feel that the facilities available with them are adequate to meet the requirements of compulsory sterilization. We are of the view that where a State legislature, in the exercise of its own powers, decides that the time is ripe and it is necessary to pass legislation for compulsory sterilization, it may do so. Our advice to the States in such cases will be to bring in the limitation after three children, and to make it uniformly applicable to all Indian citizens resident in that State without distinction of caste, creed or community.

16. Some States have also introduced a series of measures directed towards their employees and other citizens in the matter of preferential allotment of houses, loans, etc. for those who have accepted family planning. In this sphere also we have decided to leave it to each individual State to introduce such measures as they consider necessary and desirable. Employees of the Union Government will be expected to adopt the small family norm and necessary changes will be made in their service/conduct rules to ensure this.

17. In order to spread the message of family planning throughout the nation, a new multi-media motivational strategy is being evolved which will utilize all the available media channels including the radio, television (specially programmes aimed directly at rural audiences), the press films, visual displays and also include traditional folk media such as the jatra, puppet shows, folk songs and folk dances. The attempt is to move from the somewhat urban-elitist approaches of the past into a much more imaginative and vigorous rural-oriented approach. In this context my Ministry is working in close coordination with the Ministry of Information and Broadcasting, and is also trying to draw the best media talent available in the country into the structuring of the new programme.

18. This package of measures will succeed in its objective only if it receives the full and active cooperation of the people at large. It is my sincere hope that the entire nation will strongly endorse the new population policy which as part of a multi-faceted strategy for economic development and social emancipation is directed towards building a strong and prosperous India in the years and Decades to come.

Appendix VI

Family Welfare Progrmame—A Statcment of Policy (29th June, 1977)

The President in his address to Parliament on March 28, 1977, stated that, "Family Planning will be pursued vigorously as a wholly voluntary programme and as an integral part of a comprehensive policy covering education, health, maternity and child care, family welfare, women's rights and nutrition." The Prime Minister has on a number of occasions underlined the vital importance of family planning as a means of individual and national development and well-being. The Government is totally committed to the Family Welfare Programme and will spare no efforts to motivate the people to accept it voluntarily in their own interest and in the interest of their children as well as in the larger interest of the nation.

2. Family planning has, however, to be lifted from its old and narrow concept and given its proper place in the overall philosophy of welfare. It must embrace all aspects of family welfare, particularly those which are designed to protect and promote the health of mothers and children. It must become a part of the total concept of positive health. At the same time, it must find meaningful integration with other welfare programmes, viz., nutrition, food, clothing, shelter, availability of safe drinking water, education, employment and women's welfare. It will be our endeavour to bring about this integration in a greater degree. We expect the States to do the same.

3. The change in the name of the programme from family planning of family welfare is a reflection of the Government's anxiety to promote, through it, the total welfare of the family and the community. It is our intention to take the programme forward in the real sense as an investment in man. We wish to make it abundantly clear that in this task there is no room for compulsion, coercion or pressures of any sort. Compulsion in the area of family welfare must be ruled out for all times to come. Our approach is educational and wholly voluntary. There will however, be no slackening of our efforts in this direction.

4. The Government attaches the highest importance to the dignity of the citizen and to his right to determine the size of his family. We have no doubt that by and large the people of India will become conscious of the importance of responsible parenthood; given the necessary information and adequate services, they will accept the small family norm. We will promote all methods with equai emphasis and it will be left to every family to decide what method of contraception it will like to adopt. Employees of the Union Government, State Governments autonomous bodies, local bodies, etc., will be expected to set an example and to adopt the small family norm.

5. We are totally against any legislation for compulsory sterilisation either at the Central level or by the States. Sterilisation, both male and female, is a terminal method and suitable for those couples who have reached the optimum family size. Services for sterilisation will be offered free of cost to those who voluntarily wish to adopt this method. Similarly other services under the programme will be available to the people free of charge. The acceptance of voluntary sterilisation and IUD involves to and fro travel to a clinic, a brief stay in the hospital, resulting in possible loss of wages which the majority of our people cannot easily afford. In view of this, it has been decided to retain the provision for monetary compensation. Any medical complication resulting from a voluntary sterilisation operation will be attended to free of cost; and if in an unfortunate case recanalisation becomes necessary, this facility will also be offered to the individual concerned under the best possible professional care without any charge.

6. Nearly 80 per cent of our population lives in villages. Medical services are not able to reach them in an effective way. An integrated rural health scheme is on the anvil and will be implemented shortly. It is of the utmost importance that adequate ante-natal, natal and post-natal care is made available to pregnant mothers. To this end a comprehensive scheme of training of indigenous mid-wives (dais) will be implemented. Under it maternity services will be made available to all mothers who may need them. The programme of immunising children against common diseases such as whooping cough, diphtheria and tenanus will be expanded further. We expect that the State Governments will give necessary cooperation and assistance in this direction.

7. The direct correlation between illiteracy and fertility and between infant/maternal mortality and the age at marriage is well established by demographic studies. While on the one hand the Government will pursue its policy of according high priority to the improvement of women's educational level, both through formal and non-formal channels, it will also bring legislation for raising the minimum age of marriage for girls to 18 and for boys to 21.

8. In a federal system the sharing of Central resources with the States is a matter of considerable importance. In all cases where population is a factor as in the allocation of Central assistance to State Plans, devolution of taxes and duties and grants-in-aid, the population figures of 1971 will continue to be followed till the year 2001. Family Planning and population control is a subject in the Concurrent List, yet the implementation of the Family Welfare Programme is very much the responsibility of State Governments. Assistance for the implementation of the Programme is provide by the Central Government to the States on cent-per-cent basis. In order to ensure a purposeful implementation of the Family Welfare Programme, the principle of linking 8 per cent of Central Assistance to the State Plans with their performance and success in Family Welfare Programme will be continued.

9. Population education has so far not received the attention it deserves. The NCERT have developed some models for the introduction of population education in the school education system. These models have already been adopted by the Central Schools Organisation. We would urge that the departments of education in the States should adopt these models, or their modified versions, in the syllabus in the schools. Forty-two per cent of our population is below the age of 15 years. It is this population which will soon be entering in the arena of matrimony. We must take steps without any further delay to see that the youth receive population education as part of their normal course of study.

10. The population of India has been increasing at the rate of about one million every month. It has increased by nearly 270 million since 1947 and is today estimated to be 615 million. If the present rate of growth continues, we will be touching the one-billion mark by the end of the century. This rate has to be arrested. The birth rate targets of 30 and 25 per thousand by the end of the Fifth and Sixth Plans respectively can be achieved only with the total and willing participation of the community in the family welfare programme. For this purpose it is important that all media of publicity, including motivation through the extension approach, should be utilised fully by the Central and the State Governments. We would very much expect that just as at the Centre we have involved all media units of the Ministry of Information and Broadcasting in the motivational campaigns, in the States also the State

Departments of Public Relations and other departments having their own publicity set-ups would be totally associated with the motivational effort.

11. It is of equal importance that trade unions, chambers of commerce, cooperative societies, organisations of women, federations of teachers, village panchayats and all other institutions which can influence public opinion should be associated intimately with the educational campaigns. The village panchayats can play a significant role in this task. Their potential as change-agents needs to receive greater recognition and attention.

12. No programme will succeed unless voluntary organisations particularly youth and women's organisations participate in its implementation fully and extensively. So far this participation has been very limited. The Government wishes to invite the suggestions of voluntary organisations and such public bodies as are engaged in the general task of Family Welfare for evolving suitable patterns of cooperation and assistance. Full rebate will be allowed in the income-tax assessment for amounts given as donations for Family welfare purposes to Government, local bodies, or any registered voluntary organisation approved for this purpose by the Union Ministry of Health.

13. While the existing methods of contraception will continue to be available to the people, it is important that the search for newer methods should be intensified. The Government will give special attention to the necessary research inputs in the field of reproductive biology and contraception.

14. The Programme and the approach for implementation of the Family Welfare Programme as outlined in the above paragraphs will succeed only if there is willing cooperation from all in full measure. The Family Welfare Programme embraces all the principal areas of human welfare. It will be wrong to leave it only to the Ministry of Health and Family Welfare in the Centre and their counterparts in the States. It is essential that all Ministries and Departments of the Government of India as well as of the States give due importance to this Programme and work for its furtherance. The performance of Family Welfare in the States will be intensively and carefully monitored and the Union Cabinet will review the situation in depth at least once a year. Suitable machinery for ensuring coordination with other connected programmes of welfare may be set up in the States also.

18

The Particulars of Health Care Delivery

From the community surveys we have ascertained the characteristics and health needs of the populations studied as well as the sources, quantities, and costs of health services they received. Those surveys revealed that village communities use many providers of care in addition to the government health center system which was defined from the beginning as the decision making focus of our research and recommendations. In the present chapter, therefore, we concentrate upon the particulars of government health center activity but not to the exclusion of other providers of health services. Health center information was collected from a staff perspective, principally through work sampling observations and the compilation of routine service statistics, and from a patient perspective, largely through patient flow analysis. The data were collected along three dimensions to provide measures of: (1) the types of client contacts provided and services rendered, (2) staff activities in specific categories of direct and supporting services, and (3) the costs incurred through these activities in rendering services. As in the case of the community surveys, the description of methods employed in the measurement of health care delivery will focus primarily upon the more comprehensive and complex research design employed in India.

I. SOURCES OF DATA

A. Work Sampling Observations

Activity patterns of the health center staff were assessed both at the center and in the field by means of periodic intermittent instantaneous observations, following the schedule. On the days of health center assessment, observations were made at two-minute intervals. The relative frequency of observation was predetermined for each worker according to his relative contribution to the provision of services and the variety of his activities. Thus the nurse was observed frequently because she provided a wide range of direct services, whereas the clerk was observed infrequently because his duties were largely in support of direct services. Once the relative distribution of obsrvattons was established, the selection of a worker to be observed at a given instant was determined from a table of random numbers.

In the field it was obviously impossible for an observer to switch back and forth between workers. Instead he trailed a particular worker throughout an entire workday and logged all of the service contacts provided by the worker. Field activity patterns were ascertained by means of instantaneous observations made at five-minute intervals. Because of the importance of the physician's role, he was also periodically trailed at the health center for one-and-one-half hour periods in order to obtain sets of ninety instantaneous observations recorded at one-minute intervals.

Although most of the health center service activities were associated with the medical relief function, provision was also made on the observation forms for noting activities in connection with the personal preventive, maternity, and family planning functions. Twelve categories of activities were identified within five broad classifications as follows:

Direct Service

- Patient Consultation
- Dispensing
- Injection
- Other Treatment
- Laboratory

Supportive Service

- Records and Reports
- Preparation, Maintenance, and Cleaning
- Communication, Education, and Supervision or Assisting of Staff
- Liaison with Other Agencies
- Other
- Transit
- Personal

Non-professional Activity

- Absent
- In Field

The observation forms were constructed so that the observer merely checked off the worker being observed, the function involved if any could be isolated, and the specific activity being conducted. It was possible to record multiple functions or activities observed at a single instant.

A similar recording format was employed in the field work sampling except that a wider range of functions was involved and the nature of direct service activities required a different classification scheme to include: inquiry (analogous to history taking as a part of medical consultation in the health center), examination, advice, and treatment or action (in relation to functions other than medical relief).

An enumeration of the various types of patient contact in the health center itself was provided by the patient flow analysis described below. In the field, however, it was necessary to employ a special form for the logging of worker contacts according to function and according to whether they were for direct service or were indirect. A well-child visit was classified as direct service, for example, whereas discussion with a school teacher to identify student health problems was noted as an indirect contact.

B. Patient Flow Analysis

Measurements of patient flow were restricted to the scheduled clinic hours of the particular health center and included all patients attending the clinic during these hours. One observer stationed at the health center entrance gave each patient a five-by eight inch piece of cardboard with a large identification number written on both sides. The patient was instructed to retain the caid throughout his stay at the health center so that information recorded at each of the stations subsequently visited could be associated with an individual patient. For actual recording, additional observers were stationed at the consultation room, the pharmacy, the treatment area, the area for injections, and at the exit. In addition there was usually a floating observer who recorded other types of activity such as laboratory work, special examinations, and MCH and family planning work.

The forms for recording patient flow information were constructed so that non-medically trained individuals could be taught to make the observations. Thus project physicians were available to resolve difficult questions rather than for making routine observations. With experience these exceptional cases became extremely infrequent.

The form exployed at each station included a checklist of relevant activities as well as means for recording the time spent by the patient in receiving services at that station. At the medical consultation station, for example, the observer ascertained whether a history was taken, the duration of the illness was determined, pulse or blood pressure was measured, auscultation was performed, laboratory examinations were ordered, and the patient was given the diagnosis and an explanation of the prescribed treatment.

In all, up to six sets of information were compiled for each patient, depending upon the particular stations visited. One was a record of his important characteristics, including age, sex, village of residence, and diagnosis. Others summarized the medical consultation information; the pharmacy, injection, and dressing experiences; and other services. Each of the summaries included a notation of the type of worker performing the recorded activities.

C. Other Health Center Studies

1. Health Center and Subcenter Statistics

All health centers and subcenters keep records and generate service reports which are aggregated at district and state levels. Since much of this information can be useful for our purposes, we summarized such data from each of the study areas along six lines.

a. Total attendances at outpatient clinics plus the total number of inpatients and impatient days by month.

b. The number of patients with each of the ten most common diagnoses.

c. Numbers of selected services provided, including home visits, vaccinations, health talks, and IUCDs inserted, among others.

d. Quantities of drugs received and used by type.

e. Capital costs, salaries, travel allowances, and other operating expenditures.

f. Total numbers of reports by type and person responsible.

While one is attracted by the availability of such relevant information, certain precautions are necessary. In the first place we must recognize that little supervision or checking goes into the compilation of these reports; therefore, even if the health center recorders are conscientious in compiling them, there is still abundant opportunity for incompleteness, errors, and misunderstandings of interpretation. Secondly, substantial amounts of our own staff time were required in extracting the information desired due to the many report sources, lack of uniformity in reporting, the variety of languages used and the illegible handwriting typically found in the original reports. As a result about four or five full man-months of effort was required in one state to transfer the report data into useable form.

2. Health Center Staff Interviews

During the course of the year-long health center observation period each of the staff members was interviewed with the aid of a structured questionnaire. Information of a personal as well as professional nature was derived from these interviews.

On the personal side the worker was asked about his family and living conditions and the distance from his residence to the health center. His length of service with the health center, previous employment, and his general education and professional training were ascertained. Next, he was asked about his reasons for joining the health center and his job and salary satisfaction.

On the professional side, knowledge about his duties, orientation, and relationship to other staff was determined. In summary fashion a profile of a full week's work was built up by asking the worker to estimate the amount of time he spent in various activities and in various places. The person's opinion about his present ability to use his skills and the possibilities for future advancement were established. Finally, questions were raised pertaining to the various functions of the health center and their relationship to the surrounding community and to other providers of health services.

Because of the central role of the health center doctor, he was asked several additional questions. The answers provided insight into his referral practices, his assessment of the adequacy of drug and equipment supplies, and the ability of patients to pay for a portion of their care. He was asked to make suggestions about possible administrative changes that would improve the functioning of the health center. Then he was queried about his career plans and factors that led him to the medical profession.

3. Patient Follow-up

About 350 of the patients treated on days of patient flow analysis were contacted the next day to ascertain their compliance with medication instructions, their general health status, and the extent of their satisfaction with the care and treatment received at the health center.

Another potentially important aspect of follow-up relates to patient referrals. However, only one of the four health centers in the present study had a significant quantity of referrals. About fifty cases from that health center were checked to establish whether the patient had actually gone to the referral center.

D. Other Government Data

Additional information was obtained from public sources at five levels: public institutions in the study areas; other health centers in Punjab and Mysore; and district, state, and national offices. Within the study areas the registers and reports of dispensaries operated or supported by the government provided data comparable to that described in relation to the health centers themselves.

With the help of the state health directorates a questionnaire was mailed to all of the health centers in the two states in which the study was conducted. This request for information came officially from the health directorate and was signed by one of the deputy directors. It mainly required information to be abstracted from various records and reports in the health center itself and in many ways paralleled the aforementioned data collected in an intensive manner in each of the study health centers from their records.

By the use of repeated reminders and the support of the district health officers, responses were obtained from approximately 97 per cent of all the health centers in Mysore and 70 per cent in Punjab. Although the problems of the reliability of the data are great, as mentioned previously, the fact that such a large number of health centers responded makes these data very useful in permitting certain generalizations to be applied in the states in which the studies were performed.

From a questionnaire sent to district headquarters information was obtained regarding the numbers of district staff posts sanctioned and filled and the salaries. Other expenditures of the district were also estimated. Additional descriptive information was obtained by discussion with the district officials, particularly in the district in which the study health centers were located.

Information at the state level was obtained primarily from statistical compilations made by the state health services. These were supported by the summaries from the health center and district questionnaires and by interviews and discussions with various state officials.

At the national level in India information was obtained from the staff of the Director General of Health Services. Items of information included patient loads, staffing patterns, major functions, health centers using UNICEF vehicles and equipment, and morbidity patterns. These were primarily estimates on an India-wide basis and were not broken down by state. Other information collected included institutions other than health centers supported by the government, financing mechanisms, quantities of services provided in certain categorical programs such as family planning, and some general statements about policies and plans for national health programs. This information, although general in nature, permits certain applications of the analysis to be made to the entire Indian scene.

E. Sources of Private Health Care within the Study Areas

We have already reported that the private sector of medicine is an important factor in all of the study areas. In particular, three types of private practitioner deserve attention. First, the large numbers of indigenous medical practitioners (IMPs) giving services in the study areas needed to be surveyed. Secondly, the few Western-oriented practitioners had to be included since they provided a large segment of private services in comparison to their numbers. Thirdly, the indigenous midwives (the dais) were studied since they provided the bulk of maternity services in the villages.

1. Indigenous Medical Practitioners (IMPs)

In Punjab the feasibility study had already supplied data on about sixty IMPs and 542 of their patients. During the definitive study, therefore, it was necessary only: (1) to identify and interview practitioners whom respondents in the study and consulted, and (2) to reinterview the practitioners in the original survey in order to gain additional information, notably family planning data, of concern to the definitive study.

Corresponding information was obtained from all full-time and almost all part-time practitioners working in the two Mysore development blocks included in the definitive study. This amounted to 30 full-time and nearly 600 part-time practitioners. Furthermore, data were collected from the observation of about 200 patient visits to these practitioners.

The practitioner interview schedule first dealt with his personal attributes, such as his general education and professional training, as well as the hereditary occupation of the family. Then he was asked about his patient load and schedule of charges and the geographic spread of his influence. Enquiry was made into the special systems of medicine practiced, the types of drugs used, and the kinds of equipment and facilities available. Additional factors of interest concerning his practice included the extent of his contacts with allopathic practitioners, his reading of medical literature, and his referrals to fellow practitioners. We attempted to learn something of his knowledge about certain communicable diseases and family planning. Further we asked about his willingness to participate in family planning programs, especially with the government.

Patient interviews and observations were directed to eight major areas: (1) demographic characteristics of the patient, (2) his major complaints; (3) the way in which the practitioner elicited the history and carried out the medical exam; (4) laboratory examinations performed, if any; (5) details of the treatment, including types of medicines or injections given; (6) recommendations or advice, including referral, if any; (7) the method and amount of payment if any; and (8) the total time spent by the practitioner on a particular patient.

2. Qualified Allopathic Practitioners

There were relatively few full-time Western-trained medical practitioners in the areas being studied. In Punjab the respondents in the six study villages identified sixteen such practitioners who had been consulted for an illness. All sixteen were then interviewed, even though many practiced outside the community development blocks studied. In Mysore only the six allopathic practitioners actually practicing within the study area were interviewed.

Each allopath was asked many of the questions posed to the indigenous practitioners. In addition we sought to determine the reasons for his chosen location of practice and to establish any connections he had with the government's work. We also asked about areas of specialization, the use of assistants, laboratory tests performed, and immunizations given.

3. Indigenous Midwives

A limited study of 17 indigenous dais was carried out in Punjab during the feasibility study. Although no further information was gained about midwives in India during the definitive phase, we did collect data on 53 of the 97 indigenous midwives found to be working in the 27 Turkey study villages.

The data gathered included: (1) characteristics of the midwife and the family ; (2) her training and the number of years of experience in total and in her present village; (3) how she identified pregnant women in the village and how often her services were sought during the previous year; (4) details of the way she handled and treated pregnant women before, during and after deliveries; and (5) the types of advice and medicines she prescribed.

II. PRACTICAL FIELD CONSIDERATIONS

To conduct an analysis of activities performed or services provided one can obviously rely either upon existing records or upon specially collected information. While the first approach is intuitively more appealing, it requires ready access to data that are reasonably complete, correct, and in a form suitable to project purposes. Since we found these conditions inadequately fulfilled in our study, we built a substantial amount of our own data collection into the research design. Such an approach produces its own set of problems, however, and these need to be reported before we proceed to a discussion of findings.

The patient flow analysis required the presence of several observers in the health center, and this was not only relatively costly, but it endangered the normal routine of patient-staff encounters. It was necessary, therefore, to stress to the observers that they must operate inconspicuously so as not to bother the staff or interact excessively with the patients. At the beginning of the study, for example, patients departing from the health center were questioned about their understanding and satisfaction with the services just rendered, but this interview procedure was dropped when it was found that the value of the information obtained did not warrant the irritation provoked from patients who felt that they had already been unduly delayed from their normal activities.

The major difficulty with work sampling studies is the possible distortion of normal work habits produced by outside observers. This was minimized in the present study by extensive early efforts at establishing rapport with health center staff, coupled with the fact that observations continued through a full year. Bias in the observations at the health center was undoubtedly minimized by the fact that measurements were spread over several workers, and the timing of observations for a particular worker was determined randomly.

Practical considerations of field work sampling, on the other hand, required that a single worker be trailed continuously, so that he was necessarily more conscious of the presence of the observer. There were other logistical problems as well. Large geographical areas had to be covered and problems in the scheduling of meeting places and in providing transportation had to be resolved.

Observations outside the government health center system involved especially delicate relationships; in fact we initially questioned whether indigenous practitioners could be observed at all. Although it developed that IMPs seemed to appreciate a fair hearing, success was achieved only as a result of patience and careful negotiations on the part of our social scientists. In retrospect we feel that the use of social scientists as observers was essential, for the indigenous practitioners were much less threatened by their visits than they would have been by the sort of peer review clearly associated with health worker observers.

III. THE HEALTH RESOURCES BASE

Health services utilization and activity patterns depend partly on existing levels and distribution of facilities and manpower. It is appropriate, therefore, to preface a discussion of services and activities with a brief inventory of the health resources available in the various study areas.

In both India and Turkey the geo-political boundary of each study area was well defined. In India it was the community development block; in Turkey villages were explicitly assigned to each health unit. In both countries service areas were approximately 100 square miles each. Populations served by the health centers varied greatly, however, averaging 10,000 in Turkey, 64,000 in mysore, and 85,000 in Punjab.

Such artificial boundaries do not necessarily coincide with natural service or catchment areas. It was found, for example, that approximately fifteen per cent of practitioner consultations recorded from Punjab study households and ten percent of those in Mysore were outside the study block. In spite of such discrepancies an account of resources according to politically defined service areas is not only the most feasible approach but it is also relatively satisfactory.

When the various types of full-time private practitioners were added to the health center, subcenter, and government dispensary staff who provide some form of direct health service, the total personnel per study area was approximately 100 in Punjab, 50 in Mysore, and 8 in Turkey. The part-time practitioners identified in each of the areas would also contribute a substantial, though not easily measured, number of additional full-time equivalents to the health care picture.

A. Primary Health Center Configuration

Each Indian study area contained five or six subcenters in addition to the primary health center. The subcenters were staffed by auxiliary nurse-midwives, sometimes supplemented by trained dais. Mysore Area. A maintained three additional clinic subcenters, which were visited weekly by the health center physician. Three other villages served as headquarters for the activities of male basic health workers, each serving a population of approximately 10,000.

The main centers typically included limited facilities for inpatient care, but only Punjab Area A had an active inpatient service. This exception was due to the presence of a physician with considerable interest and experience in surgery, particularly cataract surgery.

The total complements of staff, recommended and actual, are shown in Table 18.1. The recommended Punjab levels are nearly twice those of Mysore. Actual differences were even greater, with Punjab Area A employing on the average three times as many personnel as Mysore Area B. The relationships were not constant, however, since staff turnover was as much as one-fifth of the total during the study year.

Due to strong central control in Turkey, health center standardization in the socialized provinces was much greater than in India. Typically the 10,000 population served by the system was distributed among 30 or more villages. The main center tended to be located in the area's largest village, which housed an average of 1,700 residents. Under the jurisdiction of the main center were three to five midwife stations, where trained midwives were permanently posted and in which weekly clinics were held by the physician when weather permitted.

The staff recommended in Turkey consisted of a doctor, nurse, sanitary technician, four midwives, a clerk, a driver, and a janitor-handy man. In some cases special technicians for trachoma or malaria were also assigned to the health center. The health centers studied were usually fully staffed except for nurses, who were present in only four of the nine centers studied. This reflects the general shortage of nurses in Turkey.

B. Other Formal Health Institutions

Only in India did facilities other than government health centers and individual practitioners' offices provide health services in the study area. Each of the Punjab areas had four government supported dispensaries, three of the western type and one Ayurvedic. Each of the Mysore areas had two government dispensaries. Clinically these public institutions functioned independently, but they relied to some degree on funds and direction provided by the district health officers who also had administrative control over the primary health centers. As part of the national family planning campaign, attempts have increased to coordinate government dispensary and PHC activities.

Each of the Punjab study areas also had an MCH center receiving Red Cross support and district health funds. Although officially supervised by the chief medical officer of the district, in practice they were treated by the primary health centers very much like additional subcenters, especially for family planning work.

One of the study areas in Punjab and one in Mysore contained a privately operated facility. The Mysore facility was owned and operated by a Buddhist religious order. It provided mostly curative services. The Punjab facility was a teaching health center which undertook community activities in the half dozen villages immediately adjacent to it. During the study year the same Punjab Area B witnessed the introduction of MCH and family planning services in six villages included in two other Johns Hopkins research projects.

Qualified allopathic physicians in solo practice represent another kind of private health resource, and our sample households identified eight such practitioners in the Punjab study

Table No. 18.1:
Recommended and actual staffing levels - Primary Health Centres in India, 1968-69

Type of Staff	*Government of India Recommended*	*Punjab*			*Mysore*		
		*Rec.**	*Actual*		*Rec.*	*Actual*	
			PHC A	*PHC B*		*PHC A*	*PHC B*
Doctor	2	2	2	1	2	2	1
Public Health Nurse (PHN)							
Lady Health Visitor (LHV)	2	2	4	1	1	1	1
Nurse (NUR)							
Midwife (MWF)	10	8	8	6	7	7	4
Auxiliary Nurse Midwife (ANM)							
Pharmacist (PHARM)	1	2	2	1	2	1	1
Laboratory Assistant (LAB)	1	1	1	1	1	1	0
Clerk-Computor	2	2	2	2	2	2	2
Block Extension Educator (BEE)	1	1	1	1	1	1	0
Family Planning Worker (FPW)	4	4	2	3	2	1	0
Health Inspector (HI)	3	2	1	2	1	1	1
Basic Health Worker (BHW)	8	8	6	6	5	5	5
Trained Dai (DAI)	8	8	5	4	0	0	0
School Health Assistant (SHA)	0	0	0	0	1	1	0
Vaccinator (VAC)	0	3	2	4	0	0	0
Trachoma Worker (TRAC)**	0	4	4	5	0	0	0
Driver	1	1	1	1	1	0	0
Dresser, Other	3	8	10	4	3	3	2
Total	46	56	51	42	29	26	17

* Recommendations depended upon size and location of PHC; those listed are estimated averages.

** Trachoma campaign discontinued in February, 1969 and workers transferred to other positions.

areas and six in the Mysore areas. One of the former stated that he had 18 inpatient beds and did a considerable amount of surgery.

C. Indigenous Resources

In a rural society which has always had to depend on its own resources to meet its health needs, full acceptance of modern services will not come easily. These services are not being introduced into a vacuum but into a social context (a traditional system of medical aid) which already has an established set of values, norms, and expectations which may contradict those of the modern practitioner. The doctor finds himself in competition with the indigenous practitioner and is frequently at a disadvantage within the traditional frame of reference.

Thus our inventory of resources cannot overlook the 200 or more indigenous medical practitioners based in each of the India study areas or the 135 estimated to be practicing in a typical study area of Turkey. Although most of these devote only a portion of their time to health matters, we did identify at least 50 full-time practitioners in the Punjab study areas and 30 in Mysore.

Most indigenous medical practitioners had some type of training usually as an apprentice, in one of the well-developed traditional medical systems, such as Ayurveda or Unani. In Punjab, however, more than half of these providers included allopathic treatments, notably antibiotics, in their practice. Their place of practice was most frequently in or near the practitioner's home village. Two-thirds of the villages in the Punjab study areas and one-half of those in Mysore were served by indigenous practitioners. Thus the India setting was characterized by the availability of locally known providers of health care whose form of practice did not differ from that of the health center doctor as much as one might at first suspect.

Because indigenous medical practitioners had been outlawed in Turkey by Attaturk, all of them had other occupations. In their medical practice, however, some followed long traditions, though none were as highly developed as in India. Thirty per cent of the Turkey practitioners specialized in bone-setting. One-fourth were religio-magic healers, and these tended to be older men, averaging 52 years of age. Needlemen were the next most common group, and they were all males under the age of 40. Typically they had learned something about medicine by working as hospital attendants or as medical corpsmen during military service. This exposure had prepared them especially for satisfying the demands of villagers for the quick results possible from injections, especially of penicillin which was available without prescription.

Indigenous midwives were common in both India and Turkey. The latter study areas averaged almost four per village of 600 population, while Punjab and Mysore villages averaged one or two resident midwives each. They tended to be women between the ages of 40 and 60 with considerable experience in delivering children. In addition to midwifery, some attended to various female medical complaints and childhood illnesses.

IV. SUMMARY OF HEALTH SERVICES PROVIDED

Within the preceding framework of service capacity we move on to an accounting of the actual utilization of resources. Summarizing first the rather gross service statistics obtained from existing records, we next review the more specific measures of service contact provided by the patient flow and work sampling studies. Finally, the work sampling observations afford a still more detailed activity analysis which gives a basis for understanding staff roles in providing services and the calculation of real program costs. Though this sequence of analysis causes other data sources to be considered first, we consider the work sampling studies to be the core of the health center analysis, and accordingly the main source of essential summary data presented in the concluding section of the chapter.

A. Routine Service Statistics

From routine records of health facilities estimates of patient care services were derived to supplement the information obtained from household surveys. These service statistics are summarized in Table 18.2.

We observe first the marked difference between India and Turkey in the use of private practitioners. This is because the Turkey study was conducted in poorly served provinces where nationalized health services were specifically designed to make care available within the government health center system.

In India the amount of services provided by the health centers and other facilities combined appeared essentially equivalent in the two states investigated. Examination of the distribution of visits among the different facilities shows, however, that there tended to be more than twice as many patient visits to other government facilities as to health centers and subcenters. This was especially true for Area B in Mysore, where two active government local fund dispensaries were located. By contrast, in Mysore Area A the health center served almost as many patients as other government facilities. The importance of these other government facilities certainly should not be overlooked in planning curative services for rural India.

In India, where data were available on the utilization of subcenters for patient care, results are quite varied. Differences between the subcenters in Punjab are probably related directly to staff effort and rapport with the community. A porbable explanation for differences between Punjab and Mysore is that patients only visited Mysore subcenters to see the physician when he came on routine clinic visits, whereas in Punjab the resident auxiliary nurse midwife (ANM) had a routine time every day in which patients could come for minor complaints.

The volume of services provided in India by private practitioners, mostly indigenous, was estimated from statements given by the practitioners about average patient loads (Table 18.3) to be more than double that listed in Table 18.2 for organized facilities and institutions. Among sixty practitioners identified as having been used during the two-week reference period by 870 Punjab study households, ten practitioners accounted for nearly half of the total consultations; one-fourth of the consultations were provided by two practitioners. By contrast, the relatively few private allopathic practitioners accounted for only a small proportion of patients seen.

Table No. 18. 2 :

Total Annual Outpatient visits to the Health Centers, Subcenters and others* facilities in the study areas

(From Each Institution's Records, August 1968-July, 1969 in India, Spring 1968 through Winter 1968-69 in Turkey)

	Total Visits	*Visits per Year per 100 Population*
INDIA		
Punjab - Area A		
PHC	22,271	26
Subcenters	4,666	5
Other Facilities	50,502	58
Total	77,439	89
Punjab - Area B		
PHC	23,989	29
Subcenters	7,636	9
Other Facilities	65,121	79
Total	96,746	117
Mysore - Area A		
PHC**	30,144	43
Subcenters**	1,700	2
Other Facilities	37,594	53
Total	69,438	98
Mysore - Area B		
PHC**	13,023	22
Subcenters**	1,500	3
Other Facilities	50,565	89
Total	65,088	114
TURKEY		
Average per Health Center	2,370	24

* Other facilities are primarily dispensaries as described in the previous section of this chapter.

** Separate statistics not available for PHCs and subcenters in Mysore. Subcenter figures are estimates.

Table No. 18.3:
Total Annual Patient visits to Private Practitioners in the study areas-estimates from practitioner interviews and community surveys

	Indigenous Medicine Practitioners		*Allopathic Practitioners*		*Indigenous Midwives*	
	Visits	*Per 100 Population*	*Visits*	*Per 100 Population*	*Deliveries*	*Per 100 Population*
Punjab	384,000	227	23,500	14	3,600	2.1
Mysore	300,000	234	22,000	17	2,600	2.0
Turkey	575	6	0	0	360	3.6

Consultations to indigenous practitioners were less common in Turkey than in India, a finding that was influenced undoubtedly by the legal constraints in Turkey in contrast to India's official support of the indigenous revival. The role of the indigenous midwife, on the other hand, appears to be more important in Turkey, but since Turkey has a higher birth rate the proportion of all deliveries performed by indigenous midwives was quite similar in the two countries.

In view of the lack of private services in Turkey, one might have expected greater health center utilization. When visits per 100 population per year to public facilities in India and Turkey were compared, however, the utilization rate in Turkey was less than one-fourth that in India. Even when the comparison was limited only to health centers the rates were still higher in India than in Turkey.

The health center records yielded only scattered information about the volume of services provided in functional areas other than patient care. Illustrative statistics for India, presented in Table 18.4, give evidence of the importance attached to communicable disease control and family planning in contrast to the relative neglect of environmental sanitation services. These comparative differences will be documented more fully in the subsequent discussion of the field activity analysis portion of our study.

Administration is a health center function that takes a greater input of time than it deserves (Table 13.4). The Mysore health center doctor was responsible for forwarding nearly one report per day, and his Punjab counterpart was even more heavily burdened. Moreover, this does not include local record-keeping requirements involving budgets, drug and equipment indents, and salary requisitions. With such a volume of records and reports, the quality of information they contain must be suspect, and they are undoubtedly little used even after the laborious recording by hand.

Although not directly related to actual service units, one additional piece of useful information obtained from the health center records is the annual total mileage travelled by health center vehicles in health center work. The information, available only for Punjab and Turkey, indicated that the typical health center in both places logged six to nine thousand vehicle miles per year. In Punjab additional information was available for the types of work for which the health the largest patient volume in Mysore was during the first half of the year. In both states patient volume tended to be heaviest on Mondays and lightest on Tuesdays.

1. Problems Presented

Patient visits were classified in several ways, including age and type of problem presented. We found that diagnoses made by the health center staff were primarily in the form of complaints or presenting symptoms, in terms similar to those used by the villagers themselves in reporting their problems in the household survey. For the patient flow analysis, therefore, we employed the same broad categories that were used for the community data. The resulting rankings of problems are presented in Table 18.6, along with rankings prepared from questionnaires filled out by health center doctors from all of Punjab and Mysore.

Respiratory diseases ranked first in all the health centers studied. The statewide surveys of doctors' estimates showed a higher ranking for infectious and parasitic diseases than was actually observed. Another finding of interest was the reversal in Punjab Health Center A of the relative positions of infectious and parasitic diseases and eye diseases (the predominant group under sensory and nervous system), which was undoubtedly due to special selectivity because the physician at this health center had particular interest and competence in treating eye diseases. Nutritional and skin problems were not ranked as high in the Mysore study areas as in the statewide questionnaire estimates. On the other hand, accidents and injuries were more common in the study areas than in the statewide reports. In general, however, the health centers studied appeared to present a relatively uniform pattern of problems and are probably more accurate than the doctors' estimates of statewide experience. Moreover, a rough comparison of Turkey and India data revealed that the only striking difference was the virtual absence of accidents and injuries among health center patients in Turkey, probably because such cases are typically taken to bone setters and other indigenous practitioners.

When we examined problem patterns within individual age groups, respiratory ailments invariably ranked first, accounting for at least one-fifth of the patient complaints in every age group. The only other conditions approaching this level of frequency were diarrhea in children under the age of five and skin conditions in Punjabi children between the ages of 5 and 14. Apart from respiratory illness, no other single problem category could be singled out as being unusually common among adults.

2. Health Center Services Provided in Response to Problems Presented

A review of health center activities in response to specific patient problems was first directed to the basic question: Who provided what services to the patient, and how long was the patient detained in the process? Then these quantitative data were supplemented by a more qualitative appraisal of service content. Since the answers varied more by state than by health center, the tabulations which follow are consolidated summaries by state.

The total time spent by patients per outpatient visit was found to vary substantially (Table 18.7). In general, however, Mysore patients were processed much more rapidly (9 minutes) than Punjab patients (19 minutes). Although 95 per cent or more of health center

Table No. 18. 5:
India Health Center
Patient Visits Sampled and in Total

	Punjab		*Mysore*	
	PHC A	*PHC B*	*PHC A*	*PHC B*
Total Patient Visits in Study Year	22,271	23,989	30,144	13,023
Number of Patients in Patient Flow Analysis	1,498	1,650	2,174	933
Percent Patients Sampled	6.7	6.9	7.2	7.2

Table No. 18. 6:
Rankings of Diagnostic Categories among Patient Flow Patients and From Statewide PHC Doctor Questionnaire responses in India

	Punjab			*Mysore*		
Diagnostic Category	*PHC A*	*PHC B*	*State*	*PHC A*	*PHC B*	*State*
Infectious and Parasitic	5	2	1	2	2	1
Nutritional and Blood	7	8	6	9	9	3
Sensory Organs and Nervous System	2	6	3	5	5	6
Circulatory and Respiratory	1	1	2	1	1	2
Digestive	4	4	4	3	4	5
Genito-Urinary	8	9	8	7	8	9
Skin	3	3	5	8	6	4
Musculo-Skeletal	9	7	9	6	7	8
Accidents and Injuries	6	5	7	4	3	7

visits were for medical relief, the few patients coming for maternity or family planning services were detained about twice as long on the average (Table 18.8). Regardless of how long a patient had to wait at the health center for whatever purpose, however, he could count on no more than four to six minutes of direct service attention. In fact, the usual pattern involved a sick patient who spent one-fourth to one-half hour at the health center in order to receive three or four minutes of medical care.

This leads to the original question concerning the specific medical relief service activities provided during this brief encounter. Table 18.9 provides the specific activity and personnel breakdown which emerged from the patient flow studies. In Punjab, 2,127 services were provided per 1,000 patients, i.e., 2.1 activities per patient. These almost always included a consultation plus some form of treatment, most frequently the dispensing of drugs. Laboratory services are excluded from the table since they were performed for only 2 percent of the patients in Punjab and 5 per cent in Mysore, and in any event consumed little of the patient's visit time. The average Mysore patient received somewhat fewer (1.8) services compared with the Punjab (2.1), due in part to a lower consultation rate and in part to a more sparing use of drugs and injections than in Punjab.

The pattern of providing services also differed in the two states. Specialization tended to be the theme in Mysore, where the doctor almost always performed the consultations and injections, the pharmacist dispensed the drugs, and the dresser carried out most of the other treatments, usually the dressing of wounds. In Punjab, on the other hand, the pharmacist frequently served as consultant during the doctor's absence and did most of the injections.

Table No. 18. 7: Distribution of Patient Visits by total Time Spent at Health Centers in India Patient Flow Study

	Punjab	*Mysore*
Total Number of Patients Studied	3,133	3,107
Percentage with Total Stay		
(In Minutes)		
0-2	0.9	9.3
3-4	2.9	16.9
5-9	14.7	32.9
10-19	35.3	24.9
20-29	21.2	8.4
30-44	14.3	4.2
45-59	4.8	1.6
60-89	3.7	1.1
90 or more	2.2	0.7
Median Time	19	9
Time Exceeded by Only 5% of Patients	67	39

Indeed, the pharmacist's multi-purpose role in Punjab caused him to provide nearly one service contact per patient, compared with a rate of 0.6 for the doctor. The Mysore doctor and Pharmacist both averaged about 0.7 service contacts per patient.

One thing which Table 18.9 cannot reveal is the effect which staff composition has upon the role assumed by a particular member of the team at a point in time. For example, in Punjab Health Center A, which generally had two physicians and a nurse on its staff, the nurse served as consultant for one patient in seven, whereas the pharmacist seldom assumed this role. In Punjab Health Center B, however, which normally operated with a single doctor and no nurse, the pharmacist consulted with nearly as many patients as the doctor. These important differences between centers serve to reinforce one of the main conclusions from Table 3.9, namely that if personnel such as the Punjab pharmacist are to be called upon to serve as multi-purpose workers they should be trained accordingly.

When several categories of workers are engaged from time to time in the provision of a given service, as in the case of medical consultations in Punjab, one may wonder whether the time devoted per contact varied substantially among workers. If it did one might ask further whether the use if more time resulted from lower efficiency or more thoroughness. In practice, we found little difference in consultation time, regardless of who was involved; the Punjab doctor averaged 2.2 minutes per consultation, the pharmacist 1.8, and the nurse 1.6. It seems

Table No. 18.8:
Mean Total Time and Service Time per patient according to function - from India patient flow study

Function	Punjab			Mysore		
	Number of Patients	Mean Time (Min.)		Number of Patients	Mean Time (Min.)	
		Total	Service		Total	Service
Medical Relief	2,984	24	4	2,978	12	3
Personal Preventive	56	24	6	4	9	2
Maternity	50	36	4	74	27	6
Family Planning	43	39	4	51	38	4

Table No. 18. 9:
Service Activities per 1,000 patients seen for medical relief in India patient Flow Study

Staff Category	*Punjab*					*Mysore*				
	Consul-tations	*Injections*	*Drugs Dispensed*	*Other Treatment*	*Total*	*Consul-tations*	*Injections*	*Drugs Dispensed*	*Other Treatment*	*Total*
Doctor	583	4	31	4	622	613	63	15	2	693
Nurse, LHV, ANM	59	35	133	23	250	56	1	19	4	80
Pharmacist	253	95	565	45	958	68	1	597	32	698
Dresser	2	0	6	201	209	30	0	22	289	341
Other	7	2	57	22	88	15	1	8	2	26
Total	904	136	792	295	2,127	782	66	661	329	1,838

safe to say, therefore, that about 2 of the 4 minutes service time provided per Punjab patients is devoted to consultation, regardless of who the consultant may be.

3. Appraisal of Services Content

With a measure of the quantities of services provided, and an indication of who the providers were, we could move on to an attempt, even though crude, to form more qualitative judgments of the content of the services rendered. Checklists wer constructed for use by the observes as they noted a service being provided. For example, whenever a medical consultation took place the observer determined whether a history was elicited, whether any type of physical examination was performed, and whether the patient was offered any explanation of the consultant's findings.

Even though caution must be exercised in the interpretation of service content, especially when all diagnostic categories are pooled, Table 18.10 provides a helpful initial overview of the manner in which services are provided. It is apparent, for example, that communication with the patient in the form of explanation and advice was generally better in Punjab than in Mysore, but even in Punjab such communication would probably be considered by most to be inadequate, except perhaps in connection with the dispensing of drugs. Incidentally, a special follow-up study of a sample of patients 24 hours after their health center visit revealed that most had used at least some of the drugs provided, although we cannot be sure that they were taken appropriately. Referrals represent another facet of communication, and not only were they virtually non-existent in both states, but another special study showed that any referrals that were made were unlikely to produce any return flow of information to the health center.

Having already noted the brevity of the typical medical consultation, we see in Table 18.10 further evidence of its superficiality. In fairess, however, it should be pointed out that many of the patient encounters were return visits merely to get approval for continuing medication. In Punjab it was possible to separate "new" patients from return visits, and it was found that in only 63 per cent of the former cases was a history elicited.

One item which can hardly be subject to misinterpretation or qualification is the use of sterile injection techniques, and the findings in this regard were disturbing, especially in Punjab. Thus we conclude that even the gross and crude measurement of service content we have employed can be useful in documenting some of the major deficiencies which evidently exist in the type of field setting we have studied.

In Turkey the content of the health center doctor's activities was always assessed by a physician observer; hence the measurement system employed was somewhat more sophisticated than that reported for India. During each physician-patient contact the observer noted those activities on a prepared checklist that in his judgment were appropriate to that patient and his circumstances. Such activities were in turn state "performed adequately" or "performed inadequately or not at all." These ratings, aggregated over a series of patients, produced activity scores as the percentage of occasions on which a needed activity was in fact performed adequately.

Table No. 18.10:
Content of Patient Services - From India Patient Flow Study

	Punjab	*Mysore*
Consultations - Total Number	2,790	2,403
Percent Having -		
History Elicited	48	34
Examination - Affected Area	22	19
Examination - General	2	7
Vital Signs Checked	11	6
Explanation and Advice	34	14
Prescription Given for Outside Purchase	13	5
Referral	2	1
Injection - Total Number	421	167
Percent Having -		
Medication Brought by Patient	21	25
Sterile Equipment Used	9	36
Drugs Dispensed - Total Number	2,472	2,043
Percent Having -		
Explanation and Advice	84	17
Other Treatment - Total Number	879	986
Percent Having -		
Explanation and Advice	25	33

The results from a total of 675 doctor-patient contacts are summarized in Table 18.11. The doctors usually established good rapport with the patient and performed the history-taking and physical examination activities adequately. However, they seldom made use of available laboratory tests or referral procedures, and they failed to communicate well with the patient following the consultation except to explain the recommended treatment. The poor communication carried over to record-keeping, where the only items written down in a majority of instances were the patient's diagnosis and the type of drugs given.

Because Indian nurses and pharmacists, as well as doctors, performed consultations, it is useful to compare the three categories of workers along the lines we have been discussing. Five important items were selected from the checklist for this purpose. Results for each of the

Table No. 18.11:

Physician's performance of Selected items related to patient care. Cumulative scores from Observations made of 675 Doctor-Patient contacts in Nine Turkish health Centres

Items Assessed	*Score**
Rapport	
Doctor established rapport with the patient	82
Preparation	
Auxiliary prepared the patient for the doctor, vital signs taken (BP, temperature, pulse)	23
History	
Patient permitted to describe complaints	84
History elicited by the physician's questions	81
Adequate history taken before the exam	70
Physical Examination	
Patient undressed when necessary	50
Patient examined lying on a table	64
General systems examination conducted	42
Affected area examined, including use of special procedures	73
Laboratory	
Necessary laboratory examinations ordered and performed	6
Referrals	
The health center's diagnostic and therapeutic facilities. appropriately used before the referral	54
Complete findings sent with the patient	20
Referral explained to the patient	43
Referred to auxiliary staff for special advice	25
Instructions and Advice	
Cause and diagnosis explained to patient	38
Prescribed treatment explained	83
Duration and outcome (prognosis) explained	16
Return visit instructions mentioned	22
Record Keeping	
Symptoms and duration of illness recorded	3
Vital signs recorded	19
Positive physical signs recorded	21
Treatment recorded	69
Drug dosage recorded	48
Duration of therapy for each drug recorded	16
Medical diagnosis (not symptoms) recorded	89
Multiple or alternate diagnosis recorded	17
Interruptions	
No interruptions by other staff during consultation	47

* Maximum score for each item = 100. See text for definition.

**Table No. 18.12:
Overall Performance Scores for selected patient care items in India and Turkey by Health Center Staff performing the consultation**

	Scores*				
		Turkey	India		
Items Assessed	*Weights Given*	*Doctors*	*Doctors*	*Pharmacists*	*Nursing Staff*
History Elicited	4	81	54	39	20
Physical Examination of at Least the Affected Area	3	73	34	8	3
Vital Sings Checked	1	23	10	14	4
Appropriate Laboratory Tests Ordered	1	6	32	14	27
Treatment Explained to the Patient	1	83	29	16	15
Total Weighted Score		66	39	22	14

* Maximum score for each item or total = 100. See text for definition.

five are listed in Table 18.12, and a weighted score has also been computed for illustrative purposes. In addition the table shows comparative scores for the Turkey doctors, who scored highest on every item except laboratory tests. The Indian doctors' performance was generally superior to that of the pharmacists, who in turn rated higher than the nursing staff. The most striking difference among the three categories of the Indian health center staff was the low score for pharmacists and nurses in the performance of physical examinations. In their consultations they appear to have depended primarily upon patients' descriptions of complaints.

Further comparisons were made with individual diagnostic categories such as respiratory illnesses, diarrhea, and undiagnosed fevers. The results tended to produce few additional insights and in any case had to be considered tentative because of the limited numbers of observations in any one category.

In closing the present discussion we must underscore the fact that measurement of the quality of medical care is generally conceded to be exceedingly difficult, especially when one tries to relate care provided to alteration of health status. Moreover, in view of the many ramifications of quality, we must recognize that subjective value judgments have strengths in summarizing multiple complex variables in addition to the obvious weaknesses. Our findings show that the assessment of service content can be an important, though admittedly limited, aspect of the total quality issue, and furthermore that content analysis based upon the employment of simple checklists can be fruitfully carried out by non-professional observers.

C. Analysis of Field Service Contacts in India

In the part of functional analysis which was carried out from the perspective of the health center staff rather than the patient, we relied mostly upon work sampling of staff activities. During the field work sampling, however, each observer made a complete tally of the observed worker's service contacts according to functional area. This information was designed to complement that obtained from the patient flow analysis in the health center itself. Whereas the health center services were almost exclusively devoted to medical relief, however, the field services covered the spectrum of functions.

The tally of service contacts of each category of worker over the varying periods of observation was translated into annual estimates by function. The assumption was that each worker, except the doctor, was active in the field about 260 days per year. Since the doctor usually spent about twenty per cent of his time in the field, annual estimates of his field time were based upon 52 days of field activity. The results of these calculations are presented in Table 18.13, in which data from individual health centers have been consolidated to produce state averages for Punjab and Mysore. Then, taking existing staffing levels into consideration, weighted totals of annual service contacts have been estimated for each functional area at the bottom of the table. Finally, the annual estimates have been converted to a daily basis in order to provide a comparison of field activity patterns on a typical day. For a total of all services then these figures should be added to the roughly 20,000 outpatient visits annually generating about 40,000 service contacts, mostly for medical relief, in the health center itself.

It is clear that every category of worker was multi-functional (Table 18.13). Each worker in Mysore tended to have more service contacts than his Punjab counterpart, but since staffing

Table No. 18.13: Estimated Annual Volume of Field Service contacts by staff type and function - State averages compiled from field worker observations in India

Staff Category	Punjab							Mysore						
					Communicable Diseases Control							Communicable Diseases Control		
	Medical Relief	Personal Preventive	Maternity	Family Planning	Immuni-zation	Malaria/ Trachoma	Env. Sanitation	Medical Relief	Personal Preventive	Maternity	Family Planning	Immuni-zation	Malaria/ Trachoma	Env. Sanitation
Doctor (DR)	130	6	60	220	60	190	0	470	210	30	60	110	90	2
Lady Health Visitor (LHV)	510	460	260	850	990	0	0	1,680	660	760	800	270	0	6
Auxiliary Nurse Midwife (ANM)	990	300	290	760	480	5	0	1,400	1,500	960	820	1,020	0	20
Trained Dai (TD)	830	250	210	480	160	0	0	—	—	—	—	—	—	—
Health Inspector (HI)	210	30	0	230	1,280	1,130	340	320	580	90	410	2,340	740	120
Block Extension Educator (BEE)	60	10	5	2,150	80	70	80	260	60	6	1,870	160	70	6
Family Planning Worker (FPW)	20	30	30	2,570	10	10	10	100	80	0	2,110	40	10	0
Base Health Worker (BHW)	130	0	0	10	210	10,080	20	650	820	70	400	3,430	7,510	60
Trachoma/Plague Worker (TPW)	0	0	0	30	60	23,460	60	—	—	—	—	—	—	—
Vaccinator (VAC)	10	40	0	40	4,310	20	0	—	—	—	—	—	—	—
Weighted Estimate Annual of Total	25,800	8,800	7,200	47,200	51,800	305,200	1,900	22,500	22,100	9,700	18,700	44,500	69,400	1,000
Service Daily Contacts	99	34	28	182	199	1,174	7	87	85	37	72	171	267	4

levels were higher in Punjab, the total volume of services was rather similar in the two states. The functional balance was quite different, however. The Punjab workers tended to emphasize malaria and trachoma control, and to some extent family planning contacts, whereas Mysore workers spent more time in the provision of MCH services. (Very little other than well-child care was noted under personal preventive services.) Neither state provided much environmental sanitation. Both had something over half as many illness service contacts in the field as were provided in the health center.

Field medical relief and MCH services were largely the domain of the nursing staff, but in Mysore the basic health worker was also important in these areas. In Mysore doctors were much more active in providing medical care and well-child services than in Punjab.

Family planning contacts were distributed among many staff categories, but family planning workers and block extension educators tended to focus more exclusively than others in this area, as one might expect.

Among the large volume of Punjab contacts in communicable diseases control, apart from immunizations, about one-third were associated with the trachoma control program, and two-thirds were for malaria control. This does not reflect the balance of time in these areas, however, for the trachoma worker often served many children in a short period of time. In Mysore there was no trachoma program, and therefore no specialized worker on the health center staff. In both states the basic health worker did most of the malaria work, but the malaria control program was much less active in Mysore than in Punjab.

V. Findings From the Analysis of Work Sampling in India

Standard methods of work sampling, as described earlier, were employed at the health center and in the field in order to generate activity profiles: (1) to appraise the appropriateness of existing work patterns; (2) to link service statistics to specific activities; (3) to identify staff training priorities, both in regard to skills required and functional areas to be emphasized; and (4) as a basis for determining health services costs along functional lines. In order to satisfy these aims it was necessary to classify and analyze the observations in two ways; first, according to the manner and extent to which the observed activity contributed to the health center's basic community service mission; and secondly, wherever possible, according to the specific service function being advanced. In connection with the first approach, we classified activities as: direct service, support, travel, or personal. For purposes of the discussion to follow, five functional groupings appear adequate. Since personal preventive services were found to be made up largely of well-child care, these have been combined with maternity services to form a consolidated maternal and child health (MCH) function. The other four functions which appeared often enough to be included here are those noted in previous sections: medical relief (Med Rel), family planning (Fam Plan), communicable diseases control (CDC), and environmental sanitation (Env San). In the figures and tables which follow, information from individual health centers in each study region has been combined to form state averages. These, of course, must be considered illustrative rather than representative in view of the non-random manner in which study health centers were selected.

A. Overall Activity Profiles

In preparing health center activity profiles with a service orientation, as in Figure 18.1, one might have in mind an inverted triangle as an ideal. A very substantial direct service component should be supported by the necessary, but ideally lesser, components of administrative and other supporting activities. Staff travel time is unavoidable, especially in connection with field work, but obviously output would increase if greater efficiency in travel could minimize the time invested. Finally, it is apparent that personal time is by its very nature unproductive and should therefore be a negligible factor in the activity profile.

To anyone holding such an image as an ideal, the findings summarized in Figure 18.1 are disappointing indeed. In the Punjab the greatest time investment is in administrative support and personal activities, while in Mysore the largest block of time goes into travel. The mere presentation of such activity profiles, however, without further analysis and interpretation does little to indicate whether performance can be improved by manipulating present conditions or whether the ideal itself is unrealistic. Nevertheless these activity profiles serve as useful starting points for consolidating large quantities of data compiled from observations of all categories of staff, each engaged in separate and varied activities. Each manpower category was assigned a weight in the overall profile in accordance with the relative manhour contribution it made to the total health center operation.

Only about one-sixth of the total health center effort went into direct service in Punjab, compared to one-fourth in Mysore. Moreover, in Punjab supporting activities consumed more than twice as much time as service efforts. Virtually all service activities are function-specific, and this further breakdown reveals that the Mysore health centers were more active than the Punjab centers in every functional area except environmental sanitation, which received little attention in either place. The state differences are especially noteworthy in the MCH area, where Mysore devoted three times as much effort as Punjab. While these differences might not hold up with a wider sampling of facilities in each state, the point is that the approach used in Figure 18.1 provides clear evidence, reported simply, of dramatic differences that would not be readily apparent in the subjective impressions of an intermittent visitor, such as the state director of health services. The objective findings are also interesting in comparison to the responses of the workers when they were asked to list the major functions of health centers. While they gave lowest priority to environmental sanitation in accordance with their observed behavior, they attached more verbal importance to both medical relief and family planning than to communicable diseases control, which is in clear contrast to actual practice.

Most of the supporting activities cannot be allocated readily to specific functions; many accourting activities, for example, support the total health center operation rather than contributing directly to particular functions. For this reason the "Support" blocks of Figure 18.1 have been divided according to activity content rather than purpose. The first two categories, records-reports and preparation-maintenance-cleaning (P/M/C), are self-evident. Staff interactions are defined as on-the-job relationships that involve communications, in-service training, supervision, or assisting. General meetings less directly associated with specific service activities have been included in the fourth category of support, along with other non-written administrative tasks and a few miscellaneous activities that are difficult to

Figure 18.1
Health Center Activity Profiles (% Time Distribution) From India Work Sampling

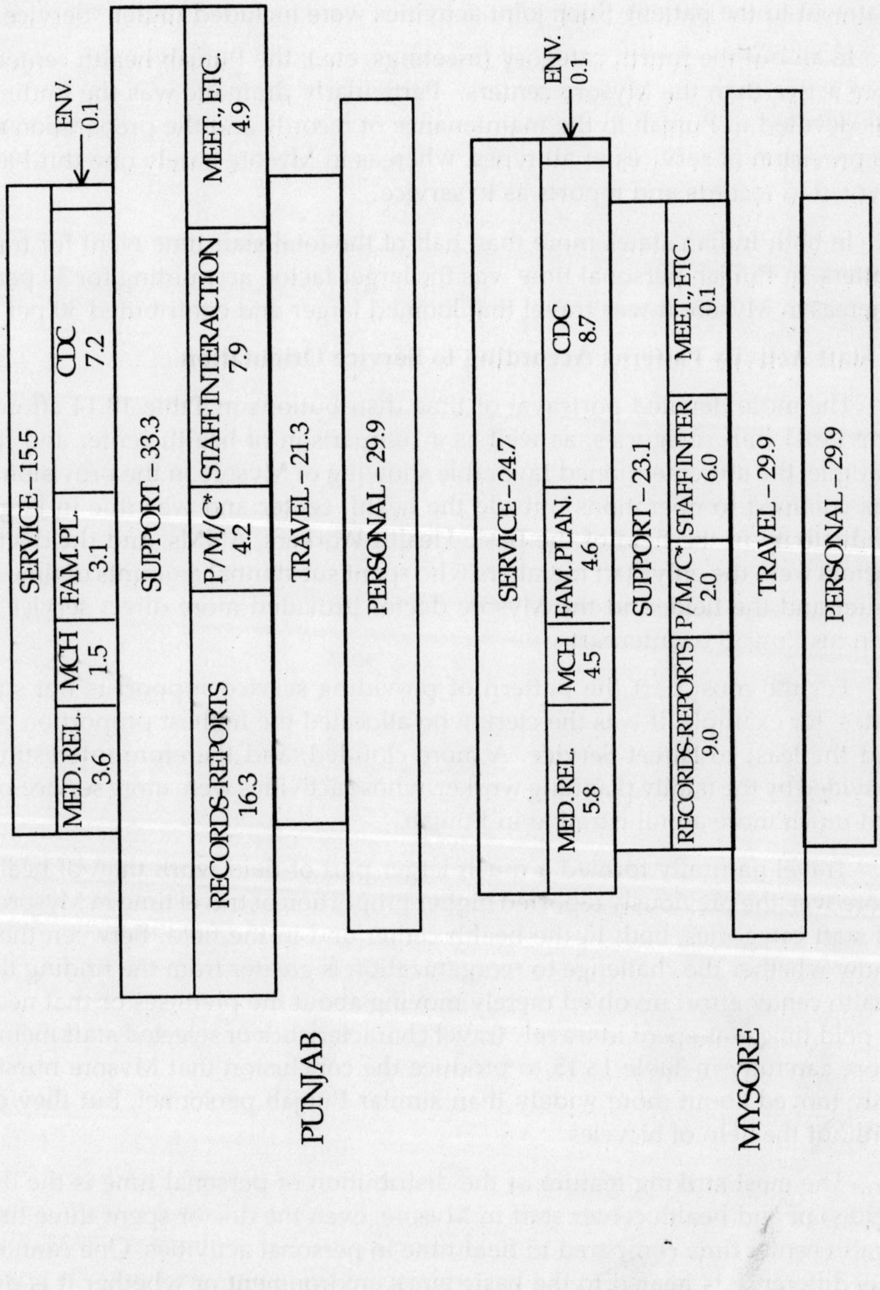

* P/M/C – Preparation, Maintenance, Cleaning

classify elsewhere. Occasionally supporting tasks were carried out simultaneously with service activities, as when the doctor recorded a patient's diagnosis while explaining the recommended treatment to the patient. Such joint activities were included under "Service."

In all but the fourth category (meetings, etc.), the Punjab health centers were relatively more active than the Mysore centers. Particularly dramatic was the finding that more time was devoted in Punjab to the maintenance of records and the preparation of reports than to the provision of services of all types, whereas in Mysore barely one-third as much time was devoted to records and reports as to service.

In both Indian states more than half of the total staff time went for travel and personal matters. In Punjab personal time was the larger factor, accounting for 30 per cent of the total, whereas in Mysore it was travel that loomed larger and contributed 30 per cent to the total.

B. Staff Activity Patterns According to Service Orientation

The more detailed portrayal of time distributions in Table 18.14 affords an analysis by individual staff categories, as well as a comparison of health center and field patterns. For example, the aforementioned favorable showing of Mysore in the provision of direct services was confined to operations outside the health center and was due in large measure to the productivity in the field of the Basic Health Workers, ANMs, and the doctor. In both states doctors were the only staff members who spent substantial amounts of time in both the health center and the field, and the Mysore doctor provided more direct service in both locations than his Punjab counterpart.

For the most part the pattern of providing service support is not surprising. In both states, for example, it was the clerk who allocated the highest proportion of time to Support and the least to Direct Service. A more clouded, and therefore interesting, exception was provided by the family planning worker, whose activities were more service-oriented in Mysore and much more administrative in Punjab.

Travel naturally formed a much larger part of field work than of health center activity. Moreover, the previously reported higher proportion of travel time in Mysore held for virtually all staff categories, both in the health center and in the field. Between the two it is hard to know whether the challenge to reorganization is greater from the finding that ten per cent of health center effort involved merely moving about the premises or that nearly forty per cent of field time was spent in travel. Travel characteristics of selected staff member are examined more carefully in Table 18.15 to produce the conclusion that Mysore nursing personnel not only moved about more widely than similar Punjab personnel, but they did so completely without the help of bicycles.

The most striking feature of the distribution of personal time is the difference between field staff and health center staff in Mysore; even the doctor spent three time as much of his health center time compared to field time in personal activities. One cannot be sure whether this difference is related to the basic work environment or whether it is due to the fact that field workers were followed continuously by our project observer, whereas health center observations were made in a random manner. If the latter factor caused a departure from normal behavior on the part of the Mysore field staff, the Punjab field staff must for some

Table No. 18.14:
Staff allocation of time according to service Relationship - from India work Sampling

Staff Category	Percentage Distribution - Punjab					Percentage Distribution - Mysore				
	Number of Observations	Direct Service	Support	Travel	Personal	Number of Observations	Direct Service	Support	Travel	Personal
HEALTH CENTER										
Dr.	1,714	27	43	4	26	1,666	32	20	10	38
Nurse	688	13	36	5	46	586	17	32	19	32
Pharmacist	1,677	29	33	9	29	1,750	19	24	19	38
Dresser	1,122	22	26	6	46	958	15	31	12	42
Lab Tech.	375	44	21	3	32	417	28	25	4	43
Clerk	608	4	65	3	28	635	1	38	3	58
Total PHC		22	40	5	33		18	29	10	43
FIELD*										
Dr.	262	13	39	37	11	754	24	15	49	12
LHV	2,278	17	32	19	32	1,890	15	32	39	14
ANM	4,060	15	28	22	35	1,733	32	11	42	15
TD	1,408	9	14	23	54	-	-	-	-	-
HI	2,141	9	37	35	19	1,872	11	31	51	7
BEE	2,828	19	23	29	29	1,891	16	28	42	14
FPW	1,138	8	38	27	27	1,077	16	13	48	24
BHW-TVS**	1,812	17	37	24	22	2,186	35	24	32	9
Total Field		14	32	24	30		28	21	39	12
Grand Total		16	33	21	30		25	23	30	22

* Abbreviations used in this and subsequent tables are as follows: LHV - lady health visitor; ANM - auxiliary nurse - midwife; TD - trained dai; HI - health Inspector; BEE - block extension educator; FPW - family planning field worker; BHW - basic health worker.

** Data for Trachoma Workers and Vaccinators in Punjab and School Health Assistant in Mysore combined with Basic Health Worker information.

Table No. 18.15:

Travel Characteristics of LHV and ANM Staff - from India work Sampling

State	*Staff Category*	*Villages per Day*	*Miles of Major Travel per Day*	*Per cent of Observations in Major Travel*	*Percent of Time Major Travel by -*		
					Foot	*Bicycle*	*Other*
Punjab	LHV	0.6	4.6	11	47	29	24
	ANM-Center	0.8	7.6	15	35	30	35
	ANM-Subcenter	0.9	2.9	10	72	6	22
Mysore	LHV	1.2	10.8	23	36	0	64
	ANM-Center	1.1	3.1	11	78	0	22
	ANM-Subcenter	1.5	8.0	33	64	0	36

reason have felt less threatened, since they, like the health center staff, consumed nearly one-third of their work day in personal time.

In Table 18.14 each category of staff is considered separately, meaning that the row percentages add to 100. A corollary summarization format is provided by Table 18.16, in which the column percentages total 100. Hence the latter table identifies, for example, the extent to which each staff category contributed to the total health center service effort. Similarly, contributions to supporting activities and total travel are also shown. We find that more than three-fourths of all direct service activities took place in the field and that these were supplied largely by Basic Health Workers and ANMs, partly because each health center had large numbers of these workers. Their contribution to the total service effort was especially large in Mysore, however, because in that state these workers devoted an unusually large proportion of their time to direct service activities, as noted in Table 18.14. Consequently Table 18.16 serves to combine the quantitative and qualitative contributions of the various staff categories.

C. Staff Patterns of Direct Service Activity by Function

The next stage of the activity analysis focussed upon the Direct Service component and explored variations among the staff categories in their functional roles. Referring to Figure 18.1 as a basic model, Tables 18.14 and 18.16 examined the Direct Service, Support, Travel, and Personal bars of the figure as they related to individual staff categories. Now, in Tables 18.17 and 18.18 the functional subdivisions of the Direct Service bar are examined as they relate to individual staff categories. As in earlier tables, Table 18.17 treats each staff category independently, so that row percentages add to 100, while Table 18.18 treats each function separately, with column percentages totalling 100.

The tables provide the expected evidence that health centers are mainly bases for medical relief, except for the work of the laboratory technician who examines blood Smears for malaria control. It is interesting to note, however, that at least one-third of all medical care services were provided outside the health center. The field staff are also active in providing MCH and family planning services and especially in communicable diseases control, so that field work is clearly more multi-functional than health center work. Some of the workers , notably the doctors and the nursing personnel, are themselves multi-functional with respect to personal health services. On the other hand, the Block Extension Educators and Family Planning Workers are essentially single-purpose family planning worker, and Basic Health Workers are almost entirely engaged in communicable diseases control. More detailed analysis reveals that in Punjab some centered their attention upon immunization programs, while others concentrated on malaria or trachoma control. As supervisors of the Basic Health Workers, the Health Inspectors were also active in communicable diseases control, and in addition they were the only ones to spend a rather substantial amount of time in environmental sanitation. Overall the two states wee remarkably similar in functional balance, except that MCH services were stressed more in Mysore and communicable disease control was emphasized more in Punjab.

Table 18.18 shows that many individuals contributed to the medical relief and family planning functions. However, MCH services could largely be attributed to the ANMs and communicable diseases control was the domain of the BHWs. The contribution to

Table No. 18.18:
Service Contributions by Staff Category to selected functions - from India Work Sampling

Staff Category	Percentage Distribution - Punjab					Percentage Distribution - Mysore				
	Medical Relief	*MCH*	*Family Planning*	*CDC*	*Environmental Sanitation*	*Medical Relief*	*MCH*	*Family Planning*	*CDC*	*Environmental Sanitation*
HEALTH CENTER										
Dr.	16.0	1.0	2.6	0	0	29.7	3.6	1.5	0	0
Nurse	3.6	0.7	0.6	0	0	5.2	0.7	0.2	0	0
Pharmacist	25.2	0.2	1.4	0	0	17.4	0.1	0.2	0	0
Dresser	13.9	0	0.5	0	0	13.3	0	0	0	0
Lab Tech.	1.7	0	4.0	10.7	0	1.2	0	0	13.2	0
Clerk	0	0	4.4	0	0	0	0	0	1.2	0
Total PHC	60.4	1.9	13.5	10.7	0.0	66.8	4.4	1.9	14.4	0.0
FIELD*										
Dr.	0.3	0.5	0.7	0.5	0	2.9	1.9	1.5	0.2	0
LHV	3.8	16.0	12.9	0.9	0	2.8	4.0	7.4	0.4	2.2
ANM	24.1	61.4	21.8	2.0	0	17.6	63.6	45.0	8.7	21.8
TD	9.8	18.6	7.4	0.2	0	—	—	—	—	—
HI	0.5	0.3	0.7	2.8	40.0	0.6	1.0	3.4	3.1	41.4
BEE	0.1	0.7	13.8	0.2	5.6	0.7	0.4	14.8	0.2	0
FPW	0.5	0.6	26.1	0.3	0	0.3	0.4	12.4	0	0
BHW-TVS**	0.5	0	3.1	82.4	54.4	8.3	24.3	13.6	73.0	34.6
Total Field	39.6	98.1	86.5	89.3	100.0	33.2	95.6	98.1	85.6	100.0
Grand Total	100.0	100.0	100.0	100.0	100.0	100.0	100.0	100.0	100.0	100.0

environmental sanitation was split because large numbers of BHWs were each doing a little in this area, and a small number of Health Inspectors were each doing a fair amount.

D. Staff Patterns of Work in Supporting Activities

While the question of functional mix is most meaningful in relation to service activities, some consideration should be given to supporting activities as well. The problem is that the majority of study observations on supporting activities were classed as non-function specific. One possibility is to assume that all Support time had the same functional distribution as observations found to be function-specific. We made this arbitrary functional assignment and combined Direct Service time with Support time, obtaining the functional mix shown in the lower portion of Figure 18.2. Compared with the distribution of Direct Service Only time (upper portion of Figure 18.2), family planning was then calculated to be much more important in the functional balance in both states. Because of the arbitrariness of the functional assignment, it is impossible to place much reliance in this broader-based functional alignment, but it certainly suggests that the family planning function has a much larger supportive element within it than the other functions have. For this reason we next looked carefully at the content of supportive activities for staff members who devoted substantial portions of their time to family planning.

Table 18.19 offers such an analysis in that it portrays for each staff category the distribution of Support time along activity content lines, much as Table 18.17 presented Direct Service time along functional lines. Both the Block Extension Educator and Family Planning Worker, who spent most of their Direct Service time on family planning, also spent exceptional amounts of their Support time in Staff Interactions. The same was true of the field nursing staff, who also contributed materially to the Family Planning function (Table 18.18). Another staff member to be specially mentioned is the Clerk, for although he provided little Direct Service, nearly all of his Support time that was function-specific was related to the Family Planning function Table 18.19 shows that much of this activity involved the maintenance of records and the preparation of reports. In summary, then, we conclude that family planning activities required a large element of Support in addition to Direct Service and that much of this support took the form of Staff Interactions and Records-Reports, the value of which may bear further investigation.

Also in Table 18.19, it can be noted that, apart from the Clerk, the workers with the highest proportion of Support time devoted to Records-Reports were the Health Inspector and the BHW, both of whom were mainly engaged in providing communicable diseases control services. While this attention to reporting might be legitimate for the Health Inspector in his capacity as a supervisor, the need for the BHW to spend so much time in these activities might be questioned.

E. Activity Profiles of Specific Staff Categories

Work sampling measurements provide opportunities for aggregation and analysis at a number of levels and along several dimensions. One extreme of aggregation is exemplified by activity profiles for entire health centers or states, as illustrated by Figure 18.1. At the other extreme we can now construct profiles for each staff category. Such special analyses are illustrated in Table 18.20 for one member of the health center staff, the Pharmacist, and in

Figure: 18.2

Distribution of Staff Time among Functions: with and without Support Time Included -- from India Work Sampling

Direct Service Only	Punjab	MED. REL. 23	MCH 10	FAM. PLAN. 20	COM. DIS. CONT. 46
	Mysore	MED. REL. 23	MCH 18	FAM. PLAN. 19	COM. DIS. CONT. 39
Direct Service Plus Support	Punjab	MED. REL. 15	MCH 10	FAM. PLAN. 34	COM. DIS. CONT. 41
	Mysore	MED. REL. 19	MCH. 15	FAM. PLAN. 33	COM. DIS. CONT. 33

* ENVIRONMENTAL SANITATION – 1% or less

Table No. 18.19:
Staff Allocation of Support Time by Activity class—from India Work Sampling

Staff Category	Percentage Distribution - Punjab					Percentage Distribution - Mysore				
	Number of Observations	Records Reports	Preparation Maintenance Clearning	Staff Interactions	Meetings, etc.	Number of Observations	Records Reports	Preparation Maintenance Cleaning	Staff Interactions	Meetings, etc.
HEALTH CENTER										
Dr.	617	34	3	27	36	284	25	5	32	38
Nurse	265	21	34	13	32	228	27	16	48	9
Pharmacist	587	34	23	31	12	444	36	21	13	30
Dresser	332	1	79	11	9	287	1	27	19	53
Lab Tech.	138	35	23	30	12	138	48	7	23	22
Clerk	377	60	3	15	22	242	50	2	24	24
Total PHC		35	23	22	20		32	11	25	32
FIELD										
Dr.	103	32	1	46	21	110	13	8	26	53
LHV	737	44	8	38	10	602	31	3	43	23
ANM	1,155	49	9	31	11	193	32	11	34	23
TD	202	7	37	42	14	–	–	–	–	–
IU	791	56	5	24	15	582	41	3	29	27
BEE	643	33	8	40	19	532	26	0	36	38
FPW	429	38	11	35	16	139	32	0	36	32
BHW-TVS	673	72	6	9	13	524	58	9	14	19
Total Field		52	10	24	14		42	7	27	24
Grand Total		49	13	24	14		39	9	26	26

Table 18.21 for one member of the field team, the ANM. At this level of summarization it has seemed most appropriate to display the data in terms of minutes per typical workday devoted to various activities.

Since nearly all of the health center service time is for the Medical Relief function, the Pharmacists's Service time, as well as his Support time, has been broken down according to content areas within that function. Table 18.20 reveals that the Punjab Pharmacist spent more time in Service and Support than his Mysore counterpart, while the latter was spending larger portions of his time in less-productive Travel and Personal activities. Moreover, the Service activities of the Punjab Pharmacist were more varied than those of the Mysore pharmacist, who was mostly engaged in the dispensing of drugs. In both states most of their Support time was devoted to Records and Reports.

A comparison of Punjab and Mysore ANMs produced quite different conclusions. The Mysore ANM devoted nearly twice as much time as the Punjab ANM to Direct Service, notably in MCH and Family Planning. She also spent more than two hours of her five-hour workday in Travel. On the other hand, the Punjab ANM devoted three times as much effort as the Mysore ANM to Support activities, and she consumed nearly two hours per day in Personal time.

VI. COST ACCOUNTING OF HEALTH CENTER EXPENDITURES[1]

Cost accounting is an essential ingredient in the assessment of health center resources utilizaiton. Linked with studies that generate information about the performance of activities by the staff, it provides a means for determining how these resources are related to the various health center services. The intent, therefore, of the cost analysis in this study was to develop an accounting procedure that would highlight the distribution of health center costs by functions and activities. Even a relatively simple method, such as the one described in this section, would be of immense use to health administrators if it were applied on a continuing basis over a period of time and in a representative sample of health centers. If would permit the comparison of expenditures within the health center system and the monitoring of trends in these expenditures. Specifically the application of this procedure would:

(a) assist in controlling health center expenditures;

(b) provide a better basis for preparing adequate health center budgets;

(c) facilitate the distribution of expenses and thus permit calculations of costs of specific programs such as family planning;

(d) permit the derivation of unit costs for services rendered; and

(e) contribute to decision-making in the planning of health center programs.

A. Summary of the Method[2]

The procedures outlined here are designed to derive cost figures for each function by cumulating the money value of all resources, including the workers' time, utilized in performing the various activities within each function. The distribution of staff time obtained

Table No. 18. 20:
Pharmacist's Typical Day in the Health Center—From India Work Sampling

Activity	*Time in Minutes*			
	Punjab		*Mysore*	
SERVICE		99		68
Consultations	29		9	
Injections	21		1	
Drugs Dispensed	34		52	
Other Treatment	15		6	
SUPPORT		114		87
Records, Reports	39		32	
Preparation, Maintenance, Cleaning	28		17	
Staff Interactions	34		11	
Meetings, etc.	13		27	
TRAVEL		30		69
PERSONAL		102		136
GRANT TOTAL		345		360

from work sampling was extensively used in distributing expenditures by function. Information collected directly from health center records or other sources[3,4], included capital expenditures appropriately depreciated (buildings, furniture, equipment and vehicles), annual fixed recurring expenditures (maintenance of buildings, furniture and equipment), annual variable recurring expenditures (vehicle running costs and maintenance, drugs, other expendable supplies, and special family planning incentives) and salaries and allowances. Except for information on salaries, allowances, incentives and vehicle costs, which were readily available from accounting records, all other expenditure information was obtained with some difficulty, often requiring estimates by knowledgeable officials. This lack of precision precluded the development of a method with a high level of sophistication. The latter is seldom achieved, however, even by the most refined accounting procedures (American Hospital Association, 1962, and Green, 1969). A differentiation between variable and fixed costs was attempted for certain recurring expenditures. Capital costs and salaries may be considered fixed up to a certain point depending on the system's ability to improve the coverage of a defined population with available facilities and to increase staff members' productivity. Beyond these limits capital and staff costs obviously cannot remain fixed. Data for determining the current limits could be estimated from the findings on geographical coverage and distribution of staff time. Indirect costs of administration such as those incurred for supervisory efforts made by district, state or national health officials towards health center programs are not included in this method.

Table No. 18.21:

ANM's Typical Day in the Field — from India Work Sampling

Activity	Punjab						Mysore					
	Medical Relief	*MCH*	*Family Planning*	*CDC*	*Not Function-Specific*	*Total Minutes*	*Medical Relief*	*MCH*	*Family Planning*	*CDC*	*Not Function-Specific*	*Total Minutes*
SERVICE	16	18	13	3	0	50	14	40	29	12	0	95
SUPPORT	6	15	24	5	45	95	1	3	6	6	17	33
Records, Reports	4	9	13	4	17	47	0	2	0	2	6	10
Preparation, Maintenanee, Cleaning	1	1	1	0	5	8	0	0	1	3	0	4
Staff Interactions	1	4	9	1	14	29	1	1	3	1	6	12
Meetings, etc.	0	1	1	0	9	11	0	0	2	0	5	7
TRAVEL						73						125
PERSONAL						115						46
GRAND TOTAL						333						299

B. Findings

1. Function and Activity Costs

The actual results obtained by applying the cost accounting procedure to the data available showed that the average health center in Turkey and Punjab incurred approximately twice the expenditures of a similar facility in Mysore. The total annual expenditures per health center expressed in U.S. dollars were about $21,000 in punjab, $11,000 in Mysore, and $25,000 in Turkey (Tables 18.22-18.24). The annual per capita expenditures for the defined service area of the health centers were $0.25, $0.17, and $2.50 respectively. All expenditures are obviously much higher in Turkey, but the differences in India are primarily related to salaries and recurring expenditures. A larger complement of staff and higher salaries in Punjab explains the salary difference in India while much greater expenditures on drugs and family planning incentives in Punjab produces the major difference in recurring costs. As an example, the drug costs averaged $2,300 in Punjab $1,100 in Mysore, and $2,400 in Turkey.

The method permits separation of expenditures incurred by work within the PHC headquarters itself (PHC) and work in the geographic area assigned to the PHC (Field). The percentage distribution of PHC-expenditures, Field-expenditures and combined expenditures by functional categories are shown in Tables 18.25 and 18.26. Such a distribution of expenditures by functions is not readily possible with standard accounting procedures. In this example, health centers in India spent about one-third of their resources on medical relief and on family planning (Table 18.26), whereas the Turkish health centers used almost three-fourths of their expenditures for illnesses and very little for family planning. Proportionately, expenditures on MCH were similar in Mysore and Turkey and Punjab spending somewhat less for this function. Punjab spent the largest proportion for communicable disease control and in all the areas very little was spent for environmental sanitation. In Table 18.25 it can be seen that communicable disease control, MCH and family planning generally involved greater expenditures in the field, while medical relief was primarily a PHC cost. Using such information about health center expenditures, questions can be raised about the appropriateness of the distribution of resources in terms of their probable effectiveness as well as efficiency.

Table 18.27 demonstrates the proportions of the total expenditures related to direct service, supportive services and non-productive activites. Fifty percent of costs in Turkey are related to direct service, but in India the largest share of the expenditures was for supportive services, which amounted to over 40 per cent of the total expenditures in both Punjab and Mysore. It can be argued that travel expenses or certain other expenditures might be removed from supportive services expenditures and allocated to direct services. Be that as it may, it would still be appropriate for health officials to account for these expenses as well as non-productive expenditures in the interest of increasing the efficiency of health centers and releasing more of the staff time and resources for generating direct service.

In recent years increasing emphasis has been placed on the importance of the PHC subcenters for the delivery of MCH and family planning services. In India the individuals who provide most of these services at the subcenter level are the Auxiliary Nurse Midwives (ANMs). By using a profile of the ANM's activity time, all expenditures related to subcenters except drugs and supplies were apportioned to the various functions carried out there. Drug and supply expenditures were allocated by examining subcenter registers. The capital and

Table No. 18.22:

Annual PHC and Field Expenditures by functions, average expenditures (Rs.) per health Center in Punjab, 1968

Item	*PHC Expenditures*						*Field Expenditures*						
	Med. Rel.	*MCH*	*Fam. Plan.*	*CDC*	*Env. San.*	*Total*	*Med. Rel.*	*MCH*	*Fam. Plan.*	*CDC*	*Env. San.*	*Total*	*PHC & Field Total Expenditures*
Capital Expenditures (Amortized)	1,169	587	833	55	0	2,644	162	174	1,532	606	25	2,499	5,143
Recurring Expenditures (Fixed Costs-Maintenance)	565	350	430	0	0	1,345	83	89	208	306	7	693	2,038
Recurring Expenditures (Variable Costs-Drugs, Supplies, Vehicle Running, Incentives)	14,160	199	2,588	453	0	17,400	511	940	11,895	3,632	347	17,325	34,725
Salary and Allowances of Staff	19,732	1,088	7,122	2,989	0	30,931	9,701	12,061	29,325	34,984	820	86,891	117,822
Total Expenditures	35,626	2,224	10,973	3,497	0	52,320	10,457	13,264	42,960	39,528	1,199	107,408	159,728 ($21,300)

Table No. 18.23:

Annual PHC and field expenditures by functions, Average expenditure (Rs.) per Health Center in Mysore, 1968

Item	PHC Expenditures						Field Expenditures						
	Med. Rel.	*MCH*	*Fam. Plan.*	*CDC*	*Env. San.*	*Total*	*Med. Rel.*	*MCH*	*Fam. Plan.*	*CDC*	*Env. San.*	*Total*	*PHC & Field Total Expenditures*
Capital Expenditures (Amortized)	692	448	570	86	0	1,796	101	187	1,377	357	21	2,043	3,839
Recurring Expenditures (Fixed Costs-Maintenance)	204	183	183	0	0	570	31	68	78	105	3	285	855
Recurring Expenditures (Variable Costs-Drugs, Supplies, Vehicle Running, Incentives)	7,695	1,090	856	347	0	9,988	484	1,204	3,991	846	472	6,997	16,985
Salary and Allowances of Staff	12,658	1,282	5,426	3,100	0	22,466	4,569	8,346	14,768	11,068	493	39,244	61,710
Total Expenditures	21,249	3,003	7,035	3,533	0	34,820	5,185	9,805	20,214	12,376	989	48,569	83,389 (US $11,100)

Table No. 18.24:
Annual PHC and Field Expenditures by functions, average expenditure (T.L.) per Health Center in Turkey, 1968

Item	*PHC Expenditures*						*Field Expenditures*						
	Med. Rel.	*MCH*	*Fam. Plan.*	*CDC*	*Env. San.*	*Total*	*Med. Rel.*	*MCH*	*Fam. Plan.*	*CDC*	*Env. San.*	*Total*	*PHC & Field Total Expenditures*
Capital Expenditures (Amortized)	4,950	3,798	396	990	0	10,134	4,896	1,539	90	2,124	945	9,594	19,728
Recurring Expenditures (Fixed Costs-Maintenance)	1,665	1,440	144	360	0	3,609	1,557	486	45	675	297	3,060	6,669
Recurring Expenditures (Variable Costs-Drugs, Supplies, Vehicle Running, Incentives)	21,501	486	738	1,710	0	24,435	8,010	2,511	153	3,456	1,575	15,705	40,140
Salary and Allowances of Staff	81,666	1,917	2,385	4,284	0	90,252	42,867	18,063	603	4,149	2,232	67,914	158,166
Total Expenditures	109,782	7,641	3,663	7,344	0	128,430	57,330	22,599	891	10,404	5,049	96,278	224,703 (US $25,000)

Table No. 18.25:
Percentage distribution of Annual Health Center expenditures by functions, average per Health Center in Punjab, Mysore and Turkey, 1968 (PHC and Field Separated)

	Area	PHC Expenditures						Field Expenditures						
		Med. Rel.	MCH	Fam. Plan.	CDC	Env. San.	Total	Med. Rel.	MCH	Fam. Plan.	CDC	Env. San.	Total	PHC & Field Total Expenditures
PHC Distribution	Punjab	68	4	21	7	0	100	–	–	–	–	–	–	–
	Mysore	61	9	20	10	0	100	–	–	–	–	–	–	–
	Turkey	85	6	3	6	0	100	–	–	–	–	–	–	–
Field Distribution	Punjab	–	–	–	–	–	–	10	12	40	37	1	100	–
	Mysore	–	–	–	–	–	–	11	20	42	25	2	100	–
	Turkey	–	–	–	–	–	–	60	23	1	11	5	100	–
PHC and Field Distribution	Punjab	22	1	7	2	0	32	7	8	27	25	1	68	100
	Mysore	26	4	8	4	0	42	6	12	24	15	1	58	100
	Turkey	49	3	2	3	0	57	26	10	1	4	2	43	100

Table No. 18. 26:

Percentage Distribution of Annual Health Center Expenditures by Functions. Average per Health Center in Punjab, Mysore and Turkey, 1968 (PHC and Field Combined)

Area	*Med. Rel.*	*MCH*	*Fam. Plan.*	*CDC*	*Env. San.*	*Total*
Punjab	29	9	34	27	1	100
Mysore	32	16	32	19	1	100
Turkey	74	14	2	8	2	100

Table No. 18. 27:

Percentage Distribution of Annual Health Center Expenditures for Direct Services, Supportive Services, and Non-Productive Activities. Average per Health Center in Punjab, Mysore and Turkey, 1968 (PHC and Field Combined)

Area	*Direct Services*	*Supportive Services*	*Non-Productive Activities*	*Total*
Punjab	36	44	20	100
Mysore	40	43	17	100
Turkey	50	32	18	100

Mysore and Punjab. With an average of 5.5. ANM subcenters per PHC in Punjab and 5 in Mysore the subcenter proportions of total PHC functional expenditures were determined as in Table 18.29. Some interesting comparisons emerge from the data when related to activity times. Approximately 80 per cent of all MCH activities in Punjab occurred at the subcenter level and an almost identical proportion of MCH expenditures were attributable to these subcenter activities. The situation was different in Mysore with 48 per cent of all MCH activities provided by subcenters and 59 per cent of MCH expenditures being related to these subcenters. These data suggest that in Punjab, subcenter MCH services are as costly as those in the PHC headquarters. This does not appear to be the case in Mysore where subcenter services are relatively more expensive than PHC services.

Another important observation is that all the subcenters and their related activities consumed only a quarter of the total expenditures of each health center in both States. This

Table No. 18.28:

Average Annual Expenditures (Rs.) by function per ANM Subcenter in Mysore and Punjab, 1968

		Expenditure by Function					
Type of Expenditure	*Study Area*	*Medical Relief*	*MCH*	*Family Planning*	*CDC*	*Environmental Sanitation*	*Total*
Capital Expenditures*	Punjab	46	64	72	18	0	200
	Mysore	26	78	62	34	0	200
Recurring Expenditures	Punjab	182	304	270	36	0	792
	Mysore	122	349	213	114	0	798
Salaries and Allowances**	Punjab	1,360	1,900	2,140	530	0	5,930
	Mysore	360	1,080	850	470	0	2,760
Total	Punjab	1,588	2,268	2,482	584	0	6,922
	Mysore	508	1,507	1,125	618	0	3,758
Percentage Distribution	Punjab	23	33	36	8	0	100
of Expenditures	Mysore	14	40	30	16	0	100

* Approximately Rs. 150 could be excluded from this total if subcenter buildings were donated by the villages.

** Staff per subcenter are: 1ANM, 1 trained dai (Punjab only), 25% of an LHV and 4% of a physician (Based on an estimate of the time they spend at subcenters).

Table No. 18.29:

Percentage Distribution of Health Center Expenditures by functions attributable to ANM-Subcenter Activities in India, 1968

Study Area	*Total Subcenter Functional Expenditures* Stated as Per cent of Total Health Center Functional Expenditures*					
	Medical Relief	*MCH*	*Family Planning*	*CDC*	*Environmental Sanitation*	*Total*
Punjab	19	81	25	8	0	24
Mysore	10	57	21	19	0	23

* Total subcenter expenditures are derived by summing the experience of all of the subcenters linked to one PHC.

would amount to approximately Rs. 40,000 per health center in Punjab, an amount somewhat less than the average expenditure of Rs. 54,000 related specifically to the PHC headquarters services. State in another way, it would cost less to double the number of subcenters in a community Development Block than to add another PHC headquarters to each block. The latter assumes that the present supervisory staff to field staff ratio is considered adequate and is not changed when more subcenters are added to an existing PHC. Finally, since recurring costs are relatively small in subcenters, increasing the volume of services in the existing subcenters by improving staff productivity would not require much additional expenditures.

2. Cost of Services

Expenditures for specific units of service can also provide useful information for assessing the relative efficiency of facilities delivering health care. As an example, the expenditure per outpatient visit was estimated as shown in Table 18.30. Table 18.31 then illustrates the components of this average expenditure. In these calculations inpatient expenditures were considered to amount to a very minor fraction of medical relief expenses in the PHCs studied and therefore were not excluded. Expenditures on drugs, injections, and other treatments were based on direct observations of patients that were treated.

The results illustrate the usefulness of this procedure for comparing different health facilities. In addition, the proportion of the expenditures that were used for drugs, injections and treatments is clearly highlighted. Since these latter variable expenditures are proportionately small, increasing the volume of patients seen by the health centers would markedly reduce the cost per visit. This however assumes current expenditure on drugs per patient is adequate, a judgment which obviously may be in error.

For comparison with the health center costs per patient visit, data from the community survey concerning the expenditures incurred by patients for practitioner consultations are shown in Table 18.32. By adding the patient's out-of-pocket expenses for a PHC consultation and the government's costs per visit, the total expenditure per patient visit to a PHC can be estimated (in this case Rs. 2.08 in Punjab and Rs. 1.51 in Mysore).

Another unit of service is the "service-contact". The total annual counts of contacts made by health workers with individuals or groups were utilized. These contacts were grouped by major functions. Dividing these into the total health center expenditures per function, the average expenditure per service-contact was obtained. Table 18.33 summarizes this information for India and illustrates the wide variation in service-contact expenditures depending on the PHC or the function. Since it is difficult to compare two different types of service-contacts because of considerable variation in content, the more fruitful use of these data is to compare the variations in expenditures for each type of service-contact between the health centers being studied.

The expenditure per therapeutic injection is an example of an expenditure item that is attributable to a more specific service. All possible expenditures related to injections were consolidated as outlined in the detailed methodology (Appendix). The cost per injection in Punjab was Rs. 0.69 (0.27 for drugs and 0.42 for staff service time), and Rs. 1.27 in Mysore (0.63 for drugs and 0.64 for staff service time). The differences between the two areas for

Table No. 18. 30:
Average Health Center Expenditure per Outpatient Visit, 1968

	Study Areas		
	Punjab (Rs.)	*Mysore (Rs.)*	*Turkey (T.L.)*
Annual Expenditures for illness care in the average PHC	35,600	21,200	109,800
Total Annual Outpatient Visits in the Average PHC	23,100	21,900	2,400
PHC Expenditure per Outpatient Visit	1.54 ($0.21)	0.97 ($0.13)	45.75 ($5.08)

Table No. 18. 31:
Expenditure Components of an Average Health Center Outpatient Visit, 1968

	Study Areas					
	Punjab		*Mysore*		*Turkey*	
	Amount (Rs.)	%	*Amount (Rs.)*	%	*Amount (T.L.)*	%
Total	1.54	100	0.97	100	45.75	100
Drugs	0.15	15	0.12	20	5.95	13
Injections and other treatments	0.08		0.07			
Staff and Supportive Services	1.31	85	0.78	80	39.80	87

Table No. 18.32:
Average Expenditure* (Rs.) per patient visit by type of practitioner - Data from Punjab and Mysore in India

Study Area	*Type of Practitioner*				
	Practitioner, Unqualified	*Non-allopathic Practitioner, Qualified*	*Allopathic Practitioner, Private, Qualified*	*Government Dispensary*	*Primary Health Center***
Punjab	1.56	2.80	3.33	2.01	0.54
Mysore	2.00	2.32	2.98	3.07	0.54

* Expenditures related to the visit including consultation, drugs, travel, diets and other expenses.
** Except for Rs. 0.10 per new patient in Punjab, this amount represented money spent outside the PHC (drugs, travel etc.).

which data were available are obvious. The factors that contribute to such differences may be identified, as in this case, by making use of other information from the PHCs. For instance it was found that Mysore PHCs administered more of the expensive types of drugs such as antibiotics and required that only physicians give the injections, both of which contributed to a higher expense per injection.

A similar analysis of smallpox vaccinations revealed that it cost Rs. 0.77 and Rs. 0.53 in Punjab and Mysore respectively for each vaccination. While it cost only Rs. 0.05 in each area for the vaccine itself and materials necessary for each vaccination, the other costs for staff services were different in the two states (Rs. 0.72 in Punjab and Rs. 0.48 in Mysore). Clearly for smallpox programs the major health center expenditure involves manpower.

Finally, an example of expenditures incurred for family planning services would be the amount spent by the health center per acceptor of a family planning method. With the data available, a number of assumptions had to be used for these calculations. Indirect estimates showed that actual service time related to family planning (such as an IUCD inserted or a sterilization procedure) amounted to less than 5 per cent of the total time spent by the health center staff for family planning. Motivation, travel time, record keeping, and other administrative activities consumed the rest of the time. For illustrative purposes, therefore, the overall cost for one acceptor, no matter what method was adopted, was assumed to require about the same amount of motivation, record keeping etc., and was treated as a homogenous service unit. In addition, every 100 condoms distributed was equated to one IUCD or sterilization acceptor for the year in consideration. The total family planning expenditure per health center was therefore simply divided by the total acceptors of vasectomies, tubectomies, IUCD insertions and condoms (as defined above) for the same year to ascertain the average annual expenditure per family planning acceptor. The figures obtained from Mysore and Punjab are in Table 18.34. These results provide an interesting contrast to the expenditure per family planning service contact in Table 18.33. It is evident that the cost of contacts need not necessarily indicate the cost per acceptor.

Many other service-unit costs could have been calculated, or the above examples could have been done more precisely if specific units of services generated by health center staff were more readily available. It is hoped that administrators will recognize the value of collecting service-unit information in order to make the fullest use of the cost accounting procedures that have been described.

Besides permitting the estimation of a greater variety of service-unit costs, detailed data would greatly assist the development of a scale of relative values (Gray, et. al., 1967) that might then be useful for rapid cost accounting of services. For example, within the function of family planning, the various activities carried out by the staff such as group meetings, home visits for motivation, distribution of condoms, insertions of IUCDs, and sterilization procedures could be given different unit values depending on their relative use of resources. For purposes of illustration, if one could establish through work sampling and other observational studies that distribution of one condom would require 1/100th of the resources that are necessary for a vasectomy, then a relative value of 1 to a condom distributed and 100 to a vasectomy could

Table No. 18.33:
Average Expenditure per Service-contact by function in four Health Centers in Punjab and Mysore, 1968

Item	Area	Functions: Med. Rel.	MCH	Fam. Plan.	CDC	Env. San.	Total
Total Annual Expenditures per Health Center (Rs.)	Punjab	46,083	15,488	53,933	43,025	1,199	159,728
	Mysore	26,434	12,808	27,249	15,909	989	83,389
Total Annual Service-Contacts Per health Center	Punjab	75,650	16,150	47,600	357,000	1.700	498,100
	Mysore	60,800	32,000	18,560	113,920	1,280	226,560
Expenditure per Service Contact (Rs.)	Punjab	0.61	0.96	1.13	0.12	0.71	0.32
	Mysore	0.43	0.40	1.47	0.14	0.77	0.37

be imputed. Aggregation of such units of activities would enable one to derive a unit cost for a family planning program. Similarly, relative value scales for other services would permit the calculation of unit costs for all service units generated by a health center.

VII. SUMMARY OF HEALTH CENTER OPERATIONS

After assembling the various elements of community information in the preceding chapter, we found that meaningful interpretation required selective consolidation of data and the calculation of certain statistical indices. Fortunately, problems of data reduction are not as severe in the handling of health center service, activity, and cost statistics. Information is collected along only a limited number of dimensions and is classified rather simply, so that the list of tabulations already presented might be considered a manageable summarization of health center operations, except for two types of service outreach indices to be introduced in the concluding section of this chapter. Nevertheless a brief recapitulation seems desirable as a succinet statement of the important relationships to be considered.

A. Overall Comparisons by Function

First, within five major functional areas we have indicated in Table 18.35 the estimated annual volume of service contacts per 100,000 population compared with the amount of effort and cost going into these areas. The service contacts were derived by projecting the estimates of Tables 18.2, 18.9, and 18.13 onto a population base of 100,000 in order to make the two states more comparable. Time and cost distributions were taken directly from Tables 18.14 and 18.26 respectively.

By putting all these factors into a single table it becomes clear that CDC work is relatively inexpensive, while family planning is relatively costly when measured either per unit of staff service time of per service contact. The table also reveals that the substantially larger numbers

Table No. 18. 34:
Average Health Center Expenditure per Family Planning Acceptor, Based on Data from four Health Centers, Punjab and Mysore, 1968

	Study Area	
	Punjab	*Mysore*
Total Annual Family Planning Expenditures Per Health Center (Rs.)	59,933	27,249
Average Annual Number of Family Planning Acceptors Per Health Center	685	273
Average Expenditure per Acceptor (Rs.)	79	100

of Punjab CDC and family planning contacts compared with Mysore did not consume correspondingly more staff time or budget. Similarly the relatively large volume of MCH contacts in Mysore was achieved with a less than proportionate increase in resources over Punjab.

B. Activity Summaries

The next five summaries present the most important features of staff time allocation, starting in Table 18.36 with the health center and field staff division of effort among direct service and supporting tasks, travel, and Persom time. The direct service time is allocated by function in Table 18.37, drawing upon earlier Tables 18.17 and 18.18. The further breakdown of supporting activities is reported in Table 18.38, which is a capsule version of Table 18.19.

The activity summaries presented here differ from earlier ones in that the contributions of individual staff categories are submerged in the totals. While the decision maker using these reports may or may not accept this level of aggregation, he should in any case insist upon the two summaries by staff category shown in Tables 18.39 and 18.40. The former gives a quick indication of the range of efficiencies at which various staff groups are operating. The table clearly reveals, for example, that the Mysore ANM was more often engaged in productive work than the Punjab ANM, and further that productive time was much more often direct service oriented in Mysore. Table 18.40 shows who are the key contributors to each of the service functions and therefore suggests areas of competence required of particular worker categories.

C. Cost Summaries

The proportional cost distribution among functions has already been summarized in Table 18.35. The actual amounts expended are shown in Table 18.41 to indicate that the Punjab health center costs were much higher than those in Mysore. The relative difference between states was especially marked in communicable diseases control and was quite small for the MCH function.

Table 18.42 allocates capital and operating costs in the two India study sites, indicating that the former represent a much larger proportion of the total in Mysore, although in absolute terms capital investment is larger in Punjab. In both locations, however, salaries and allowances are the dominant component of costs.

Table 18.43 is a recapitulation of Table 18.27 to show the distribution of expenditures for direct service and other activities.

Table 18.44 summarizes information contained in Table 18.33 depicting average expenditure per service contact within each of the functional areas. Recognizing that the content of such contacts varies considerably among services, Table 18.45 was constructed to show the unit cost of each of four illustrative specific services.

D. Indicators of Service Outreach

While the preceding sections have illustrated ways of measuring the quantity and types of services provided by the primary health center and how they are provided, they have

Table No. 18.35:

Gross Comparisons of Service Contacts, Time and Cost by Function – Based mainly upon India Work Sampling

Functions	*Estimated Annual Service Contacts per 100,000 population*		*Distribution of Service Time (%)*		*Distribution of Total Cost (%)*	
	Punjab	*Mysore*	*Punjab*	*Mysore*	*Punjab*	*Mysore*
Medical Relief	89,000	95,000	23	23	29	32
MCH	19,000	50,000	10	18	9	16
Family Planning	56,000	29,000	20	19	34	32
CDC	420,000	178,000	46	39	27	19
Environmental Sanitation	2,000	2,000	1	1	1	1

Table No. 18.36:

Percentage Distribution of Staff Time Among Direct Service, Supporting, Travel and Personal Activities – from India Work Sampling

Activity Category	Punjab			Mysore		
	PHC	*Field*	*All*	*PHC*	*Field*	*All*
Direct Service	22	14	16	18	28	25
Supporting	40	32	33	29	21	23
Travel	5	24	21	10	39	30
Personal	33	30	30	43	12	22
Total	100	100	100	100	100	100

Table No. 18.37 :
Allocation of Direct Service Time Among Functions—from India Work Sampling

Function	*Punjab*			*Percent of Function Time in Field*	*Mysore*			*Percent of Function Time in Field*
	PHC	*Field*	*All*		*PHC*	*Field*	*All*	
Medical Relief	64	12	23	40	70	10	23	33
MCH	1	12	10	98	3	22	18	96
Family Planning	13	22	20	86	2	24	19	98
CDC	22	53	46	89	25	43	39	86
Environmental Sanitation	0	1	1	100	0	1	1	100
Total	100	100	100		100	100	100	

Table No. 18.38:

Allocation of Supporting time among Activity Categories — from India Work Sampling

Activity Category	*Punjab*			*Mysore*		
	PHC	*Field*	*All*	*PHC*	*Field*	*All*
Records, Reports Preparation	35	52	49	32	42	39
Maintenance, Cleaning	23	10	13	11	7	9
Staff Interactions	22	24	24	25	27	26
Meetings, etc.	20	14	14	32	24	26
Total	100	100	100	100	100	100

D. Indicators of Service Outreach

While the preceding sections have illustrated ways of measuring the quantity and types of services provided by the primary health center and how they are provided, they have given little attention to the question: for whom are the services provided? In particular, we must assess the population coverage by the health center in comparison with other providers of medical care. We have devised two measures of this: the INTENSITY of services utilization and the effective RANGE of service coverage.

With respect to intensity we calculated the rate of visits made to a local practitioner. For every 1,000 residents in Punjab study villages, for example, we found that 739 visits per year were made to indigenous medicine practitioners within a one-mile radius of the patient's residence. Table 18.46 shows that residents of the health center village had an even higher rate of PHC utilization (5,438 visits per 1,000), indicating that the health center has considerably

Table No. 18. 39

Proportion of Staff Time spent in service and other Productive Activity—from India Work Sampling

	Per cent Time Productive (Service, Support, Travel)		*Per cent Time Service*	
Staff Category	*Punjab*	*Mysore*	*Punjab*	*Mysore*
Health Center				
DR.	74	62	27	32
NURSE	54	68	13	17
PHARMACIST	71	62	29	19
DRESSER	54	58	22	15
LAB TECH	68	57	44	28
CLERK	72	42	4	1
Field				
DR.	89	88	13	24
LHV	68	86	17	15
ANM	65	85	15	32
TD	46	–	9	–
HI	81	93	9	11
BEE	71	86	19	16
FPW	73	76	8	15
BHS-TVS	78	91	17	35

Table No. 18.40:
Principal Staff Categories Performing particular Service Functions – from India Work Sampling

Medical Relief			MCH			Family Planning			CDC			Environmental Sanitation		
	Present Contribution			Present Contribution			Present Contribution			Present Contribution			Present Contribution	
Staff	Punjab	Mysore	Staff	Punjab	Mysore	Staff	Punjab	Mysore	Staff	Punjab	Mysore	Staff	Punjab	Mysore
DR.	16	33	ANM	61	64	ANM	22	45	BHW-TVS	82	73	BHW-TVS	54	35
PHARM.	25	17	BHW-TVS	0	24	FPW	26	12	LAB. TECH.	11	13	HI	40	41
ANM	24	18	TD	19	-	BEE	14	15	ANM	2	9	ANM	0	22
DRESSER	14	13	LHV	16	4	BHW-TVS	3	14						
TD	10	—				LHV	13	7						
OTHER	11	19	Other	4	8	TD	7	—						
						OTHER	15	7	OTHER	5	5	OTHER	6	2

Table No. 18.41:

Summary of Health Center Expenditures (in Rupees), By functions –India

Location	Function					Total
	Medical Relief	*MCH*	*Family Planning*	*CDC*	*Environmental Sanitation*	
Punjab	46,083	15,488	53,933	43,025	1,119	159,728
Mysore	26,434	12,808	27,249	15,909	989	83,389

Table No. 18. 42:

Summary of Health Center Expenditures (In Rupees) By Fixed and Variable Categories - India

	Amount (Rs.)		*Percentage*	
Item	*Punjab*	*Mysore*	*Punjab*	*Mysore*
Capital Expenditures	5,143	3,839	3	5
Recurring - Fixed	2,038	855	1	1
Recurring - Variable	34,725	16,985	22	20
Salaries and Allowances	117,822	61,710	74	74
Total	159,728	83,389	100	100
Dollars	$21,300	$11,100		

Table No. 18. 43:
Percentage Distribution of Health Center Expenditures by Category of Services —India

Category	*Punjab*	*Mysore*
Direct Services	36	40
Support and Travel	44	43
Non-Productive	20	17
Total	100	100

Table No. 18. 44

Summary of Average Expenditures (Rs.) per Service Contact by Function —India

Function	Punjab	Mysore
Medical Relief	0.61	0.43
MCH	0.96	0.40
Family Planning	1.13	1.47
CDC	0.12	0.14
Environmental Sanitation	0.71	0.77

Table 18. 45

Summary of Expenditures (Rs.) Per Recipient of Selected Services —India

Service	Punjab	Mysore
Outpatient Visit	1.54	0.97
Injection	0.69	1.27
Smallpox Vaccination	0.77	0.53
Family Planning Acceptor	79.00	100.00

Table No. 18.46:

Health Services Utilization Intensities and Effective Service Areas —Punjab

Service Category	*Annual Visits per 1,000 Population Travel Under One Mile*	*Maximum Miles Travelled by 75% of Patients*	*Effective Service Area (Sq. Mi.)*	*Number of Service Areas Needed per CDB*	*Approximate Number of Practitioners or Facilities Available*
IMP	739	2.5	19.6	5.1	200
PHC	5,438	2.9	26.4	3.8	1
Private Allopath	7	7.2	162.8	0.6	4
Other Public	3	3.4	36.3	2.8	5

greater local attraction than the IMP. The overall utilization of IMPs, however, was greater due to the large number of these practitioners throughout the community development block. Corresponding rates for private allopaths and government dispensaries are low, but the comparison is not very meaningful because the number of villages sampled was not sufficient to assure that the general distribution of these services was adequately represented.

The effective range of service coverage was calculated from the travel radius that included three-fourths of all patient visits to a given service. For example, 75 per cent of the IMP visits in Punjab involved travel of less than 2.5 miles. The effective IMP service area, therefore, is estimated to be a circle with area:

$$\pi R^2 = (3.14)\,(2.5)^2$$
$$= 19.6 \text{ square miles}$$

Since a typical CDB contains roughly 100 square miles, it follows that:

$$\frac{100}{19.6} = 5.1 \text{ IMP service areas}$$

are needed per development block in order to permit all areas to be covered. Instead of five practicing IMPs, however, there were estimated to be about 200. The ratio

$$\frac{200}{5.1} = 39$$

gives an indication of the amount of overlap of service areas, suggesting that the typical patient has effective access to 39 IMPs within his IMP service area.

A similar analysis of PHC coverage indicates a somewhat larger radius of coverage, 2.9 miles, which provides an effective service area of 26.4 square miles. At this rate complete block coverage would require 3 or 4 health centers, or perhaps a more complete subcenter infrastructure. Even then, "coverage" only connotes accessibility, not assured utilization by everyone.

In general, then, the clinical coverage of the Punjab PHC was found to be characterized by exceptionally intensive utilization but an effective service area that is only one-fourth of the CDB.

References

1. A slightly modified version of the above chapter was published in the *Indian Journal of Medical Research*, Vol. 60, No. 12, December 1972 (pp. 1849-1863), "Cost Accounting of Health Centre Expenditures", C. Alex Alexander, et. al.

2. A step by step illustration of the methodology is provided in an Appendix.

3. Data on capital expenditures in Turkey have been taken from Goodman, N.M. "Turkey's Experiment in `Socialization'. of Medicine", *The Lancet*, January 4, 1964, pp. 36-38.

4. Administrative-costs of a planning, supervisory and evaluative nature at the district, state or national level are not reflected in this costing procedure due to the difficulty in separating out costs related only to the health center programs at these levels. The data presented, therefore, reflect as closely as possible the entire costs at the health center level.

19

Providing for Immediate felt Health Needs

MEDICAL CARE OF COMMON ILLNESSES

People seek medical care of common illnesses from the health personnel. Relief from pain and alleviation of suffering are their immediate concerns and felt-health needs. Prevention of diseases and promotion of health are in the larger interest of the community. But these are often not perceived as important as the clinical services by the people. It is far easier to provide preventive and promotive health services to the people, through their contracts with the health sector for obtaining clinical services. It may, at times, be difficult to persuade parents to bring their children to the health center for immunisation shorts, when they are apparently not ill. The prophylactic vaccination is however more easily done, when the child is brought to the health center for the relief of illnesses such as sore eyes or scabies. Medical care of common illnesses prevalent in the community is recognised as an important component of primary health care. However, it should be appreciated that medical services provided in primary health care approach, are not a substitute for services normally rendered in the hospital and that every demand made by the community on the health sector cannot be easily satisfied through primary health care. Only essential clinical care is provided mainly

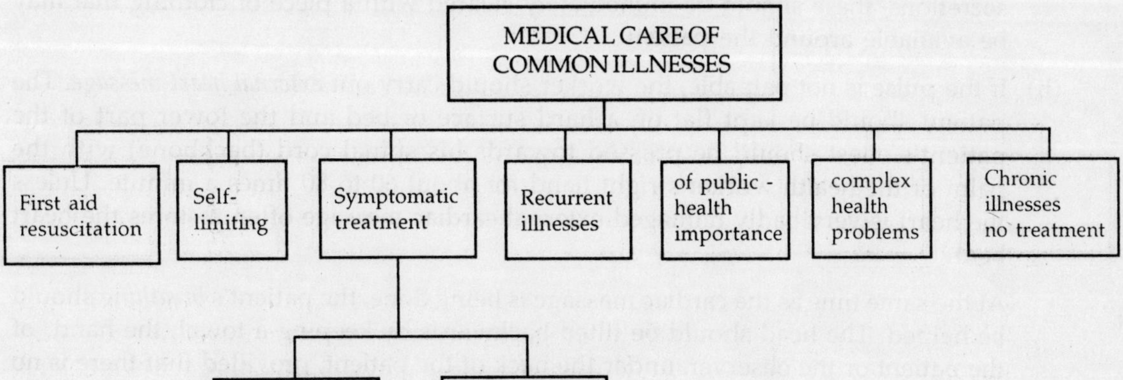

to alleviate suffering, prevent handicaps and reduce deaths. The type of illnesses for which medical care is sought by people, may necessitate different approaches according to the nature of the illness, sensitivity to the existing methods of treatment, cost of therapy and need for the most effective utilisation of the scarce available resources. Principles of organisation of such medical care and described below:

1. FIRST AID FOR LIFE-THREATENING ILLNESSES

People in the village may sustain serious injuries or may become acutely ill. Some of the life-threatening acute emergencies encountered in villages include the following: Burns in the kitchen, falls from tress or roofs, near drowning in the stream, roadside accidents, thresher accidents with amputation of hands and severe bleeding, snake bites, poisoning, high fever, coma, shock and heart failure.

The primary health care worker in the village should be competent in carrying out the first-aid measures, necessary to save the life of a patient and sustain it, till the patient can be sent to a nearby hospital or a doctor can be summoned to the village to provide specific emergency care. The health workers should be well trained to resuscitate a dying patient with minimum of facilities available to them. Her ability to revive a dying patient boosts her own morale and the confidence of people in her skills.

In most emergency situations, the condition and environment around the patient become chaotic. Family members and neighbours collect together and start crying and sobbing. The health worker's first duty is to take full command of the situation, remove all unnecessary persons from the spot and try to reassure the relations that she will do her best to revive the patient till help arrives from the health centre. Meanwhile, one of the relatives should be sent to the health center doctor for help, including the despatch of an ambulance and equipment for revival. The health worker may not be carrying tools for revival of a patient, when she is suddenly called upon to take care of an emergency. She may have to rush to the site immediately, since even a few minutes dealy may be catastorphic. She should immediately look for the following clinical features *viz. pulse, breathing, pupils and bleeding*. Whatever the cause of emergency, the following general resuscitative measures are mandatory.

(i) If the mouth cavity or the nore appear to be chocked with blood, vomitus or other secretions, these should be immediately cleared with a piece of clothing that may be available around the patient.

(ii) If the pulse is not palpable, the worker should carry out *external heart message*. The patient should be kept flat on a hard surface or bed and the lower part of the patient's chest should be pressed towards his spinal cord (backbone) with the palm of the health worker's right hand for about 60 to 80 times a minute. Unless the heart is very badly damaged external cardiac message often restores the heart beat.

At the same time as the cardiac massage is being done, the patient's *breathing* should be helped. The head should be tilted backwards by keeping a towel, the hand of the patient or the observer, under the neck of the patient, provided that there is no injury to the cervical spine of the patient. As the head is tilted backwards the tongue is lifted up and the entry to the airway (trachea) becomes patent. The worker should tear a part of her sari or robe of the patient, fold it like a handkerchief and place it in the mouth of the patient. She should pinch the nostrils of the patient, and herself take a deep breath, fill her lungs with air and then clasp the open mouth of the patient snugly with her lips. She should then forcibly exhale all the air, she had breathed in earlier, into the mouth of the patient. Meanwhile she should keep pressing the upper part of abdomen or the area of the stomach with her right hand, so that the exhaled air goes into the lungs of the patient and not in the stomach. This *mouth to mouth breathing* is the only effective method of revival of a patient in an emergency situation occurring suddenly in the community.

(iii) She should look at the *pupils* of the patient. If these appear widely dilated and do not react to light, probably the damage is extensive and nothing more can be done.

(iv) If there is any sign of *blood* on the clothes, the worker should remove the clothes of the patient and carefully look at the site of bleeding. In most cases a sustained pressure on the site of small injury is enough to stop the bleeding. Tourniquet is often not necessary. In cases of severe bleeding there is no alternative but to send the patient to the nearest hospital in the shortest possible time.

(v) In case of *falls* from trees or other roadside injuries, unnecessary movement of the patient without full and careful assessment should be scrupulously avoided.

(vi) In cases of *snake bite*, the area of bite should be examined for fang punctures, local pain, swelling, numbness or weakness appearing within 20 minutes of the bite. In the absence of these, the bite is not likely to be caused by a poisonous snake. If the bite is by a poisonous snake, a tourniquet should be applied a few cm above the site of the bite, if it is possible to do so. A handkerchief is tied round the limb and the knot is twisted round with a twig or pencil so much, that one finger of the health worker can pass beneath the tourniquet with difficulty. When the local swelling makes the tourniquet very tight, it should be slightly loosened. The area of bite is cleaned. A cruciate incision, about 0.5 cm deep should be made through the fang punctures. The blood and secretion should be sucked even by mouth if there is no ulcerated lesion in the mouth of the first-aid worker. The limb should be gently immobilised by a splint and the patient should be sent to the hospital, where further treatment such as polyvalent-antisnake-venomserum can be administered.

2. SYMPTOMATIC TREATMENT OF COMMON ILLNESSES

1. SELF-LIMITING ILLNESSES

Certian illnesses such as short fever for 1 or 2 days, mild cough, coryza, abdominal cramps or a few loose stools for a day or two are often *self limiting*, since these have a short duration and there is little disability. These do not prevent the individual from doing his normal household or vocational chores. Often a simple reassurance is all that is needed or simple symptomatic relief with aspirin may be adequate. Loose watery stools in young children are best managed with oral hydration (glucose 20 g. NaCI 3.5 g., NaIICO 2.5 g and

KCI 1.0 g in one liter of water given by spoonfuls *ad lbo*. The community health workers can easily provide this services.

2. ILLNESSES WHICH LAST LONGER THAN A WEEK OR WHICH INCAPACITATE THE PATIENT FOR MORE THAN 3 DAY

Pneumonia, accidental injuries, dysentery, persistent vomiting, specific infections of eyes, ears, throat and urinary tract, multiple boils, impetigo, scabies, intestinal parasites, pallot and malnutrition. The community health worker should refer these patients to the health center, where treatment should be provided by the regular staff such as multipurpose health workers, nurse or the doctor. *Such illnesses may or may not be presentable, but these need specific treatment* for relief of pain and suffering. Early treatment prevents complications and progression of the disease. The reader is advised to refer to standard text books of medicine or pediatrics for the treatment of such common illnesses. The following account of treatment of some common illnesses in the community relates only to primary health care by village level paramedical workers.

Skin

1. *Boils,* Small painful lumps under the skin which feel hot are treated by compresses of salty water (one tablespoon in a liter) 3 times daily and sulphadimidine 2 tablets 3 times daily. If a wide area of the skin is infected, sulphadimidine, (dose as above) co-trimoxazole (2 tablets twice daily for adults) or penicillin 5000 units IM twice daily are given. If watery blisters or scabs are present, gentian violet 1% aqueous solution may also be applied.

2. *Scabies.* Itchy shin is treated by salt water compresses if a small area is affected. Scabies is common in villages and involves large areas of the body. It is treated by application of 25 per cent Benzyl benzoate emulsion on 3 successive days. Concurrent treatment of all contacts and boiling of clothes and bed linen of all treated patients and contacts is necessary.

Eyes

Somewhere, If the eye of patient hurts, the health worker should even the eyelid of the patient with clear washed hands and look for any dust particle or foreign body and remove it with a clean piece of cloth. Thereafter tetracycline ointment should be applied two or three times daily for one or two days. If the eye continues to hurt, patient should be referred to the hospital.

2. If there is a mucopurulent discharge from the eyes or eyes becomes sticky, tetracycline ointment should be applied to eyes three or four times daily. Eyes should not be allowed to remain glued together even for more than half an hour, since this might result in corneal ulceration and permanent impairment of vision.

Abdominal pain

In case of severe abdominal pain Tincture of belladona three drops per year of age (maximum 30 drops) are given. Patient is asked not to eat or drink anything and is sent forthwith to the health centre or the hospital. If the abdominal pain is not very severe, he might be having worms in the stools or might be going for diarrhea. Abdominal pain may improve within two or three hours. If not, patient is referred to the health center or hospital.

If the pain is located in the lower part of the abdomen, during micturition or the patient appears feverish, plenty of fluids, aspirin and sulphadimiding are given for 3 days. If response if poor, send the patient to the hospital.

Joint pains

If a wound or fracture is excluded, a firm (not too tight) bandage is tied around the joint. Patient is asked to rest at home and given aspirin tablet three times a day for 3 or 4 days. If response is not adequate, send the patient to the hospital. If the patient appears feverish and joint appears hot, give 100,000 units of procain Penicillin IM for 5 days (Sulphadimidine, if penicillin is not available) and aspirin 1 tablet three times daily for 5 days. If no response, send the patient to the hospital.

Worms in stools

If the patient has passed large *roundworms,* give piperazine salt 1 g all at one go for those above 10 years of age; 3 gm for children between 4 and 10 years; 2 gm for younger children and 1 g for infants.

Tapeworms are treated with 10 tablets of 100 mg each of mepacrine given on empty stomach in the morning after a laxative given the night before. Alternatively seek help of the health center.

Threadworms are treated with lower dose of piperazine, 750 mg for those above 4 years, 500 mg for those between 1 and 3 years, three times daily for 7 days.

Weakness and tiredness

If the inside of eye, inside of lips and tongue appear pale and creases of hand are not more pigmented than the palm of the hand, give iron sulphate tablets of 250-300 mg each twice a day for one month for adult women. Smaller dose are used for children.

If the patient becomes weak all of a sudden and there is swelling of feet, refer the patient to the doctor.

Convulsions

Exclude hysteria by talking to relatives about any family quarrels, financial difficulties, or if the patient had fear of evil spirits. Reassure relations about the nature of illness. Such patients do not hurt themselves during fits and there is no involuntary passage of stools or urine. In true convulsions, patient may fall down, his body may become stiff, there may be violent movements in his arms and legs and there is foam around the mouth. The patient may pass urine involuntarily. The attacks passes off after some time but the patient usually does not remember the fit.

If the convulsions are continuous, the patient should be immediately sent to the hospital. If there is fever, aspirin ½ to 1 tablet may be given to reduce the temperature. It is useful to give chloroquine (4 tablets) as well, since these may be due to cerebral malaria, especially in many tropical countries. If a child gets several convulsions at variable intervals he should receive phenobarbitone 5-7 mg/kg of body weight per day for several months and should be under surveillance of the health-centre doctor.

3. RECURRENT ILLNESSES SUCH AS BRONCHAIAT ASTHMA, EPILEPSY, CARDIOVASCULAR DISORDERS AND NEPHROSIS.

The duration of episode is short in epilepsy and asthma but may be prolonged in cardiovascular illnesses. These illnesses cause considerable anguish, pain and disability. It is not always possible to arrest the disease or prevent its progression. Specific treatment may prevent complications and recurrences. It is advisable to refer these patients to the doctor, who should prescribe the initial treatment and review these during the course of illness periodically.

Table 19.1

Some guide lines for referring serious patients to the nearest health centre or hospital by the village level community health worker.

1. Any individual who does not improve with the symptomatic treatment in 2 days, whose condition deteriorates and who looks very sick.
2. If the village level health worker is not sure about his or her competence in providing the necessary primary health care to the individual.
3. If the patient has following serious symptoms:
   - i) Rapid feeble pulse.
   - ii) Cold limbs , blanching excessively on pressure.
   - iii) Breathing difficulty.
   - iv) Fits.
   - v) Persistent vomiting.
   - vi) Persistent headache.
   - vii) Unconsciousness.
   - viii) Unexplained weight loss.
   - ix) High fever persisting for more than 3 days.
   - x) Bone tenderness.
   - xi) Joint pains.
   - xii) Severe abdominal pain.
   - xiii) Large mass in abdomen.
   - xiv) Bleeding in sputum, urine or ear.
   - xv) Head injury.
   - xvi) Pallor not responding to hematinics.

4. ILLNESSES OF PUBLIC HEALTH IMPORTANCE

These include illnesses such as, malaria, kala azar (leishmaniasis), tuberculosis, leprosy, or other deficiency problems such as endemic goiter. The district health officer of the area should draw out a plan of action for epidemiological surveillance of the community for early detection, prompt treatment and prevention of spread of these illnesses in the area.

The primary health center doctor should undertake the follow up action and ensure compliance of patients for the treatment of illnesses such as tuberculosis and leprosy for long periods. Actual disbursement of medicines may however be done by the community-health worker under the supervision of the doctor.

It is advisable to refer to standard text books of Medicine or Pediatrics for detailed description of the diseases. The following description is given briefly only for their management in the community.

MALARIA

Intensive malaria control programmes in India during the sixties and early seventies, considerably reduced the incidence of malaria. Deaths due to malaria became rare. There was an upsurge in the incidence of malaria due to relaxation and complacence in malaria control measures, and emergence of insecticide-resistant strains of the mosquito vector recently. Malaria should be suspected in individuals, who present with high, intermittent fever, starting with chills and rigors and who have no other evidence of infection such as of urinary tract, otitis media, tonsillitis or osteomyelitis. Some patients may present with diarrhea and have persistent vomiting. In endemic or semi-endemic areas, patients develop partial immunity. In such cases chills and rigors at the onset, intermittent character of fever and its subsidence with sweating may not be seen. The character of fever may be atypical. Therefore, it is advisable to examine the blood slide for malarial parasites in all cases of fever of unknown origin especially in endemic areas.

Malaria may involve brain (cerebral malaria). These cases present with convulsions and may remain unconscious after the subsidence of convulsion. If malaria continues, spleen becomes enlarged and the patient looks pale.

Malaria is caused by mosquito (anopheles) bite, which transmits Plasmodium vivax or P. falciparum in the blood of the host. Adult patients should receive 4 tablets of 150 mg dose of chloroquine, followed by 1 tablet after six hours and 1 tablet every day for the next three days. The dosage is proportionately reduced for children. (10 mg of chloroquine base per kg of body weight per day). Malaria due to Plasmodium vivax generally relapses. The prevent relapses and to make the gametes of Plasmodium vivax in human blood non-infective, it is desirable to give a course of primaquine 15 mg a day for 7 days. The dose is proportionately reduced for children (1 year, no; 1-4 years, 2.5 mg; 5-8 years, 5 mg; 8 to 14 years, 7.5 mg). Alternatively one or two tablets of chloroquine are given every week for several months (for adults). In some parts of the country, Plasmodium falciparum has become resistant to chloroquine therapy. These patients should be treated by a combination of sulphamethoxazole or sulphadoxime 500 mg and pyrimethamine (daraprim) 25 mg. In some resistant cases, it might become necessary to use cinchona quinine (dosage 300 mg three times daily for 7 days).

TUBERCULOSIS

Tuberculosis is caused by infection with Mycobacterium tuberculosis. It spreads by droplet infection. Adults with cavity lesions in the chest expel a large number of tubercle bacilli in their cough and sputum. If a susceptible individual inhales these bacteria, these lodge in the lungs, where they set up an inflammatory response in about 6 to 8 weeks. A small primary focus is formed in the lungs, from which the infection travels to the regional lymph nodes in the hilum of the lungs; the infected lymph nodes are enlarged. The primary focus in the lung and the glands together constitute the primary complex of tuberculosis. Primary complex occurs in children who are infected for the first time. Since the body tries to overcome this infection by cell-mediated immunity, a state of delayed hypersensitivity to tubercle bacterial protein develops in 6 to 10 weeks. This is demonstrated by injecting interadermally, 0.1 mg of 1 tuberculin unit of purified protein derivative (PPD) of tuberculin. In 48 to 72 hours, the site of injection is observed for erythema and the skin is palpated for induration. In India, tuberculin reaction (Mantoux test is considered positive, if the diameter of the indurated area exceeds 10 mm. A diameter of between 10 to 40 mm. indicated hypersensitivity due to previous infection but the disease may not be active. If the diameter is above 15 mm. it is strongly suggestive but not absolutely diagnostic of active disease. If, the reaction to 1 tuberculin unit is negative, but the disease is strongly suspected, the test may be repeated with 5 tuberculin units. Absence of reaction does not necessarily rule out previous infection with tubercle bacilli, especially if the patient is markedly undernourished, had a severe infection or had a recent episode of measles.

Clinical features suggestive of tuberculosis include moderate or hectic fever, poor appetite, loss of weight, night sweats, vague feeling of being unwell and at times palpable liver and spleen. Cough with expectoration may not always be present. In children cough with expectoration is less common. Malnourished children from poor families often develop tuberculosis after debilitating illnesses such as measles or whooping cough.

Most cases of primary complex heal by themselves if the body's resistance is good. In poor undernourished children, the infection may spread to be surrounding areas of lungs. The lesion may rupture into the bronchi and spread to other parts of the lung. A tuberculous lesion just under the pleura may cause pleural effusion. The tuberculous lesions may erode into a blood vessel and the infection may be carried to distant parts of the body such as kidneys, liver, joints, brain, meninges, etc. If only a few bacteria enter the blood stream, the infection may not become generalised and remain localised in distant tissues. In case of massive seeding of the blood vessels the infection may become generalised in the entire system, resulting in small miliary (millet seed) lesions everywhere in the body. These patients become very sick and if not treated early, succumb to the generalised infection.

Tuberculosis should always be suspected in any chronic fever with or without constitutional symptoms; painless but significant enlargement of lymph nodes; effusion into joints or pleural cavity; abdominal distension with vague doughy feel and unexplained loss of weight.

Treatment: The community health worker should always seek the advice of the doctor for all suspected cases of tuberculosis, since long intensive treatment is necessary. It is advisable to treat children less than 3 years old with positive tuberculin reaction, whether they have clinical symptoms or not, with isoniazid 10 to 15 mg/kg of body weight per day orally for about one year. This is done to prevent serious complications of tuberculosis such as meningitis and miliary spread. In order children and adults, positive tuberculin reaction is not an indication for treatment, unless there are other clinical or x-ray film evidences of active disease or if their sputum is positive for tubercle bacilli. In suspected cases the mode of treatment depends on various social considerations such as distance of the health center from the place of residence of the patient, the mode of transportation, cost of travel, socio-economic status of the family and the personality of the patient with regard to compliance for treatment. The treatment could be domiciliary if it is inconvenient to bring the patient to the health center for regular treatment. Compliance of the patient should be sought by regular visits of the health worker to the home of the patient.

Domiciliary treatment: Only oral medication can be given for modiciliary treatment, several schedules have been tried in the community. In symptomatic patients two or three drugs should be given together depending on the severity of illness. Following drugs can be used orally depending on their availability and ability of the family or health centre to afford these.

Isoniazid Adults. 300 mg orally once daily for one year. Recent evidence indicates that it might be possible to get good results even with twice a week schedule.

Children. 10 to 15 mg/kg/day orally for one year.

Side effects: Neuropathy, optic neuritis, liver damage.

PAS. Para amino Salicylic Acid. Dose 200 mg/kg/day orally in 3 divided doses. *Side effects*. Vomiting, gastrointestinal upset, goiter, hepatomegaly.

Rifampicin. Dose 10-15 mg/kg/daily orally as a single dose 1 hour before meal. Total dose for adults 450-600 mg/day. *Side effects*. Jaundice, leucopenia, fever. Treatment for 3 to 6 months in adequate.

Ethambutol. Dose 20-35 mg/kg/day orally in 3 divided doses for 4 weeks. Thereafter the dose is reduced to 15 mg/kg/day and continued for about a year, *Side effects*. Retinopathy, liver toxicity.

Antitubercular drugs should always be used under doctor's supervision. Streptomycin has limited role in domiciliary treatment and can only be given at the health centre.

LEPROSY

Leprosy is a chronic infectious disease caused by Mycobacterium leprae. Skin and nerves are two most commonly affected tissues. Since the disease causes disfigurement and loss of function of limbs, most people shun contact with patients and ostracise them for fear of contacting the disease. Therefore, patients hide the disease. Unlike the popular misconception, most cases of leprosy are either non-infective or not highly contagious. Nasal secretions of infective type of leprosy or discharge from ulcers contain the organism and may transmit the disease. Rarely, even one ideal contact in a susceptible patient may lead to infection. However a large majority of people have an inborn immunity from the disease and do not suffer inspite of close contact. Leprosy is a curable disease with modern treatment and all patients can be rehabilitated to lead a useful and normal life in their own families.

A hypopigmented (lighter color) patch on the skin, which persists for several days or weeks and does not itch should arouse suspicion of leprosy. The patch shows decreased sensation for temperature, light touch and pain. Since the temperature sensation is lost first, patients may not feel pain on contact with hot objects and therefore present with burns and scalds. The cutaneous nerves supplying the area get thickened and may be tender. Ulner, median, external popliteal, posterior tibial and great auricular nerves should always be palpated. This type of leprosy is called maculoanesthetic and is non-infective.

Some patients present with a slightly thickened, pinkish areas of skin. The thickened area is well demarcated and has diminished sensations. The peripheral nerves are thickened. Trophic ulcers occur in the hypoaesthetic areas and muscles of hands and feet are paralysed due to involvement of motor nerves, resulting in deformities such as claw hands, drop foot etc. Both the above types are of tuberculoid type, and are generally not infective. These patients have some degree of inborn resistance to the disease.

Lepromatous type of leprosy is contagious. In these patients skin is infiltrated, and thickened, margins are not well defined, and skin appears shiny and erythematous. Sensations are not affected or only minimally involved. Nerve involvement occurs in late stages of the disease. Patients may develop large disfiguring nodules on the face and other parts of the body. There is widespread involvement of all body tissues. Nasal secretions are highly infective. Smears made from tissue fluids obtained after slitting the skin over the pinna show leprosy bacilli.

Lesious of leprosy may be indeterminate or borderline in some patients.

Treatment: Dapsone is the drug of choice for primary care of most cases of leprosy. Treatment should be started with a dose of 25 mg once daily, which should be increased in steps of 25 mg every week till a dose of 100 mg a day is reached. The treatment should be continued without interruption for at least 2 to 3 years in maculoanesthetic type; 5 years for tuberculoid type and 10 to 15 years for lepromatous type. It is desirable to add Rifampicin in a dose of 450 to 600 mg before breakfast once a day uninterruptedly for a minimum period of 6 months in case of lepromatous leprosy or those types of tuberculoid leprosy which develop resistance to dapsone.

CHOLERA

Cholera is endemic in eastern part of India. It is caused by Vibrio cholerae which is transmitted to the host in food and water contaminated by feces of cholera patients through flies or hands of asymptomatic carriers of cholera.

The patients develop effortless vomitting and severe watery diarrhea with an abrupt onset. Patients become dehydrated very quickly, apathetic, or even moribund. Their limbs appear cold and clammy; eyes appear sunken. Breathing is fast due to acidosis; urine is not passed for several hours. There may be high fever especially in children. Some patients develop seizures.

These patients should be treated with oral hydration as explained in subsequent section on diarrhea in the chapter on Material and Child Health. Oral rehydration solution is prepared by dissolving 20 g of glucose, 3.5 g of sodium chloride, 2.5 g of sodium bicarbonate and 1.5 g of potassium chloride in one liter of water. This solution is given ad lib according to thirst.

Since the patient vomits profusely, it is safer to give this fluid by spoonfuls rather than cupfuls. Fairly large quantities of fluids are taken by patients. After starting oral hydration, patient should be sent to the health center for further therapy. If oral rehydration solution is not available any fluids could be used till oral rehydration packets are made available. A three finger pinch of salt and four finger scoop of sugar in half liter of water may be used as a stop gap arrangement. Tetracycline 250 mg 6 hourly should be administered till the diarrhea is controlled. Dosage is reduced proportionately for children.

DIPHTHERIA

It is a highly infectious disease of early childhood, caused by Corynebacterium diphtheriae. It spreads by droplet infection from patients or carriers. Incubation period is 2 to 4 days.

Clinically, the child looks very ill and toxic. Temperature is only moderately elevated. In the commonest variety, tonsils are congested with a greyish membrane, which spreads to surrounding areas. Lymph nodes in the neck are large and painful. If the membrane spreads to larynx, the child may die of suffocation. Less often nose may be involved, causing a blood strained nasal discharge.

If the child survives the acute stage of illness, he may develop serious complications 2 to 6 weeks later. Myocarditis occurs in about 2 weeks. Child becomes restless and pale; pulse may be rapid and feeble, irregular or even slow. The child may succumb due to heart failure.

Almost at the same interval, the child may develop nasal tone in his speech and the swallowed fluids may regurgitate through the nose. Paralysis of convergence and accommodation occur after 3 weeks. Near vision becomes blurred. In 4 to 6 weeks, the patient may have general weakness of limbs due to peripheral neuritis.

Acute streptococcal follicular tonsillitis may be mistaken in diagnosis. These children have high fever and less toxemia. Thrush may present as a thick membrane, which when scrapped leaves a raw area underneath.

If a child in a school is suspected to have diphtheria, school should not be closed. District health officer should be alerted and all children who came in contact with the index case should be kept under surveillance for a week. Those with membrance and susceptibility (Schick Test negative) should be treated actively.

Diphtheria is a serious illness. It cannot be treated in ambulatory setting in the village. Patient should be isolated in primary health center or infectious disease hospital. He should be given 20,000 to 60,000 units of diphtheria antitoxin serum by injection as early as possible. Penicillin injection is given to treat the infection and to prevent its spread, but it is ineffective to abort the symptoms caused by toxins of diphtheria bacillus.

MEASLES

Measles is a common infectious disease of childhood, caused by measles virus. Infants are relatively protected from contacting this infection in the first 6 to 9 months of life because of antibodies acquired from the mother via the placenta. Incubation period is 10-14 days. Spread is by droplet infection. Patient is most infective at the onset of the illness.

Clinically, the illness starts with high fever, watering of eyes and running of nose. The peak of fever is lower on the second, third and fourth day. On the fourth day a few greyish white pinhead size spots surrounded by a red flush (Koplik spots) may be seen on the inner side of cheek or on the soft palate. On the fifth day, the fever rises again and a reddish rash appears on the skin in the following order; behind the ears, forehead, face, neck, trunk and extremities. Fever lasts for a few days and rash disappears in the same order, leaving behind a branny, pigmented desquamation for a few days.

Measles is a debilitating illness and poor undernourished children are likely to get serious complications such as diarrhea, kwashiorkor, keratomalacia, pneumonia and eventually bronchiectasis. These children are more prone to develop serious complications of tuberculosis if they are already exposed to tuberculosis or are in contact with an open case.

There is no specific treatment for measles. Personal hygiene should be maintained. Child should receive good nourishing diet. Parents should be instructed about the true nature of the illness and given appropriate health education. Antibiotics are generally not necessary except for complications such as pneumonia or suppurative otitis media.

MUMPS

Mumps is caused by a virus. Children are most commonly affected. Illness starts with fever and pain behind the lower jaw, where a tender swelling (parotitis) may be seen, initially on one side and later on both sides. These children may complain of headache, vomiting and sometimes of stiff neck and mild drowsiness (meningoencephalitis). Some children develop painful swelling of testes. Abdominal pain in not unusual. There is no specific treatment. Pain is relived by aspirin. The child should be kept away from the school, till the parotid swelling subsides.

WHOOPING COUGH (PERTUSSIS)

It is an infectious disease caused by Bordetella pertussis, common in childhood. It is most infectious in the early stage of the illness and is spread by droplet infection from nasal discharge or cough. Incubation period is about 3 weeks.

Clinically the child has cough and nasal discharge just like ordinary upper respiratory infections for a week or 10 days. Even at this stage, cough is more marked at night, and is often followed by vomiting and comes in spasms. Gradually nasal discharge disappears but the spasms become more prolonged. A paroxysm of cough is usually followed by a long whooping inspiration. This may or may not be always present. Any activity or feeding may initiate the paroxysm of cough followed by vomiting. This stage lasts for 3 to 4 weeks and thereafter the duration of spasms decreases and interval between these increase. The child recovers in 6-8 weeks from the onset of illness.

Younger babies may not have a characteristic whoop and may only get attacks of apnea which may be dangerous.

Whooping cough is early childhood is a debilitating illness with high morbidity and mortality.

Pneumonia and other pulmonary complications are common. Children may develop hernia due to excessive cough raising the intraabdominal pressure. Subconjunctival hemorrhage is not uncommon. Cerebral bleeding may cause encephalopathy and convulsions. Patients are afraid of taking food because of fear of paroxyms and become progressively debilitated. They may develop marasmus, kwashiorkor and keratomalacia.

Antibiotics (erythromycin or chloramphenicol) are useful only if given in the first week or 10 days when clinical diagnosis is not always evident. Afterward only symptomatic treatment may be done with an antispasmodic and expectorant. Phenobarbitone 15 mg. may be given at night to help the child sleep in comfort. Good nourishing food is necessary. If the food initiates a spasm, give the main portion of food soon after a spasm of cough. A second spasm may not cause vomiting.

5. MORE COMPLEX HEALTH PROBLEMS, in which progression of disease may not be easily controlled but which require definite medical care for the relief of pain and alleviation of suffering. These include *disorders of muscles and joints, other sensory and neurological disorders and malignant disorders*. Very few of these illnesses can be adequately managed in the primary-health-care setting. There should be facilities for referring these patients to the district hospital on institutions with better facilities.

6. CHRONIC ILLNESSES, with prolonged course of illness, but which do not cause significant disability need not be treated.

20

Maternal and Child Health

Introduction

According to the population projections for the year 1983 by the Registrar General and Census Commissioner of India, women in the reproductive age group (between 15 and 45 years old) and children (under 15 years) together would constitute about 60 per cent of the population. Of these 38 per cent will be children, 13.4 per cent under 5 years old, 12.8 per cent between 5 and 10 years and 12 per cent between 10 and 15 years old. Mothers and children together account for about three-fifths of the total deaths in the community. Morbidity among them is also very high. Therefore, mothers and children deserve high priority in primary health care.

Social Status of the Mother

Women in India, do not enjoy a similar social status as men because they are not considered equal economic partners in the family, since they usually do not bring cash earning for the family kitty. Women have to do hard physical work for household chores. They often share the jobs of their husbands in agricultural fields and toil nearly as strenuously as menfolk. Women bear the added burden of pregnancy, over the timing and frequency of which, they have little control. The over-worked mother is often undernourished and anemic, because she gets a disproportionately low share of the food and other nutrients available to the family. She suffers from pregnancy-related complications and medical illnesses, which adversely affect the health of the undernourished pregnant mother. The maternal mortality significantly declined from 6 per 1000 in 1916 to less than 3 per 1000 during the last three decades or so, but it is still 20 times higher than in the advanced countries of the West. A large proportion of Indian mothers suffer from serious illnesses during pregnancy, which incapacitate them for their entire life.

Cost of Upbringing of a Child

Notwithstanding, the individual variations in some families and different regions, it is estimated that an average Indian couple spends a sum equivalent to wages of an average worker for 4 to 5 years, simply for upbringing of a child from the time of birth to his maturity into adulthood. This money is spent on providing food, clothing, shelter and medical care. Besides this expenditure incurred by the parents, the government also spends on making arrangements for the health-care, education, recreation and other welfare activities for children. This amount may vary in different parts of the country. Generally an amount equal to the wages earned by a worker in one year is spent by the society for these social services for every child over a span of 18 to 20 years of childhood. If a child dies before he becomes an economically active adult, all the investment made on his upbringing is lost irretrievably. When a child falls sick, his parents stay at home to nurse him. They lose wages and there is loss of production in the fields or the factory. Children provide social security to parents in their old age. It is a wise economic policy to protect mothers and children from ill health, handicaps and avoidable deaths. Health services for the mothers and children yield maximum social and economic benefits in relation to the cost incurred.

Mother and Child Dyad

Health of the child is intimately linked to that of the mother. If the mother is malnourished, suffers from pregnancy-related complications or other medical illnesses the fetal growth and development are adversely affected. Such fetuses may be born preterm or have low-birth weight. They suffer from severe illnesses and are more prone to die in the neonatal period. If they survive, their future growth and development and compromised. Satisfactory lactation by the mother protects the infant from a variety of exteral infections. Mother suffering from infectious illnesses not only transmits these to her offspring but is often unable to look after them adequately.

Since the health of the mother and child are so intimately linked, *maternal and child health services* should also be properly *integrated and coordinated* in such a manner that the mother can obtain health care for her children at the same time as she seeks medical care or antenatal check-ups for herself. If services for the mother and children are provided at different physical settings on different days, these are not likely to be fully utilised. These should be as near her home as possible, so that a mother busy in her household chores can utilise these services. It is administratively more convenient, technically sound and socially more relevant not only to provide the maternal and child health services together, but also to link these with family planning activities. When the mother recognises that her child has a reasonable chance of survival to adulthood, she becomes motivated to limit her family size. There is less stress on the mother's health, if she has fewer pregnancies. She can look after her own and her children's health better if the family size is small.

Synopsis of principles of maternal, child health, family planning services.

1. Mothers and children are a precious resource of the country. Together they constitute 60 per cent of our population.
2. Health of children is intimately linked to the health, nutrition and social status of the mother.
3. Health of mother and child are adversely affected in large families.
4. Health services of mothers and children should be as near their homes as possible and should be available at the same physical set up-almost at the same time.

Health Status of Mothers and Children

Mothers

Although maternal mortality declined during the last three decades, it is still unacceptably high as compared to that in the more advanced countries of the West. The maternal morbidity and mortality due to malnutrition, anemia, medical illnesses and pregnancy related complications such as hyperemesis, toxemia, vascular accidents, antepartium, hemorrhage, sepsis, problems of child birth such as prolonged obstructed labor, retained placenta, placenta previa, hemorrhage and shock *etc.* can be substantially reduced by good health care during pregnancy, at the time of delivery and during the post-partum period.

Children

Infants, infant mortality rates did not decline significantly during the last three decades since independence of India. According to the data for the year 1980, for every 1000 live born infants, 114 died before they were 1 year old. About 55 per cent of these deaths occurred in the first month of life. In the corresponding period the crude death rate for the entire population (general mortality rate) of India declined significantly, largely due to eradication of small-pox and fall in death rates due to malaria, kala-azar, cholera and other infectious and parasitic diseases, mostly occurring among older children and adults. Apparent increase in the life expectancy has led to an erroneous belief among decision makers that infact mortality rates have declined substantially. Health rates among preschool children also continue to be high. In a cohort of babies born in the year 1973, 2.2 per cent died in the second year, 1.4 per cent in the third year, 1.1 per cent died in the fourth year and 0.6 per cent in the fifth year. In contrast, infant deaths in Europe and America are only 15 to 20 per 1000 live birth infants. Likewise the preschool-age deaths are minimal in these advanced countries.

Table 20.1

Infant Mortality Rates 1911-1980
(Adapted from Survey on Infant and Child Mortality 1979 Registrar General India 1981) and subsequent information

1911-15	204 (5 years average)
1941-45	161
1946-50	134
1951-1961	146 (Actuarial report)
1961-1971	129
1970	129
1972	139
1975	140
1977	130
1978	125
1979	120
1980	114

Neonatal deaths High, incidence of low-birth-weight babies (about 30-35 per cent) is the major epidemiological factor responsible for a large proportion of neonatal deaths, which are largely attributed to systemic infections, tetanus neonatorum and diarrheal disease. Respiratory distress is not an uncommon cause of death in the neonatal period and may be attributed to depression of the respiratory center in the brain due to birth injuries, interference with pulmonary ventilation due to aspiration and pneumonias *etc*. Major congenital anomalies such as congenital heart disease or neurological malformation are responsible for *less than one per cent of* neonatal deaths.

Causes of low-birth-weight, Low birth weight may be caused by maternal, fetal, placental or biological factors.

Causes attributed to mother.

These include maternal malnutrition, anemia, medical illnesses such as afflictions of heart and kidney, smoking during pregnancy and pregnancy-related complications, such as eclampsia, antepartum hemorrhage and intrauterine infections. Fetuses with congenital anomalies and with twinning have low birth weight.

Placental causes

Disorders of implantation, and placental infarcts.

Biological factors

Very young mothers below 20 years old or mothers older than 35 years bear smaller babies. Primipara or those above 4th para also tend to get infants with low-birth weight.

In the post-neonatal period of infancy (1 to 12 months) morbidity and mortality are by and large due to causes similar to those operating in the *second and third years of life. Diarrheal disease* and *respriatory infections* together account for half of the total deaths. Malnourished and anemic children are prone to suffer from more severe and more frequent episodes of these illnesses. It is difficult to estimate the direct or indirect contribution of malnutrition and anemia to early-childhood deaths but it is believed to be about 30 per cent. Other important causes of post-neonatal early-childhood deaths are tetanus, whooping cough, diphtheria and poliomyelitis, together causing about 5 per cent of deaths in that age period. Snake bites, accidental poisoning and accidents are responsible for about 5 per cent of early childhood deaths.

Table 20.2

Epidemiological Correlates of Infant Mortality in Kerala (low IMR), Uttar Pradesh (high IMR), Panjab (intermediate IMR)

	Kerala		*Uttar Pradesh*		*Punjab*		*All-India*	
	R	*U*	*R*	*U*	*R*	*U*	*R*	*U*
Neonatal mortality	27	17	93	59	60	30	80	41
Post-neonatal mortality	15	9	79	51	51	35	56	30
IMR	42	26	172	110	111	65	136	71
IMR related to female literacy								
Illiterate	55	29	188	125	128	95	145	88
Below primary	44	40	141	105	87	63	101	57
Primary or above	29	21	115	72	48	40	71	47
IMR related to mother's age at marriage								
Below 18 years	52	24	175	115	125	90	156	88
18-20 years	30	34	155	106	101	45	132	67
Above 20 years	32	14	145	46	101	41	90	46
IMR related to sources of drinking water								
Tap/handpump	-	26	140	95	108	63	112 121	66 Tap 81 hand-pump
Well/pond/tank/river	38	26	182	156	140	138	143 115	84 well pond 106 tank river

In the later part of preschool age *i.e. 4th and 5th years* of life the death rate declines. Diarrheas, pneumonias and malnutrition are prominent but relatively less important than in the earlier years. Incidence of tuberculosis, diphtheria, whooping cough, tetanus, poliomyelitis and enteric infections rises because the child is exposed more and more to environment outside his intimate family.

Parasitic infection are fairly common is preschool years and contribute significantly to ill health, pallor and malnutrition.

Table 20. 3

Social, Economic Development: Utilisation and Availability of Health Services

	Kerala		*Uttar Pradesh*		*Punjab*		*All-India*	
Medical attention at death	*R*	*U*	*R*	*U*	*R*	*U*	*R*	*U*
Medical Institution	75.1	-	18.1	42.3	50.9	66.6	30.22	56.8
Trained medical practitioner	4.3	-	15.62	24.9	34.6	28.4	11.48	13.7
Untrained medical practitioner	7.3	-	31.1	8.2	8.7	-	21.6	6.5
Others	13.3	-	35.2	24.6	5.8	4.9	36.7	22.9
Medical attention when sick								
Medical Institution	97.2	100	50.35	79.4	65.1	75	74.2	85.4
Trained medical practitioner	1.9	0	80.5	19.35	34.9	25	13.8	11.7
Untrained medical practitioner	0.5	0	19.15	4.35	-	-	12.0	2.9
Per cent infant deaths not attended by trained medical practitioners		20.6		66.3				58.3
Per cent estimated popn. by type of facility								
Less than 2 km	64.2	8.8	71.6	34.9				
2-5 km	22.6	42.9	22.0	25				
5-10 km	7.6	30.9	5.5	24.1				
Over 10 km	5.6	17.4	20.9	16.0				
Higher Secondary school								
Less than 2 km	57.1	20.7	43.2	27.4				
2-5 km	33.9	37.4	38.2	33.4				
5-10 km	8.0	33.2	18.0	29.2				
Over 10 km	1.0	8.7		15.0				
Primary school								
Less than 2 km	95.7	86.2	98.6	94.1				
2-5 km	3.7	11.1	1.0	4.4				
5-10 km	-	1.5	-	0.7				
Over 10 km	0.6	1.2	0.4	0.8				

Contd..

Bus stand					
Less than 2 km		85.5	24.5	75.5	44.7
2-5 km		6.9	36.8	18.0	26.2
5-20 km		2.7	28.6	5.6	18.8
Over 10 km		4.9	10.1	0.9	10.3
Rly. Station					
Less than 2 km		9.3	8.5	12.5	6.6
2-5 km		13.9	12.5	17.1	9.4
5-10 km		14.0	25.3	28.1	19.0
Over 10 km		62.8	53.7	42.4	65.0
Post Office					
Less than 2 km		89.1	55.5	66.3	61.5
2-5 km		10.9	36.5	26.9	27.2
5-10 km		-	7.3	6.8	7.6
Over 10 km		-	0.7	-	3.7
Literacy					
Illiterate	M	23.9	56.6	50.8	54.7
	F	35.7	85.1	66.7	79.1
Below primary	M	35.1	23.4	21.7	26.3
	F	33.4	10.3	18.0	14.5
Below Matric	M	33.5	14.2	19.3	14.6
	F	26.0	4.0	12.4	5.5
Matric and above but below graduate	M	6.6	5.0	7.3	3.8
	F	4.5	0.6	2.7	0.8
Graduate & above	M	0.9	0.8	0.9	0.6
	F	0.4	0.0	0.2	0.1
Water Supply					
Tap	R	5.11	0.9	4.9	5.6
	U	10.5	67.6	53.0	76.1
Handpump	R	0.2	23.4	83.7	17.4
	U	0.3	14.1	45.8	9.2
Well	R	88.1	70.8	9.7	67.7
	U	83.5	16.8	1.0	12.6
Pond/tank	R	3.1	0.2	0.7	3.2
	U	2.6	0.1	-	0.8
River	R	2.3	0.1	-	3.3
	U	1.9	0.4	-	0.3
Population below poverty line		47	50.1	15.1	

Maternal and Child Health Services

The major goal of maternal and child-health services in primary health care is to reduce the incidence of illnesses, disabilities and deaths among mothers by providing treatment for medical illnesses during pregnancy, preventing pregnancy-related complications and promotion of health and nutrition of mothers during pregnancy and lactation. Children are protected from illnesses, and their optimal growth and development are promoted by better nutrition, good environmental stimulation and freedom from illnesses.

Both mothers and children are protected from incapacitating handicaps and helped to play a useful role in the society. In order to achieve the above objectives the following sets of services for MCH and family planning should be provided.

For Mothers

(1) All pregnant women in the community should be indentified.

(2) They should be examined periodically during the antenatal period and helped so that,

(i) they remain healthy during pregnancy.

(ii) their anxieties associated with pregnancy, child birth and lactation are allayed.

(iii) medical illnesses and pregnancy-related complications are detected early and given appropriate attention.

(iv) mothers at high risk to develop complications are identified and protected.

(v) unforeseen complications of pregnancy receive prompt remedial measures.

(vi) position and lie of the fetus are observed and arrangements made for delivery in appropriate setting.

(vii) health and nutrition of mother is preserved and promoted.

(viii) the mother is motivated and prepared during pregnancy for satisfactory breast feeding of her infant.

(ix) she is motivated to limit her family size by spacing of pregnancies, use of contraceptives or by undergoing sterilization in the postpartum period.

(3) unforeseen complications during labor are anticipated and their hazards to the mother and fetus minimised by adequate preparatory arrangements and training of the traditional birth attendants for safe and clean midwifery practices during labor.

For Children

(1) Mothers should be encouraged to breast feed their infants.

(2) Infants and young children should be immunised against common infectious illnesses such as tuberculosis (BCG Vaccine), diphtheria, pertussis and tetanus (Triple antigen or DPT), poliomyelitis and measles.

(3) Infants and preschool children are kept under surveillance by regular health check and serial weight record to detect at an early stage, any deviation from the normal pattern of growth for the child by comparing his growth curve with the average growth curve of children. Arrested or delayed growth of a child is an early and useful indicator of undernutrition or hidden infection.

(4) Health education to the mother for personal hygiene, lactation nutrition, prevention of illnesses, domiciliary care of simple health problems and prevention of household accidents and poisoning.

For Family Planning

(1) All eligible couples should be motivated to limit their family size.

(2) Family planning education should be given to all persons at every medical contact, such as, methods of spacing the pregnancies, use of contraceptives and the possibility of sterilisation through vasectomy or tubectomy.

(3) Family planning services as outlined above, should be provided to all eligible couples, in a flexible and individualised manner, which is most convenient and acceptable to them.

(4) Identifying those members of the family and community who are decision makers, about the family size. Family planning education should be specially directed towards them.

Strategies for MCH and Family Planning Services

(1) Training of doctors, paramedicals and community health workers.

(2) House visit by health workers and identification of all pregnant women in the community.

(3) Antenatal care of the pregnant women at regular intervals.

(4) Intenatal care.

(5) Postnatal care.

(6) Perinantal care of the fetus and newborn infant.

(7) Motivation of mother and health care of the mother for satisfactory lactation. Promotion of breast feeding.

(8) Immunization of infants against communicable diseases.

(9) Health and nutrition education of the family.

(10) Surveillance of growth and development of preschool children. Early detection of deviation from the normal pattern of growth.

(11) School health services.

(12) Nutrition supplementation of pregnant, lactating mothers and children at high risk.

Home Visits by the Health Worker to Identify Pregnant Women

The village health worker should visit each household in her area regularly at predetermined interval. She should identify the mothers, who had missed their period and motivate them to visit the health center for antenatal check up regularly. She should explain to her the advantage of regular antenatal health check for her own health and that of infant. She should make a record of her observations in the specially provided registers for such domiciliary visits. If the response of the mother is lukewarm because of inadequate motivation or other household difficulties the health worker should not relax in her efforts. She should re-educate her and persuade other members of the family such as her husband or mother-in-law. Her difficulties in attending attended clinic should be identified and obviated if possible. If this is not possible the health worker may provide as much health check up as needed at home for those mothers who do not attend the clinic at regular intervals. Nutrition and health education should be imparted during home visits. Better cooperation of the mother is assured, if some multivitamin and hematinic tablets are issued to the mother at home and she is asked to replenish these and obtain further supplies from the clinic.

Antenatal Care

Under optimal conditions, a mother should have an antenatal health check every month during the first seven months of pregnancy, once a fortnight till 36 weeks and weekly thereafter. It is however, not practicable since the health centre staff will not be able to look after such a large load of work. Most mothers cannot attend the clinic that frequently because of the resulting disturbance in their household chores. Long distance of the clinic from the place of residence and the loss of work or wages are other reasons for poor attendance at clinics. It is however necessary that every mother should make at least 4 to 5 antenatal visits at around 10th, 20th, 30th, 35th and 38th weeks of gestation to the primary health center or subcenter.

First antenatal contact (Around 10th week)

During the first antenatal visit the diagnosis of pregnancy should be confirmed. Health status of the mother should be reviewed specially for any medical illnesses. Weight and blood pressure should be obtained. Blood hemoglobin level should be estimated and urine analysed for albumin and sugar. When facilities are available, Rhesus blood grouping and serological tests for syphilis should also be done. Data should be recorded on an antenatal card. Mother should receive multivitamin and hematinic tablets, if no morning sickness is present.

Second antenatal visit (Around 20th week)

In all subsequent visits, weight and blood pressure should be recorded, hemoglobin level estimated and urinalysis carried out. The skin over upper part of ankle should be gently pressed to look for edema. Even before the edema becomes evident, the mother may complain that her shoes have become tight and pinch her feet. Pallor is common during pregnancy due to increased body fluids and nutritional inadequacy. Poor rural women are often undernourished and anemic. They need hematinic and multivitamin tablets. An injection of tetanus toxoid may be given during the second visit at around 20th week of pregnancy. Abdominal examination should be done to confirm fetal parts, fetal movements and fetal heart sounds.

Third antenatal visit (Around 30th week)

Besides the routine antenatal health care as in the second visit, the mother should receive second does of tetanus toxoid. Her abdomen should be palpated for the height of uterine fundus and presentation. Fetal heart sounds should be ausenltated. Health and nutrition education should be reinforced. Mother should be motivated to breast feed her infant after delivery. She should be advised to space her next pregnancy after at least 2 years. If she already has two living children, she should receive appropriate advice to stop further increase in her family size.

Fourth antenatal visit (Around 35th week)

Besides the above mentioned measures, the mother should be subjected to obstetric examination to check for any fetal malpresentation. High risk mothers should be identified and appropriate anticipatory measures adopted. Decision should be made about the place of confinement. Third dose of tetanus toxoid may be administered during this visit.

Fifth antenatal visit (Around 38th week)

Signs of engagement of head are observed. High-risk warning indicators such as antepartum bleeding per vegina are looked for. Mother should be psychologically prepared and advised to breast feed her infant after delivery. The health worker should see that the breast nipples are supplied are not inverted and are kept clean. If these are retracted gentle manipulation with fingers from the periphery of breasts towards areola helps in improving these Pelvis examination should be done to assess the pervis and presentation of the feltus.

High Risk Pregnancies

Major factors

1. Moderate to severe toxemia of pregnancy.
2. Chronic hypertension.

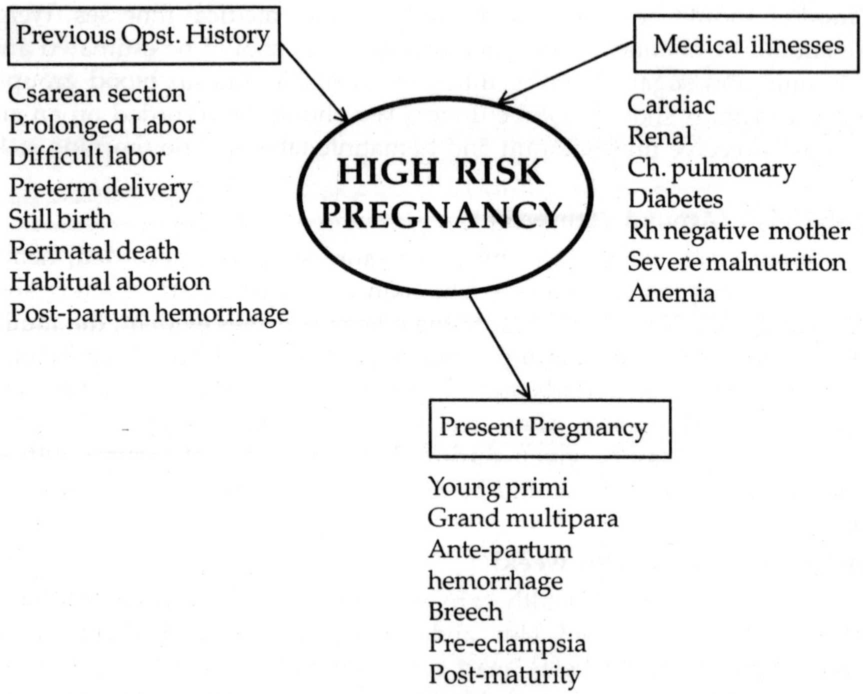

Fig. 20.2

3. Significant renal or heart disease.
4. Hydramnios or oligohydramnios.
5. Rupture of uterus.

Moderate risk factors

Maternal factors

1. Mild toxemia.
2. Prior history of urinary tract infection, eclampsia, cesarean section and still births.
3. Medical illnesses, such as without cardiacfailure heart disease, tuberculosis, diabetes mellitus and acute pyelonephritis.
4. Rhesus incompatibility.
5. Threatened abortion and antepartum hemorrhage.
6. Small deformed pelvis.
7. Short-statured, low-weight mother.
8. Primigravida mother.
9. Very young (under 20 years) or very old mother (above 35 years).

Intranatal Care

Under normal circumstances, child birth, a physiological process does not pose any serious danger to the mother or the fetus. Rarely, the labor may be complicated and hazardous for the mother or the fetus. The health worker should be able to forestall these complications and undertake preventive measures to protect the health and safety of the mother and the infant. Although some complications may be unforeseen, it is possible to anticipate most of these. Guidelines for identifying high risk pregnancies have been outliner above. Such pregnant mothers should be seen by the doctor and booked for delivery in the primary health center or the district hospital with adequate facilities. Non-high risk mothers mav be delivered at their own homes by the trained dai or traditional birth-attendant (TBA). In domiciliary midwifery, the delivery is conducted in familiar environments and the mother can soon look after her other children and participate in some simple household chores. There is lesser risk of cross infection in the home than in the institutions. The disadvantage of confinement at home is that the mother does not get adequate rest, or prompt appropriate medical care in case of unanticipated complications. It is, therefore, necessary that the TBA should be able to recognise situations, during labor, which could be hazardous for the mother and the infant. She should be able to immediately seek help of the doctor from the health center.

Table 20.4

Danger signals during labor

1. Excessive bleeding prior to labor, at the time of delivery or soon thereafter.
2. Malpresentation.

3. Premature rupture of membrane (more than 12 hours before delivery).
4. Sluggish or no pains or poor progress after good pains.
5. Rapidly rising pulse rate, shock or collapse of the mother during labor or immediately thereafter.
6. Abdominal girth of more than I meter (hydramnios).
7. Fetal distress as evidence by slow irregular or fast fetal-heart rate, exaggerated fetal movement or passage of meconium stained liquor amnii.
8. Prolonger labor (greater than 24 hours).
9. Non-separation of placenta for more than half an hour after the delivery of the fetus.

Table 20.5

Functions of Traditional Birth Attendant (TBA)

1. To conduct a normal delivery.
2. Identify high risk pregnancy and look for danger signals during labor.
3. Use a midwifery kit properly. She should be conversant with the needs for sterilisation of the instruments.(She should be able to substitute locally available, clean, preferably sterile materials in place of the midwifery kit in times of need, such as use of a new shaving blade for cutting the cord, or clean washed and sunned sari piece as pads and edge of the sari as cord for tying the umbilical stump).
4. Immediate care of the newborn infant. She should be able to cleanse from the oral cavity of the new born blood, mucus and amniotic fluid, and remove vernix caseosa from the skin. She should be able to do mouth to mouth breathing.
5. Referal of infants who develop such illnesses, which she cannot manage adequately herself, to the doctor. These conditions include severe jaundice, neck rigidity, twitchings, convulsions, rolling movements of eyes, persistent vomiting, lack of opening at the anus, cleltpalate, difficulty in breathing, refusal of the baby to suck at breast and very low-birth weight *etc.*
6. Care of the mother in the post-partum period for conditions such as, non-separation of placenta, after pains, constipation, piles, inability to pass urine for more than 24 hours after delivery, painful episiotomy and retracted or cracked nipples.
7. Surveillance of the mother for development of any postpartum complications.
8. Psychological preparation of the mother for breast feeding her infant and helping her in establishing satisfactory lactation.
9. Linkage between patients and the doctor.

Care of Common Abnormalities of Pregnancy

First Trimester

Retention of Urine

The mother may not be able to pass urine, after experiencing some difficulty in passing urine for a few days. This usually occurs suddenly at about 12 to 18 weeks of gestation. It is most often attributed to retrovetted uterus getting fixed in the pelvis. Fnlarging utterus may press on the neck of the bladder, thus causing obstruction to the urinary outflow. The bladder should be emptied gradually by a rubber catheter. Mother should be instructed to preferably lie with the ace downwards while resting at night.

Hemorrhage

Threatened abortion is a common cause of vaginal hemorrhage, but it may also be due to vesicular mole, ectopia pregnancy or ulceration of the cervix. Hemorrhage during pregnancy should be regarded as a serious complication. Such patients should be referred to the appropriate level of health care, where a detailed history and physical examination should be carried out. Blood pressure, pulse rate and hemoglobin level should be obtained. Cervix should be examined through a speculum to rule out a cervical lesion. Veginal examination should be carried out to note the size and position of the uterus, condition of os, and any render adnexal mass in fornices.

In cases of *threatened abortion,* there is little bleeding and only slight disturbance. Such patients do not go into shock. Os is closed and uterus corresponds to the duration of amenorrhea. Fornices are clear. These mother should be asked to rest. They should be given mild sedation. Most patients improve with this. It is preferable to avoid interference, unless bleeding is severe and abortion becomes inevitable such as when hemorrhage is recurrent for more than 3 to 4 days or when os is found open on vaginal examination.

If bleeding is severe, give 0.2 mg of methergin IM. Pethedine 50 to 100 mg IM may be given to relieve pain. If os is open, index finger may be inserted gently into the cavity to empty the uterine contents, followed by a second dose of methergin. The patient is referred to hospital. If bleeding continues syntocinone I.V. drip is given. In primary health center, the uterus may be emptied by suction under sedation or by dilatation and curettage under general anesthesia.

If os is closed in the presence of profuse hemorrhage, no attempt is made to open or evacuate the uterus. Blood transfusion is generally necessary. Antibiotics are given in cases of septic abortion and following evacuation of the uterine contents.

Ruptured ectopic pregnancy

Ruptured ectopic pregnancy is a major surgical emergency necessitating immediate referral to a good hospital. In such cases vaginal bleeding is generally not heavy but patient becomes very ill suddenly, goes into shock with pallor and has rapid thready pulse. Abdomen becomes full and lower abdomen is tender. On vaginal examination, a tender vaginal swelling is felt on one side or in the Pouch of Douglas. Uterine size is smaller than expected from the duration of amenorrhea. The patient should be resuscitated, laparotomy should be performed immediately and ruptured tube should be resected during the operation.

Vesicular mole

This should be suspected in cases where uterine height is more than that expected from the duration of amenorrhea. Such patients should be referred to the hospital. The principles of treatment in the hospital are as mentioned. If there is massive bleeding and vesicular mole is being expelled, the patient should be treated as for abortion with open os. If os is closed in a uterus of over 20 weeks, and bleeding is marked, syntocinone 10 units in 500 ml of 5 per cent glucose, should be given by intravenous drip. When os opens and admits one finger, uterus could be evacuated by vacuum aspiration. Blood transfusion is needed and 0.5 mg of ergometrine should be given intravenously.

Second Trimester

Bleeding

If bleeding is slight, the patient is treated with rest and sedation as for threatened abortion. When bleeding is heavy, exytocin 10 units in 500 ml of 5 per cent glucose is given by I.V. drip and spontaneous expulsion is anticipated. Digital evacuation is done. If os is closed and bleeding is heavy, oxytocin drip is given as above. Transfusion is given and antibiotics are administered, if necessary.

Third Trimester

Bleeding

Bleeding during third trimester may be due to (i) *premature separation of normally placed placenta (abruptio placenia or accidental* hemorrhage *or due to* (ii) *placenta previa i.e.,* when placema covers the lower uterine segment os. Moderate to severe accidental hemorrhage is usually painful and tends to be continuous. On palpation, uterus appears tender and hard. Fetal heart rate is altered. In case of placenta previa, bleeding is generally painless and is intermittent. Uterus appears soft and non-tender. Fatal heart rate is normal. Vaginal examination should not be done unless the patient can be shifted to the hospital, since a traumatic vaginal examination may result in severe bleeding.

Management. In cases of ante partum hemorrhage, it is desirable to avoid the vaginal examination Patient should be sedated with 1.5 mg of morphine or 100 mg of pethedine and immediately moved to the district hospital. Transfusion is necessary for severe bleeding. If bleeding continues, membrane should be ruptured below the level of presenting part to initiate labor. If the bleeding increases slow oxytocin IV drip should be started with 2 units in 500 ml of 5% glucose solution, giving 5 to 10 drops a minute initially, adjusting the rate to obtain optimum contraction of the uterus.

All cases of placenta previa should be moved to the hospital. If bleeding starts before 38 weeks, patient is sedated with 15 mg IM of morphine. Blood pressure and pulse are watched. Blood transfusion is given when possible. In cases of marginal placenta previa (only a part of placenta reaching the lower uterine segment), membrances are ruptuned below the presenting part and oxytocin drip is started to induce labor. As the descent of the presenting part starts, bleeding usually stops. In cases of complete placenta previa covering the whole of os. as detected on PV examination, cesarrean section in a hospital is unavoidable.

lower segment cesarean section operation is done. Multigravida mothers should be sterilised by ligation of the tube at the same time.

Toxemia of Pregnancy (PET)

Although pre-eclamptic toxemia cannot be prevented in all cases, its hazards can be largely minimised by good antenatal supervision, early detection and management. These patients develop swelling of legs, which may extend upto the waist. In early stages, their shoes start pinching. Blood pressure, especially the diastolic pressure rises and albumin appears in the urine. In severe cases, there may be vomiting, headache and visual disturbances.

Mild cases are managed by bed rest and mild sedation. Most patients respond in 4 to 5 days. Prognosis is good if there is no recurrence. There is some risk of bleeding until the time of delivery. Fetus is generally small in these cases.

Severe case of toxemia with high BP (150/100 or above), headache, vomiting *etc.*, should be referred to the hospital. The mother should be sedated with advice to have complete bed rest. Diet should be light. Blood pressure should be recorded 6 hourly and 24 hours urinary output should be measured. Diuretics (furosemide or hydrochlorthiazide) are given. Antihypertensive drugs are used, if diastolic blood pressure is high. A drip of 20 per cent glucose solution (maximum 1 litre in 24 hours) is given if vomiting is severe and persistent pregnancy if possible but if the condition deteriorates or no improvement is observed, pregnancy may be terminated preferably by low amniotomy. Vaginal delivery is generally safer for the mother. During labor, progress should be watched by abdominal palpation. Labor is quickened when vertex is descending. When vertex reaches the perineum, delivery may be helped by outlet forcep or vacuum extraction. Cesarean section should generally be avoided but when blood pressure remains high with unfavourable cervix, it may have to be undertaken.

In *Eclampsia* (toxemia with convulsions) mortality rates both of fetus and mother are high. These patients should be moved to the hospital where prolonged supervision is possible. These patients should receive continuous sedation such as a bolus of 50 mg of pethedine and 25 mg of promethazine IM followed by an IV drip of 100 mg of pethedine in 20% glucose solution, giving 20 to 30 drops per minute. Generally pethedine dose should not exceed 300 mg in 24 hours. Glucose infusion should be limited to 1 liter. It may be necessary to give additional promethazine hydrochloride 25 mg or chlorpromazien 50 mg IM alternately every 4 hours. If convulsions are controlled in 24 hours, the interval for these injections should be increased every 6 hours. Magnesium sulphate 25% 10 ml, was given IM or IV previously for the treatment of eclampsia.

Common Medical Illnesses during Pregnancy which may affect its Outcome Adversely

Anemia

In mothers, who appear pale, hemoglobin level should be estimated by Tehlquist scale or Sahli's method. Stoods should be examined for ova of hook worms. If hemoglobin level is upto 8 g/dl, the mother should receive 200 mg of ferrous sulphate orally 3 times a day and folic acid 0.5 mg orally once a day. If the hemoglobin level is less than 8g/dl. iron dextran (Imferon) should be given by IM injection, starting with a dose of 50 mg (1 ml) on day 1 increasing gradually to 100 mg, 150 mg, 200 mg and 250 mg IM twice a week. The total dose is calculated by the formula: wt in kg x deficit of hemoglobin expressed in g/dl x 4.

Congestive heart failure may supervene in patients with hemoglobin level less than 5 g/dl. In such cases premature labor is common. It is not desirable to interfere with pregnancy. Such patients should be referred to the hospital.

Urinary Tract Infections

These patients may have frequent micturition with painful burning sensation. In acute illness, there is high fever with shivering, which almost simulates malaria. Vomiting is not unusual. In chronic urinary tact infection there may be little discomfort but the patient generally appear off colour. Diagnosis is made by microscopic examination of the urine. These patients should be treated with sulphamezathine 2 g stat and 1 g 8 hourly. Treatment should be continued for 3 weeks after urinalysis is normal. If the response to treatment is inadequate, doxycycline 250 mg twice a day may be used. Other useful drugs are nitrofurantoin 200 mg/day oraiy for 7 days or chloramphenicol 50 mg/kg/day in divided doses orally for 7 days.

If hematuria is associated, urinary calculus should be excluded. In cases of tuberculosis of kidney, the pyuria and hematuria are painless and ordinary culture examinations of urine are sterile. These patients should be managed in a hospital.

Heart Diseases

Pregnant women with heart disease should always be referred to the hospital.

Mild cases may be treated as outpatients. Patient should take as much rest as possible, limiting her activities. She should report to the doctor if she becomes breathless or if she develops cough.

Congestive heart failure may supervene in same cases at between 30 and 34 weeks. It is desirable to hospitalise the mat at 30-36 weeks of gestation. Majority of women may have quick spontaneous delivery. Oxygen is given for the management of dyspnea. Patient should be sedated moderately. Outlet forcep may be used to expedite delivery, when the head is in the perineum. Oxytocics should be avoided in the tnird srage of labor. Heart failure should be treated appropriately with sedation, oxygen, diuretics (Furosemide 40 mg OD) and digitalis (0.004 mg/kg/orally digitalising dose followed by one quarter of this does orally in divided doses every day).

Prognosis is poor in severe cases with decompensation. Heart failure should be treated without interfering with pregnancy. Also look for bacterial endocarditis, other infections and embolisation.

Some Common Gynecological Problems of Women

Dysmenorrhea

Some women have severe pain during menstrual periods. If the paid is mild, no active treatment is necessary. In severe cases, analgesics such as aspirin and codein are given to relieve the pain. Patient is reassured. In married women, dilatation and curettage may be done. Oral administration of ethinyl eslradiol 0.05 mg daily for 14 days from the first day of the menstrual cycle and ethisteron 5 mg twice daily for 7 days often relieves the pain.

In secondary dysmenorrhea, due to organic causes such as tumors, endometriosis, pelvic infections, uterine displacement, gynecological advice should always be sought.

Menorrhagia, Dysfunctional Uterine Bleeding

Dysfunctional uterine bleeding without any organic cause is common in girls, around the time of puberty postdelivery and premenopause. Usually normal menstrual cycle is established within 2-3 months. No active treatment is necessary. The girl is reassured and iron is given for the treatment of anemia. If the bleeding continues for more than a few months the girl should be referred to the hospital. In such cases a gynaccologieal examination should exclude fibroid, functioning ovarian tumour, genital tuberculosis and malignancy. If none of these are present hormone therapy for 3 months may be tried. If this fails then histopathological examination of scraping, after dilatation of cervix and curettage of the uterine cavity should be done.

Leucorrhea

Leucorrhea or whitish discharge from the vagina is a common complaint in women. The most frequent cause is infection of the vulva or vagina. In cases of trichomonas infection, the discharge appears yellowish, watery and is profuse, vaginal mucosa is stippled with red spots. Vaginal discharge shows pus cells and mobile organisms. These patients are treated with metronidazole 200 mg given orally three times daily for 7 days. It is desirable to treat the husband concurrently to prevent reinfection.

Infection with candida is another important cause. The discharge is thick, white and curdy. The smear stained with Gram's stain shows pus cells, beside the spores and branching filaments of candida. Patients with candidiasis of vagina are treated by local application of 1/2 per cent aqueous solution of gentian violet or introduction of myscostatin vaginal suppositories every night for 14 nights.

Pruritis Valvae

Itching over the vagina is due to similar causes as in lencorrhea. Pruritis valvae is managed by ensuring good genital hygiene. Patients should be relaxed and free from worry and tension. Netrodermatitis and general diseases like diabetes should be excluded. In women beyond the age of menopause, estrogen deficiency may cause itching. In some cases application of estrogen cream over the vagina may be necessary to relieve itching.

Problems during Delivery

Management of Fetal Malpresentations

Fetal malpresentations are a common cause of prolonged labor. Malpresentations are frequently observed in early months of pregnancy, but most of these correct themselves as the gestation, advances. If these persist beyond 34 weeks of gestation the cause of malpresentations should be investigated. Mothers with malpresentation who are primigravida or multigravida with poor obstetric history should always be referred to the hospital.

Persistent Occipito-Posterior Presentation

This is a common cause of prolonged labor. In these cases the vertex does not engage easily. On abdominal palpation, back of the fetus is indistinctly felt in the flank, and limbs appear more anterior or palpation. Fetal heart is heard further away from the midline. On vaginal examination, anterior fontanel of the fetus may be felt at the anterior end of one of the two oblique diameters.

(i) In most cases of occipito-posterior presentation, the occiput eventually rotates to the front, and fetus is delivered normally, especially if it is of an average size, pelvis is adequate and uterine contractions are good.

(ii) If there is no progress in the delivery of the fetus after 2 hours of pains during the second stage of labor, vaginal examination should be carried out. If in the meanwhile, signs of fetal distress develop, rotation of the occiput should be attempted especially if it is incompletely rotated and if the head is stuck below the ischial spine, after full dilatation of the cervix. The delivery is assisted by *vacuum extraction*. If the vacuum extractor slips and occiput comes forward, delivery should be assisted by applying outlet forceps. In cases, in which the failure of anterior rotation of the occiput is attributable to weak uterin contractions, 2 units of oxytocin dissolved in 500 ml of 5% glucose solution are given by slow IV drip, provided that there is no cephalopelvio disproportion or obstruction to the delivery of the fetus.

(iii) If the fetal heart has already stopped, but mother's condition is satisfactory, time should be given for the head to descent normally. If however, maternal distress becomes evident, forceps should be applied to hasten the delivery. In such cases caput is usually formed over the occiput and therefore it is not easy to apply suction for assisting the delivery. In difficult cases, craniotomy may become necessary.

Even when fetal heart sound is audible, prognosis for the fetus remains poor. Time should always be given for spontaneous delivery. If feasible, manual rotation or forceps rotation may be done to assist the delivery of the fetus. If the fetal heart stops, craniotomy occasionally is necessary to save the mother's life.

Breech Delivery

If breech presentation is discovered after the labor has already started, the patient should be sent to the hospital. All primigravidae and multigravidae with breech and bad obstetric history also deserve referral to the hospital. If the fetus is large with expected weight of more than 3.5 kg and possibly contracted pelvis, cesarean section is unavoidable to save the life of the fetus. In case of average sized fetus and normal pelvis, vaginal delivery may be allowed, but arrangements should always be made for the management of possible fetal asphyxia.

Extended breech. If there is no cord presentation or prolapse, a patient with extended breech may be allowed to continue in labor, while keeping a vigilant watch over the fetal heart rate. Mother should be sedated. Episiotomy is often required in these cases. It is necessary to assist in the delivery of shoulders and head to the fetus. It is difficult to deliver the head and the cord pulsations stop for sometime, forceps may be applied during delivery. In hydrocephalic baby, craniotomy becomes necessary to complete the delivery. Methergin should never be administered before the fetus is completely delivered.

If there is no progress in labor despite full dilatation of the cervix and good uterine action, full breech extraction may be done under anesthesia for an average size baby. If extraction is expected to be difficult, then cesarean section may be done.

Cesarean section is necessary in cases with cord prolapse, who have strong cord pulsations and incomplete dilatation of cervix, especially if baby is big and the breech presentation is complicated such as, with placenta previa, contracted pelvis and diabetes.

Shoulder Presentation, Arm Prolapse, Oblique Lie.

These cases are difficult to manage and require highly specialised care in the hospital. Fetal and maternal mortality are generally high. Rupture of the uterus is a common complication.

Internal podalic version and extraction under anesthesia should be one by specially trained persons. If the uterus is tonically contracted but maternal pulse rate is rising and the fetal heart rate is falling, internal version should not be carried out. Instead lower segment cesarean section should be immediately done to save the life of the mother. In dead fetus delivery is possible only after the fetus is decapitated and spondylotomy is done. Chances of infection in such cases are high. Mothers should receive adequate antibiotics and should also be treated for shock. For threatened rupture of uterus or rupture of uterus immediate laparotomy should be done.

Face Presentation

If the chin is presenting anteriorly, previous obstetric history is good and pelvis size is adequate, vaginal delivery may be allowed. This may be assisted by application of outlet forceps. However if the chin is posterior, cesarean section becomes necessary to save the life of fetus, if it fails to rotate anteriorly.

Twin Pregnancy

Twin pregnancy should be considered as a possibility if the height of funds is more than that anticipated from the duration of amenorrhea. It should also be suspected, when there is hydramnios, two fetal heads are palpable or two fetal hearts with difference of 10 beats per minute can be auscultated. Diagnosis is confirmed by x-ray. Babies are generally small-for-date (low-birth weight). They are often born before term. Perinatal mortality especially for the second twin is high. Twin pregnancies are best managed by referral to the hospital. First baby is usually born normally with vertex presentation. After the first baby is born, position of the second fetus should be felt by abdominal palpation. Although the second fetus is usually vertex, but it may be breech or shoulder presentation. External version is done in cases of shoulder presentation. This is followed by rupture of membrances. If external version fails, internal podalic version may become necessary before the second baby is extracted. In case of fetal distress or prolonged second stage of labor, outlet forceps may need to be applied.

Complications of Delivery

Retained Placenta

Normally the placenta should be expelled within half an hour after delivery. If the uterine contractions are poor or the placenta is adherent to the uterus, placenta may be retained in the uterus even beyond half an hour, resulting in severe bleeding. Shock is usual and occurs even with minimal or absent bleeding. A careful watch should be kept over the blood pressure and pulse rate of the mother. If signs of separation of placenta become evident, placenta may be easily expelled by expression. In cases without evidence of separation, uterus should be massaged. If uterine contractions are poor 0.2 mg of methergin should be injected IM.

If there are no signs of separation of placenta for half an hour manual removal of placenta should be undertaken. The evacuation should be done completely despite continuous bleeding. Antibiotics should always be administered after manual removal of the placenta.

Post-Partum Hemorrhage

Post-partum hemorrhage occurs within 24 hours after delivery. It is often due either to (i) atonic uterus or (ii) lacerations.

In cases of atonic uterus, the bleeding is severe and sudden.

Uterus appears soft.

In case of lacerations or tears of cervix or vagina, uterus is well contracted and tears are easily observed through the speculum. These should be sutured.

In case of atonic uterus, bleeding is treated by injection of 5 units of oxytocin and 0.2 mg of Methergin IM Uterus should be massaged to make it contract. An I. V. drip of 20 unit of oxytocin in 500 ml of 5 per cent glucose should be started.

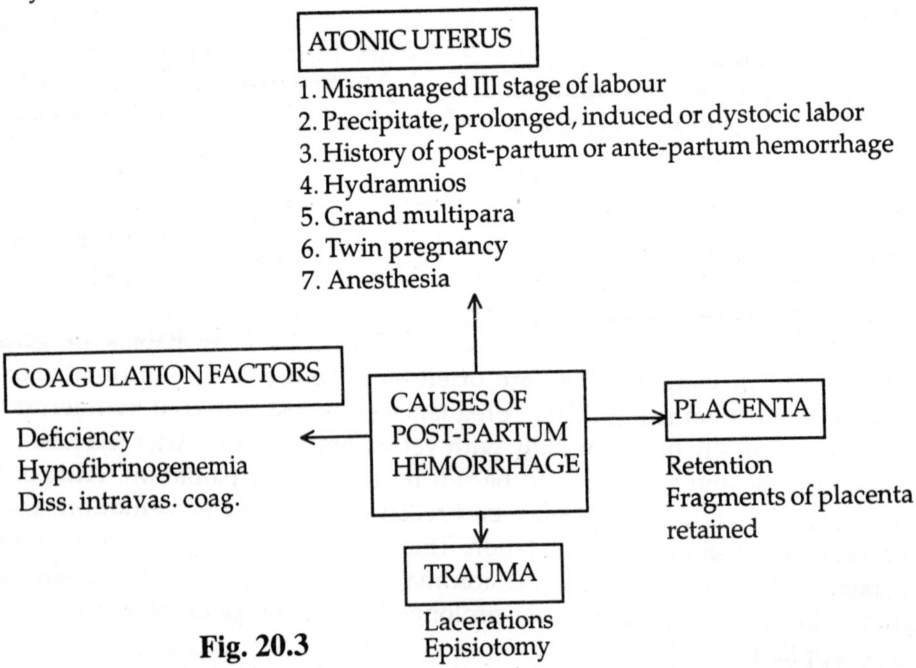

Fig. 20.3

Retained placenta should be excluded in all cases of post-partum hemorrhage. Any retained fragments of placenta in the uterus should be removed manually with fingers. Bimanual compression of uterus may be done to control the bleeding for 10-15 minutes. Blood transfusion is necessary to save the life of the mother who bleeds severely.

Shock and Collapse

Shock and collapse occurs more often in mothers with (i) severe anemia, (ii) after sudden severe blood loss, (iii) incomplete abortion, (iv) ruptured ectopic pregnancy, (v) placenta previa, (vi) antepartum hemorrhage (vii) ruptured uterus, (viii) postpartum hemorrhage (ix) embolism of amniotic fluid and following (x) severe infections.

Mothers with shock should be treated by keeping their body ward. Their head should be kept low. Plasma op 5 per cent glocose solution are infused. I.V. In cases of septic shock, antibiotics are given. Large doses of hydrocortisone (0.5 to 2 g) given I.V. are helpful in case of septic shock.

Postnatal Care

Postnatal care of the mother should aim at

(i) *Preventing complications*, such as puerperal sepsis, mastitis, secondary post-partum hemorrhage, thrombophlebitis, incontinence of urine, urinary infection and puerperal psychosis. This may be done by observing general condition of the mother, pulse rate and temperature besides the examination of vaginal pads for change of colour of lochia and other discharges.

(ii) The mother should be helped to recover to a state of optimal health, both physically and emotionally, through surveillance, good nutrition, administration of hematinics and postnatal exercises.

(iii) She should be psychologically prepared to breast feed her newborn infant. The breast nipples should be examined for retraction or inversion. The primigravida mother should be instructed about technique of breast feeding. Her fears and anxieties should be assuged and problems associated with of breast feeding mitigated.

Improved Perinatal Pediatric Supervision

1. High risk infants should be identified.
2. Multipurpose health workers should be trained in the case of preterm, low birth weight and sick neonates.
3. Breast feeding should encouraged.
4. Facilities for the transport of immature, sick and high-risk-newborn infants requiring special care to the neighbouring upgraded primary health center should be provided. It should be possible to provide some important components of perinatal care such as gavage feeding, temperature regulation and oxygen even in peripheral hospitals.
5. Low-birth weight and immature infants should be kept under surveillance by the female health worker in rural areas for identification of danger signals indicating

serious illnesses. she should refer the sick newborn to appropiate health facility in the neighborhood. This involves regionalisation of health care for these infants.

Care of the Newborn Baby

Most child births in the community are uneventful. But complications may occur at any time. Help of the doctor may not always be available on the spot. Therefore the community health worker should be able to revive a gasping or dying newborn infant and learn to do so with minimum or no aids at her command. Such a worker will earn the admiration and confidence of the mother and the community.

Traditional birth attendants practising in villages in many developing countries often cut the umbilical cord of the baby at the time of birth using dirty agricultural implements. They often annoint the umbilical stump with cow dung or other dirty pastes and use unclean household linen as dressing pads. The community health worker should consider it her responsibility to teach the birth attendant the correct use of sterile midwifery kit or alternately, substitute these kits with common household articles easily available with the village grocer, such as clean shaving blade. She should instruct her to use no medication or at the best a crude turmeric paste to annoint the stump instead of cow dung and to employ clean laundered linen as dressing pads instead of dirty rags.

The health worker should look at the baby's external orifices such as the anus, genitals and oral cavity for any evidence of congenital malformations. If these are present, the doctor should be informed immediately for appropriate action. After birth, the baby is cleansed of the vernix caseosa using clean moist pieces of cloth. The baby is then laid on a clean dry warm bed to rest for some time. Generally the baby lies quiet for several house and does not cry for food.

Although at this stage, the mother has hardly any milk in her breasts, she should be encouraged to put the newborn baby on the breast even on the first day. The mother secretes some colostrum or pre-lacteal milk, which appears cheesy, but is a useful source of anti-infective substances for the baby. The breast milk is secreted early, if the baby is allowed to suckle on the breast as early as possible.

Most village mothers can manage breast feeding adequately and well through a natural instinct. The health worker should help those mothers who are uninitiated or cannot handle the baby for breast feeding successfully. The baby should be encouraged to *draw the areola and a part of the breast tissue well in its mouth to suck the milk from the breast and not only nibble at the teats.*

While feeding the baby, the mother should be relaxed preferably in a semi-recumbent position. She should support the baby's head on her elbows and his buttocks on the palm of her hand. She should feed the baby almost as often as the child wants. If the baby cries too soon-after a feed his napkin should be checked, since the baby might have passed urine or stools. The wet napkin should be changed. The feeding schedule *should not be followed too rigidly* by the clock. Early morning feeds are generally larger in volume and richer with regard to concentration of nutrients. Therefore, the baby remains satisfied for long periods. The breast feeds in the afternoons are generally smaller in quantity and are comparatively less concentrated than those in the morning. The mother should be advised to follow a semidemand schedule. If the infant is sleeping at the expected time of feeding, he should not be aroused for feeding. If he is hungry and demands a feed before the scheduled time, the feed should not be denied.

Most babies demand a mid-night feed during the early weeks of life. Although it may be exhausting for some mothers, the baby's needs should receive due consideration. It may be possible to obviate the need for the midnight feed by delaying the last breast feed before the mother retires to bed by half to one hour, so that a more hungry baby obtains a larger feed from the mother and sleeps till early hours of the morning. Usually a satisfactory schedule is established in three to four weeks.

Some mothers may become anxious that their breast milk secretion is inadequate to meet the nutrition needs of the baby. The feeding should be considered satisfactory if the baby sleeps for 2 to 4 hours after each feed and continues to gain weight at a satisfactory rate. It is not usually necessary to do the test feeding to determine adequacy of breast milk secretion.

Children

Health Problems in the First Month

Babies who are born before full term or appear very small due to abnormally-low-birth weight as expected for their gestation period may suddenly become sick and even die. These babies should lbe immediately referred to the health center after initial help by the birth attendant and proper arrangements for transport of the baby should be made.

Babies do not tell their health problems. The health worker should *learn to recognise* the clinical signs and symptoms in the baby which imply *danger singnals*.

A sick baby develops fever or appears very cold, looks vacantly on one side, cries intermittently without apparent reason, becomes excessively drowsy and cannot be easily aroused. A baby who stops sucking at the breast for several feeds after the initial breast feeding had been established is obviously a very sick baby. Immediate attention of the doctor should be sought to help such sick babies. These babies may be suffering from generalised infection of the blood or septicemia.

Neonatal tetanus. Neonatal tetanus is a common but totally preventable cause of early infact deaths, if every mother is actively immunised against tetanus during her pregnancy or if the delivery is conducted by a trained birth attendant in a clean surrounding without exposure to the infected material, such as cow dung.

The usual age at the onset of symptoms in neonatal tetanus is 5 to 15 days (rare before 3 or after 15 days). The baby cries excessively, refuses feeds and is apathetic. Mouth appears open due to pull of facial muscles and neck becomes stiff due to spasm of neck muscles. Reflex spasm of the masseters causes difficulty in feeding. Dysphagia and choking during feeding is due to pharyngeal spasm. Lock jaw or reflex trismus is followed by spasm of the limbs, generalised rigidity and opisthotonus. These children should be immediately transferred to the community health center or the hospital.

Congenital malformations. The birth attendant should look for congenital malformations of the palate or other morphologic abnormalities and bring these to the attention of the doctor.

Health Problems of the infact after the First Month of Life

Pneumonias and diarrheal disease are the two major causes of ill health and death in infants and young children beyond the age of first month.

Respiratory infections. Avoidance of cross infection through overcrowding, better housing and improved nutrition are generally expected to result in a decline in the risk of infections of the lungs and the respiratory tract, such as penumonias and bronchitis. However, there are no specific and definite measures for prevention of pneumonias. Even healthy-well-nourished children from good homes living in good sanitary conditions suffer from these illnesses. There is a considerable morbidity and mortality due to respiratory infections secondary to measles and whooping cough especially in infants and undernourished children from poor homes. Hazards of these secondary pulmonary complications are avoidable by appropriate treatment with drugs and other supportive measures. Measles vaccine is at present not manufactured in India and many other developing countries. It is expensive and required good cold storage conditions. It is not economical and administratively feasible for the administration at the present stage of development to offer measles immunisation in the standard regimen at age one year to 15 months to all children in India. But with improved facilities and lowering of costs it will be possible to do so in the foreseeable future. Whooping cough vaccine is included in the triple antigen, which is freely available. Whooping cough component of the vaccine is not as effective as the diphtheria and tetanus toxoids included in the triple antigen. Whooping cough vaccine is known to cause neurological complication such as post-vaccinial encephalopathy. The incidence of this complication is not high (1 in 1,00,000) but the sequelae of whooping cough are devastating. Whooping cough vaccine should be avoided in children with pre-existing *progressive neuological illness* or history of febrile convulsions. Non-progressive neorological disorders are not a contraindication for pertussis vaccine.

Diarrhea. Diarrheal disease is a major killer of infants and young children in most developing countries. It is difficult to totally eliminate the diarrheal disease among infants, with the use of the presently available health intervention technologies. Improved sanitation facilities and provision of safe water supply reduce the incidence of diarrheal disease to some extent. Promotion of breast feeding is an effective measure for reducing the incidence of diarrheal disease, since the breast milk is safe and clean, with no risk of contamination. It also provides anti-infective factors, which increase the resistance of the child to infections of the gut. Most cases of diarrheal diseases are self limiting and except for those with blood and mucus in stools do not require antibiotics or chemotherapy for their treatment.

Deaths associated with diarrheal disease are largely attributed to malnutrition and to a lesser extent directly to dehydration and dyselectrolytemia, at least in the community setting.

Diarrheal diseases are most prevalent in infants around the *time of weaning*. As the child is gradually weaned from the breast, the milk offerred for artificial feeding is, in most cases, inadequate to meet the growth requirements of the baby and is often offered in contaminated receptacles resulting in recurrent infection of the gut. Undernourished children have poor resistance and are often more susceptible to develop diarrhea. During diarrheal episodes, mothers often withold feeds or dilute the milk excessively. The child becomes more undernourished; his resistance to infection is further compromised and he falls a prey to a variety of other infections, and when unable to adapt to the stress of these illnesses, succumbs. Acute attacks of diarrhea often precipitate kwashiorkor in previously marasmic children.

Table 20. 6

First Ten Causes of Infant Deaths in Rural Areas With the Cause Specific Death Rates for 1000 Infants

Kerala	*Uttar Pradesh*	*All India*
Prematurity 5.78	Tetanus 68.51	Tetanus 19.8
Other respiratory disorders 3.02	Pneumonia 24.12	Prematurity 12.48
Bronchits 2.35	Prematurity 18.00	Pneumonia 8.96
Dysentery 1.82	Dysentery 14.51	Other respiratory disorders 8.35
Gastroenteritis 1.01	Influenza 12.33	Influenza 7.10
Tetanus 0.85	Typhoid 9.41	Dysentery 6.9
Infantile liver 0.84	Diarrhea 4.94	Typhoid 5.28
Influenza 0.33	Jaundice 4.73	Malaria 5.0
Jaundice 0.66	Bronchitis 4.66	Diarrhoea 4.04
Typhoid 0.49	Diphtheria 4.2	Bronchitis 2.66

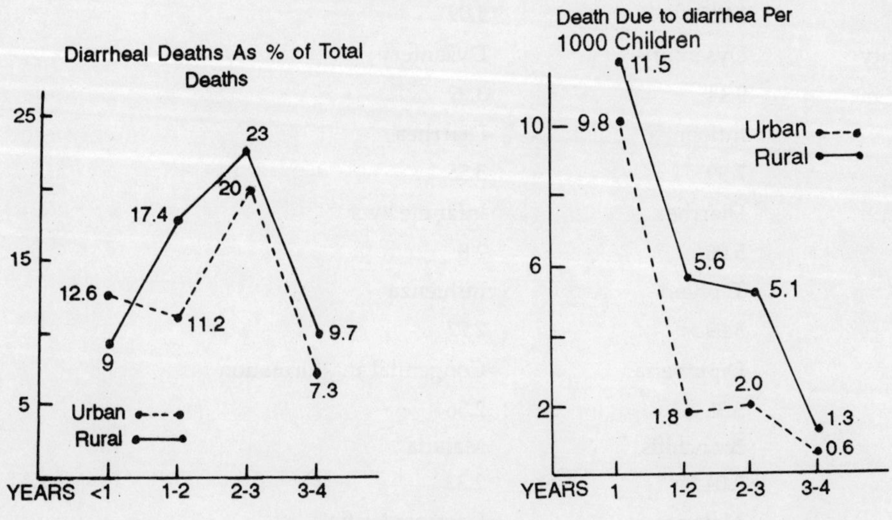

Fig. 20.4

Considerable evidence has accumulated all over the world, that deaths in infants and children due to diarrheal disease can be considerably reduced by the use of *oral rehydration*. Diarrhea due to cholera vibrio and toxigenic strains of E. coli disturbs the sodium pump mechanism at the intestinal cell level. More sodium, chloride and water are lost in the diarrheal stoods. The intestines also lose potassium. Physiologists observed that obsorption of glucose from the gut is not disturbed in cases of diarrhea. Since the absorption of glucose and sodium have an inter-linked mechanism of absorption, the absorption of glucose facilitates simultaneous absorption of sodium, chloride and also water from the gut, which is otherwise purging large amounts of sodium and water. As more sodium is absorbed more water is retained in the body. Thus oral hydration is useful not *only* to replace the losses of electrolytes and water but to actively promote their absorption. *The duration of diarrheal illness is often reduced; and the appetite of the child improves.* The child accepts more food readily and is protected from ill offects of malnutrition.

Table 20. 7

First 10 Causes of Infant Death in Urban Areas with the Cause specific Death Rate per 1000 infants.

Kerala	*Uttar Pradesh*	*All India*
Other respiratory disorders	Tetanus	Prematurity
3.64	23.86	6.98
Influenza	Pneumonia	Tetanus
2.02	16.38	5.30
Gastroenteritis	Prematurity	Pneumonia
1.31	14.67	4.09
Prematurity	Dysentery	Dysentery
1.27	9.44	3.99
Malaria	Influenza	Diarrhea
1.09	7.39	3.55
Dysentery	Diarrhea	Infantile liver
1.01	5.06	2.8
	Typhoid	Influenza
	3.69	2.77
Bronchitis	Diphtheria	Congenital malformation
0.88	3.36	2.36
	Bronchitis	Malaria
	3.04	2.33
	Malaria	Gastroenteritis
	1.96	1.85

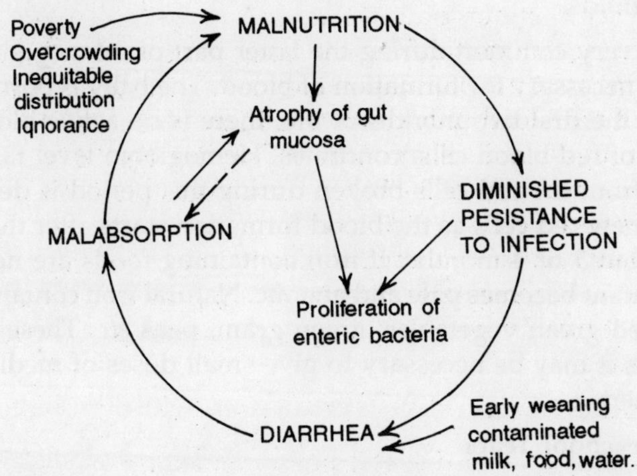

Fig. 20.6 Vicious circle of diarrhea and malnutrition.

Oral hydration is an important advance in the primary health care approach, because this can be carried out even in the remotest villages by the unskilled or semiskilled-health workers, without the umbrella of expert medical supervision. The World Health Organisation recommended the use of a solution containing glucose 20 g, sodiumchloride 3.5 g, sodium bicarbonate 2.5 g and potassium chloride 1.5 g dissolved in 1 liter of *clean water*. This solution should be administered to children with diarrhea. Rehydration should be carried out be teaspoonfuls in small sips, rather than in gulps. This is done *adlib*, according to the thirst of the child. An infant may consume fairly large quantities of oral rehydration fluids, as much as one to three liters in a day. After the initial rehydration is complete, roughly one half tumbler full of oral rehydration fluid should be offered to the child for each liquid stools passed thereafter. A three finger pince of salt and four finger scoop of sugar in half liter of water may be used as an interim solution.

Infants with diarrhea, who do not pass urine for more than 8 hours, appear cold and clammy, in shock, and are semiconscious or in a moribund state should be sent promptly to the nearest hospital or health center for further treatment, after starting oral rehydration, all the time taking care to prevent aspiration of the vomitus by the child. It is also preferable to refer diarrheal patients with marked abdominal distension or those with persistent vomiting to the nearest health center for observation and further treatment. When the standard solution for oral rehydration is not easily available, a substitute may be made locally dissolving 40 gm of sugar, molasses or jaggery and 5 g of common salt in a liter of clean potable water. Field studies in Bangladesh have confirmed that home made solutions are fairly effective in reducing diarrheal deaths. Common household measures available with the village health workers should preferably be standardised by comparison with standard measures. Milk measures in the village are generally fairly adequate for preparing home made hydration fluids.

Anemia. Anemia is very common during the latter part of infancy, since milk is a poor source of iron, which is necessary for formation of blood. The baby is born with hemoglobin level of 16-18 g/dl. For the first two months of life, there is no active blood formation, but the normal breakdown of red-blood cells continues. Hemoglobin level falls to 11 g/dl by 2 months. Iron liberated from the red cells broken during this period is deposited in tissues. This iron is utilised for new red cells as the blood formation starts after the age of 2 months. This is adequate for about 3 or 4 months. If iron containing foods are not supplied by the age of 4-5 months, the infant becomes pale and anemic. Natural iron containing foods include well cooked and mashed green vegetables, green gram, peas *etc*. These should be started gradually. In some cases it may be necessary to give small doses of medicinal iron (ferrous sulphate) to prevent anemia.

Health Problems of Preschool Years

Malnutrition, anemia, diarrheal disease, pneumonias, other respiratory illness and parasitic infections such as ascariasis, hookworm disease are common causes of morbidity in preschool children. These children are also increasiny exposed to accidental poisoning, falls burns, drowning and road accidents.

Strategies for Reduction of Early Childhood Deaths During Preschool Years

Main planks of strategy for reducing early childhood deaths are:

(i) Health and nutrition education.

(ii) Health surveillance of all children. Identification of high risk children and adequate follow up services.

(iii) Prevention of malnutrition. Nutritional supplementation of severely malnourished children. Increased food output and earning capacity of parents.

(iv) Prophylactic immunisation.

(v) Adequate and appropriate treatment of medical illness. Most early childhood deaths are caused by pneumonias and infections for which no specific primary prevention measures may be available. These should be treated adequately and promptly.

Overwhelming majority of early childhood deaths are attributed to poverty and lack of resources. Low birth weight is a major cause contributing to early neonatal deaths. Such babies are more often born to poor, undernourished mothers, who suffer from frequent illnesses, during pregnancy. Unhygienic environment of poor households contributes to the high incidence of infections. Respiratory and diarrheal illnesses are more frequent in children who do not have access to safe water supply and who live in overcrowed areas with poor sanitation and ventilation. Several epidemiologic studies correlated the high incidence of diarrhea to malnutrition and poor socio-economic status of the family.

General Consideration

1. The remarkable decline in the infant and early child deaths in the Western countries during this century was largely brought about by economic growth, better wages, ability of parents to afford good for children, safe water supply, good environmental sanitation and better housing, long before for development of immunising agents, chemotherapy and antibiotics. Therefore, it is important to recognise that non-health sectors need to contribute significantly for reducing the early childhood deaths.
2. Recommended health interventions should have a broad coverage so that their impact is wide and actively felt by the people.
3. A critical minimal level of health inputs in necessary to achieve the desired results. If the resources are spread too thin or are very much diluted, the health efforts may be totally wasted. If resources are limited, these should preferentially be expended on the *high vis k groups* and on those activities which are more amenable to available preventive and therapeutic approaches and are of low cost.
4. Health interventions should be scientifically sound and should be based on a good data base, such as the pattern of diseases causing infant and early childhood deaths, their incidence, amenability to available technologies, nutritional profile, social cultural milieu, available health facilities, budgetary appropriations by the Government and contributions from the voluntary agencies.
5. The existing health facilities should be fully utilisd instead of creating new categories of workers and new schemes. Alternate strategies introduced too frequently may become the biggest deterrant to effective health-care-delivery system because large proportion of available meager funds are diverted to new projects of unproven value. Furthermore these lead to duplication of work, overconcentration in certain geographic areas, rivalaries between categories of workers in different schemes, trade unionism and exploitation.
6. Strategies for reducing early childhood deaths should be developed by reinforcing the health infrastructure and not be replacing it.

Specific Activities

Neonatal Period

Neonatal Tetanus. Neonatal tetanus accounts for 5 to 30 per cent of infant deaths in different parts of India. Its prevalence can be greatly reduced by active immnisation of the mother with at least 2 injections of tetanus toxoid during the later part of pregnancy so that tetanus antibodies are transplacentally transferred to the fetus, who will then be protected from tetanus in the neonatal period. The infant should be further protected by training of traditional birth attendants on principles of asepsis, use of sterile equipment such as new shaving blade for cutting the umbilical cord, using clean thread for tying the umbilical stump and prohibiting annointing of the stump with cow dung or other unhygienic practices. Facilities for treatment of tetanus neonatorum should be provided at the upgraded health centers.

Table 20. 8

Specific Possible interventions to Reduce Infant Mortality

	Measure	*Cost*	*Constraints in organisation*	*Vulnerability and Effectiveness*
A.	*Tetanus Neonatal*			
	Tetanus toxoid to mother	Moderate	Moderate	High
	Training of midwives	Moderate to high	Moderate	Locate high
	Supply of obstetric kits to midwives	High	Moderate	
	Substitutes for obst. kits (new blades and clean thread)	Low	Low	Moderate
	Health Education	Moderate	Moderate	Moderate
B.	*Prematurity and low Birth Weight*			
	Nutritional supplements for mothers during pregnancy	High	High	Low
	Good medical and antenatal care during pregnancy	Moderate	Moderate	Moderate to High
	Institutional delivery	Moderate	Moderate	Moderate
	Premature nursery care	High	High	Moderate to High
C.	*Panumonia, Bronchitis, Respiratory Disorders*			
	Immunization	High	High	Low
	Treatment in OPD	Moderate	Moderate	Moderate to High
	Treatment in			High
	medical institution	High	Moderate	High
		Moderate		Moderate to High
D.	*Dysentery, Diarrhea Gastroenteritis*			
	Environmental sanitation	High	High	Low to moderate
	Piped water supply	High	High	Low to moderate
	Fly control	High	High	Low
	Prevention of food contamination	Moderate	High	Moderate
	Rehydration with home	Low	Low	Moderate

Contd.

	made solutions			
	Ready made WHO formula	Moderate	High	High
	Use of antibiotics	High	High	Low
E.	*Malaria*			
	Mosquito control	Moderate	Moderate	Moderate
	Treatment	Moderate	Low	High
F.	*Other Infections*	Moderate	High	Moderate
	Immunization			
	Treatment	Moderate	Moderate	High
G.	*Congential Malformations and Metabolic Disorders*			
	Prenatal diagnosis	High	High	Low
	Neonatal screening	High	High	Low
H.	*Protein Energy Malnutrition*			
	Nutrition supplementation	High	Moderate	Low
	Socio-economic development	High	High	Moderate to High

Low birth weight. There is no effective method of eliminating birth of preterm babies. Epidemiological studies in Guatemala and India showed that average birth weight was higher in babies born to mothers given nutrition (energy giving) supplements during the last trimester of pregnancy. Magnitude of the problem is large and the available food resources are limited. Therefore, nutritional supplementation of all mothers during pregnancy is not practical. This facility needs to be restricted to high-risk mothers *i.e.* very poor, emaciated women, weighing less than 40 kg. of height less than 145 cm, young primipara, mothers with anemia, heart disease or those with pregnancy-related complications such as toxemia and antepartum hemorrhage. It is presumed but as yet no convincing evidence is available that a moderate increase in the average birth weight of babies of mothers on nutritional supplements, does contribute to the reduction of morbidity or mortality in the neonatal period. Mothers should be advised not to smoke during pregnancy since smoking during pregnancy, by the mother results in birth of small-for-date infants.

Care of High-Risk Infants. High risk infants cannot be cared for adequately through primary health care. There should be facilities for referring and transporting these babies to an institution for intermediate level health care in the taluk or district hospital. Tertiary level health care for very sick newborn babies is not feasible even in the district hospitals. Such babies, requiring intensive care should be referred to a regional-center for intensive care of highrisk-newborn babies. The main responsibility of the primary health care worker is to identify highrisk babies and refer these to an appropriate institution.

Birth Injuries and Asphyxia Neonatorum. Morbidity and mortality due to these can be considerably reduced by training of birth attendants, basic health workers and augmenting facilities for better care of mothers during delivery.

Post Neonatal Period

Deaths of infants in the postneonatal period are more amenable to the recent technical developments in the field of public health and pediatrics. Widespread use of triple antigen in some parts of the country has already resulted in a marked decline in the prevalence of diphtheria, whooping cough and tetanus. Three doses of this vaccine are given at monthly intervals from the age of 3 months onwards. Protection from whooping cough by this antigen is not complete. Whooping cough is a cause of some deaths in infants due to pulmonary complications, malnutrition and encephalopathy.

Infants are relatively protected from measles in the first few months of life. Measles is a serious illness in the later part of the first year. Measles causes serious respiratory complications encephalitis and adversely affects the nutritional status of infants. It can be prevented by measles vaccination, which is usually given between the age 9 and 15 months. It is an expensive imported vaccine and requires good cold chain for its storage.

Pneumonias and other respiratory infections take a heavy toll of the life of infants and young children. There is no effective strategy for preventing most of these infections but deaths and long term complications due to these can be significantly reduced by prompt and adequate treatment even at primary health care level.

incidence of *Diarrrheal Diseases* may be reduced by (i) health education (ii) improved sanitation (iii) safe water supply (iv) protection of food from contamination by dust, flies, cockroaches (v) by keeping the food containers clean, (vi) exclusion of carries of intestinal infections from the preparation of food and (vii) improving the nutritional status of children.

It may not be possible to drastically reduce the prevalence of diarrheal disease by the above measures, which are difficult to implement fully because of the high cost involved but the *number of deaths due to diarrheal disease can be significantly reduced by oral hydration*. For details see under health problems in the post neonatal period (vide supra).

Strategies for Nutrition Education

As a general rule, nutrition education conducted by simple transmission of information, which does not fit with the cultural norms of the community is ineffective.

(a) *Mothers meetings*. In some rural areas, the village ladies meet together in common community areas for gossip and recreation. This opportunity may be utilised for imparting health education. Though a public health nurse or physician ma address the group of mothers on nutrition education, a more desirable approach is to encourage discussions in groups of mothers, so that they can bring up problems of child rearing and feeding and seek solutions from amongst their own group. The physician and nurse should intervene only for purposeful direction of the discussion. These group meeting are likely to be more successful if some mothers with healthy children and others with undernourished children are included in the group, because the former may be able to lead the discussion by demonstrating how they were able to bring up healthy and well nourished babies with the use of locally available resources. Mothers prefer to learn from example of persons of their own group.

(b) Participating of mothers in the preparation of weaning foods for their children.

(i) In some community health projects raw ingredients of the suggested weaning food are given to a group of mothers and the method of preparation of the weaning food from the ingredients is explained to them. They are paid a small remuneration for processing the 'take home' packets of weaning foods. The packets are then distributed free to be used as nutritional supplements for their own children. Participation of mothers of malnourished children in the preparation of weaning foods becomes a good educational experience for them. These mothers continue to use similar weaning food for their children when distribution of free food packets is discontinued.

(ii) In several Indian projects, parents are encouraged to grow leguminous plants which are cheap source of protein and carotene in the diet. The mothers participate in cooking of food for their own children in the demonstration kitchens and nutritional rehabilitation centers.

(iii) Malnourished children have been treated in their own homes with locally available food supplements. Since the mothers are involved in the dietary treatment of their children, they easily learn the principles of nutritional care of their children.

(c) The recipes for preparing weaning foods may be practically demonstrated by the health worker to the group of mothers.

(d) Visits of the health worker to be households in the community, for observation and personalised discussion with the mothers is a useful traditional method of nutrition education.

(e) In many nutrition education programmes, great reliance is placed on these. To what extent, these methods help in change of attitudes of the target population is not very clear. Documentary films, television, posters, newspapers and other media of mass communication may be used for nutrition education but these have a limited role.

(f) Preserve and reinforce local culturatly practices such as breast feeding and an-prasan (introduction of cereals in the diet of infant) ceremony as in several seets of Hindus in India.

Prevention of Malnutrition

Malnutrition causes a variety of metabolic disturbances. Resistance to infections is decreased, gastrointestinal functions are disturbed and learning abilities are adversely affected. The growth of children is retarded and there is higher morbidity and mortality among malnourished individuals.

Improvement of nutrition of people is, therefore, an essential component of primary health care. It is necessary to keep the community under nutritional surveillance, so that appropriate decision can be made whenever required to prevent malnutrition and improve the nutritional status of people.

Nutritional surveillance involves the following steps:

1. To define the character and magnitude of nutritional problems as prevalent in the community and any observed changes in these over the course of time.
2. To analyse causes of these nutritional problems and identify any other associated factors.
3. To select appropriate preventive measures to counteract these problems. The strategies may be nutritional or food related or may be in economic, social or cultural domains.
4. To assist the government in formulating the nutritional policy.
5. To help in the planning, development and implementation of projects for the improvement of nutrition of people and to participate in monitoring and evaluation of such programmes.

Nutrition Problems

1. Type of Malnutrition

(a) Protein energy malnutrition. This may result from acute deficiency of food or may be attributed to chronic deprivation.

(b) Deficiency of micronutrients, such as, vitamins, iron, iodine and other trace elements.

2. Groups of Population Most Affected

The groups of population may be most affected because of their,

(a) biological vulnerability as in infants, preschool children and pregnant mothers;

(b) socioeconomic factors (poor, socially deprived orphans) or

(c) habitat such as those living in inaccessible remote areas, thick forests and mountainous regions e.g., tribal population and nomads.

3. Causes of Malnutrition

Malnutrition may be attributed to:

(a) low food consumption.

(b) poor health (infections, infestations, recurrent diarrhea, malabsorption.

(c) lack of awareness of nutritional qualities of food, irrational beliefs about food, inappropriate child rearing and feeding practices and

(d) socio-cultural and economic factors such as inequitable distribution of food either among different members of the community or the household and

(e) poor quality of housing, sanitation and water supply, which contribute to ill health.

Strategies to Prevent Malnutrition and Improve Nutrition

The nutrition of people can be ameliorated by two major approaches *viz. nutritional planning* and *direct nutrition* and *health interventions*. Both strategies need to be carried out concurrently, since the former result in long-term-permanent benefits and the latter provide immediate relief to those who need help.

Nutritional Planning

Nutritional planning involves a political commitment by the government, formulation of a nutrition policy and overall long term planning to improve production and supplies of food, ensure its equitable distribution and increase the purchasing power of the people. Since long-term projects might be badly planned and poorly executed at times, results might be uncertain and benefits might not become evident immediately. If properly planned, long term benefits for accelerating the development processes are more rewarding and permanent. As already stated, nutritional planning involves the following activities.

(i) *To stimulate increased food production*

(a) Land reforms should be carried out, so that the person who tills the farm also has a chance to own it. This gives him added incentive to increase the yield, output and earnings from his own land holdings.

(b) Guidance of farmers in the scientific method of agriculture, such as, efficient use of high yielding seeds and fertilisers to increase the output and appropriate use of pesticides to prevent the damage to crops from pests and plant disease.

(c) Establishment of cooperative agencies for marketing of agricultural produce, creation of post-harvest-storage facilities for the food grain, rational prices for crops and supply of animal foods to farmers at subsidised prices.

(ii) *Increasing the capacity of people to buy nutritious food in adequate quantity*

(a) Income generating activities for the economically weaker section of the community.

(b) Making stocks of staple food available in the area, throughout the year.

(c) Building up of buffer stocks of food grain, to tide over the periods of scarcity and maintaining the supply line.

(d) Distribution of food at fair prices through chain of retail outlet.

(e) Subsidised marketing of less-preferred staple foods.

Direct Nutrition and Health Interventions

(a) Integrated health package. Infections such as malaria, measles and infective diarrheas are widely prevalent in several developing countries. These have adverse effect on the nutritional status of people, especially of infants and children. These often precipitate acute malnutrition. Therefore primary health case package should also include preventive immunisation chemo-prophylaxis, oral hydration, periodic deworming, early diagnosis and prompt treatment of common illnesses.

(b) Nutrition education. Apart from the inability to procure nutritious food in adequate quantity due to poverty, other factors such as lack of awareness among the people of the nutritional quality of common foods, irrational beliefs and cultural practices of feeding significantly contribute to the development of malnutrition. Thus nutrition education is of paramount importance in strategies for the control of malnutrition. People should be informed of the nutritional quality of various locally available and culturally accepted low cost foods. Nutrition education should be specially directed to those members of the family who make decisions who can influence other persons in the family.

(i) Iatrogenic restriction of feeding in fevers and diarrhea should be discouraged, (ii) Breast feeding of infants should be vigorously promoted and encouraged, (iii) Nutrition supplements should be introduced in the diet of infants by the age of 3 to 5 months, (iv) Weaning foods should be based on a judicious mixture of staple cereal and legumes, so that the deficiency of a limiting amino acid in one is compensated by the extra quantity of specific amino acid in the other food, (v) As much milk, meat, eggs or foods of high biologic value as the family can afford should be offered with the weaning food mixtures to enhance their Net-dietary-protein value.

(c) *Early detection of malnutrition and intervention.*

It is extremely expensive to provide nutritional supplements to all the preschool children in the community so as to raise their nutritional status to an optimal level. This will require very large financial inputs, which can only be provided by massive diversion of the funds from projects for economic development of the country. Therefore, alternate approaches should be sought. Thus nutritional supplements may be provided only for the severely malnourished children and the moderately undernourished children may be kept undernuitional surveillance. Efforts should be made to prevent these children from becoming severely malnourished by nutrition education, health check, early intervention and control of infections.

Growth Cards

Children should grow continuously from birth to adolescence at the average rate expected for the age. It is desirable to record their growth periodically on growth cards. If the growth of the child is slowed or is arrested, as shown by a flat curve on the growth card, the physician should be immediately alerted. He should examine the child for any hidden infections and nutritional deficiencies, evaluate the dietary history and provide the appropriate treatment.

Velocity of growth is more important than the actual weight at a given time. Thus a child whose weight was above average, but whose growth was slowed or arrested recently is at greater risk than the child who started with a lower weight but whose growth curve is parallel to or better than the average.

The mother in the developing countries often do not remember the correct age of their children. Therefore, weight of the child cannot always be compared to the expected weight for the age. The difficulty can be circumvented by requesting the mother to relate the date of birth of the child to some important events or village festivals. Age is then estimated by referring to the calendar of important festivals or events in the village.

Table 20. 9
Physical Growth of Children. Percentiles of Selected Measurements.
Birth to 15 years.

Percentage for Boys					*Weights in kg. & Lengths in cms*	*Percentage for girls*				
10	*25*	*50*	*75*	*90*	*Age*	*10*	*25*	*50*	*75*	*90*
					AT BIRTH					
2.42	2.68	2.98	3.24	3.48	Weight	2.26	2.55	2.76	3.02	3.32
45.90	46.70	47.96	49.90	51.70	Crown heel length	45.90	46.90	48.00	49.30	50.60
30.10	31.33	32.45	33.57	34.55	Crown rump length	30.00	30.72	31.65	32.86	33.86
29.73	30.40	31.20	32.35	33.70	Chest circumference	29.46	30.00	30.75	32.00	33.30
32.60	33.30	34.10	35.00	35.60	Head circumference	32.00	32.80	33.50	34.40	35.30
					1 MONTH					
3.10	3.52	3.92	4.38	4.77	Weight	3.22	3.41	3.82	4.20	4.55
51.20	52.55	53.85	55.66	57.30	Crown heel length	48.10	51.10	53.20	54.95	56.60
33.85	34.82	35.68	37.10	38.58	Crown rump length	33.15	34.12	35.25	36.80	38.20
33.20	34.25	35.55	36.72	38.00	Chest circumference	32.34	33.33	34.60	35.80	36.80
34.60	36.00	36.90	37.80	38.40	Head circumference	34.30	35.50	36.40	37.30	37.80
					2 MONTHS					
3.79	4.25	4.65	5.20	5.73	Weight	3.57	4.00	4.30	4.75	5.20
53.20	55.00	56.75	58.80	80.60	Crown heel length	52.00	53.90	55.60	57.40	59.10
35.70	36.85	38.20	39.59	40.39	Crown rump length	34.50	35.75	36.80	37.72	38.65
34.28	36.20	37.02	39.30	41.40	Chest circumference	33.66	34.95	36.35	37.86	39.35
36.90	37.80	38.60	39.40	40.20	Head circumference	36.40	37.00	37.80	38.80	39.50
					3 MONTHS					
4.75	5.18	5.63	6.23	6.82	Weight	4.55	4.98	5.25	5.50	6.23
57.12	58.50	59.90	61.20	63.80	Crown heel length	53.80	56.80	58.80	59.80	61.65
37.90	39.12	40.10	41.30	42.72	Crown rump length	36.50	37.75	39.15	40.13	40.95
36.90	38.00	39.90	41.12	42.00	Chest circumference	36.00	37.40	38.40	39.05	40.80
38.80	39.90	40.30	40.90	42.30	Head circumference	37.60	38.50	39.30	40.10	41.50
					6 MONTHS					
5.54	6.35	7.14	7.81	8.35	Weight	5.54	6.19	6.83	7.32	7.90
61.50	63.40	65.10	66.70	66.45	Crown heel length	59.70	63.10	63.90	65.75	67.70
40.50	41.70	42.50	43.90	46.10	Crown rump length	39.85	41.90	42.56	43.70	44.48
39.65	40.00	42.40	43.80	45.00	Chest circumference	38.70	40.40	42.00	43.10	44.30
40.40	41.40	42.60	43.80	44.60	Head circumference	40.00	40.80	42.00	43.20	44.00

Contd.

					9 MONTHS					
6.50	7.35	8.05	8.72	9.64	Weight	6.48	6.90	7.37	8.02	9.00
65.30	67.00	68.95	70.90	72.45	Crown heel length	64.00	66.70	68.40	70.10	71.60
42.10	43.85	45.80	46.15	47.45	Crown rump length	42.10	43.30	44.33	45.22	46.32
41.10	42.80	44.20	45.40	47.20	Chest circumference	41.20	42.20	43.10	44.00	45.60
42.80	43.80	44.70	45.40	46.00	Head circumference	42.10	42.80	43.40	44.10	44.60
					1 YEAR					
7.25	8.00	8.90	9.85	10.84	Weight	6.85	7.65	8.45	9.27	10.05
69.60	71.40	72.90	75.50	78.30	Crown heel length	69.00	71.20	72.80	74.50	76.60
44.60	45.50	46.42	48.08	49.57	Crown rump length	43.40	45.00	46.00	47.10	49.10
42.80	44.70	46.00	47.88	49.40	Chest circumference	42.20	43.95	44.90	46.05	47.40
43.60	44.60	45.60	46.30	47.30	Head circumference	43.50	44.40	44.90	45.80	46.70
					1½ YEARS					
8.15	9.15	10.05	10.80	11.60	Weight	7.75	8.78	9.55	10.15	10.95
73.00	76.00	89.00	81.30	84.40	Crown heel length	74.50	77.00	79.10	80.20	81.4
46.30	47.86	49.36	50.30	51.60	Crown rump length	45.40	47.55	49.73	50.60	51.40
45.00	46.10	47.70	49.90	51.20	Chest circumference	45.15	45.45	46.25	48.70	49.4
45.30	46.00	46.8	48.20	49.00	Head circumference	44.40	45.30	46.30	47.40	48.30
					2 YEARS					
10.05	10.85	11.53	12.10	13.10	Weight	9.10	9.66	10.30	10.88	11.45
80.50	82.05	84.10	86.20	88.72	Crown heel length	80.25	81.40	82.40	83.30	84.75
48.60	50.20	51.30	52.15	53.30	Crown rump length	48.12	49.60	50.40	51.00	51.85
46.50	48.20	49.80	50.90	51.60	Chest circumference	45.90	46.85	48.25	49.20	49.85
46.40	47.70	48.40	49.10	49.80	Head circumference	45.20	46.00	47.30	48.00	49.20
					2½ YEARS					
10.22	10.95	11.80	12.50	13.45	Weight	10.05	10.47	10.92	11.53	12.50
82.50	84.42	86.65	89.30	92.60	Crown heel length	81.90	83.00	86.80	88.70	90.00
49.00	50.28	51.70	53.20	56.90	Crown rump length	49.10	50.00	51.20	52.80	53.95
47.30	48.50	49.80	50.70	51.70	Chest circumference	47.00	48.50	50.10	50.80	51.40
47.00	47.70	48.40	49.20	49.90	Head circumference	46.20	47.10	47.70	48.50	50.20
					3 YEARS					
10.86	11.63	12.50	13.60	14.55	Weight	10.35	11.20	11.90	12.90	13.60
84.20	87.60	90.80	92.20	94.20	Crown heel length	82.00	85.00	87.80	89.60	91.20
48.90	50.20	52.00	53.40	56.05	Crown rump length	48.76	49.68	50.70	52.40	54.30
46.64	48.00	49.55	50.80	52.30	Chest circumference	46.64	48.00	49.45	50.80	52.30
47.50	48.10	49.00	49.60	49.90	Head circumference	45.50	47.50	48.00	49.10	49.40
					3½ YEARS					
11.40	12.15	13.15	14.34	16.45	Weight	11.55	12.35	13.26	14.20	15.28
87.20	89.40	91.7C	94.60	97.50	Crown heel length	85.60	88.50	91.50	93.65	95.20
49.00	50.00	52.70	55.60	56.50	Crown rump length	48.60	52.20	53.90	56.30	57.00
48.20	49.60	50.80	52.60	53.90	Chest circumference	47.80	49.20	52.20	53.50	54.10
47.60	48.70	49.70	50.10	50.60	Head circumference	48.30	48.80	49.70	50.50	50.80

Percentage for Boys					Weights in kg. & Lengths in cms	Percentage of girls				
10	25	50	75	90		10	25	50	75	90
					4 YEARS					
11.70	13.00	14.60	16.70	18.60	Weight	12.90	14.00	15.10	16.40	18.10
92.20	93.70	95.00	98.20	101.20	Standing height	92.50	94.00	96.60	100.80	102.20
51.80	53.82	55.95	57.00	58.00	Sitting height	53.60	55.10	56.80	58.10	58.90
48.90	50.30	52.00	53.00	54.00	Chest circumference	49.60	51.10	53.80	54.20	54.50
48.60	49.20	49.90	50.50	50.80	Head circumference	47.80	48.60	49.80	50.50	50.90
					4½ YEARS					
12.20	13.50	15.22	17.60	20.25	Weight	13.60	14.40	15.20	16.85	18.80
95.70	97.10	100.40	105.00	107.40	Standing height	96.00	97.65	99.15	102.20	104.92
53.10	55.60	57.30	57.92	59.53	Sitting height	53.90	54.60	56.80	58.40	62.50
49.20	50.90	52.70	53.42	54.00	Chest circumference	51.00	52.80	54.00	54.60	55.00
48.80	49.30	50.10	50.60	50.90	Head circumference	47.60	48.30	50.20	50.40	51.30
					5 YEARS					
14.50	15.00	17.60	19.95	21.85	Weight	14.85	15.86	17.00	18.30	19.40
98.80	100.80	104.00	109.50	110.80	Standing height	100.10	101.20	103.00	106.00	108.80
53.10	54.70	58.30	59.74	61.00	Sitting height	53.12	54.80	56.90	50.30	61.00
51.55	53.20	53.88	54.42	55.40	Chest circumference	52.40	53.60	54.02	55.10	56.20
49.20	49.60	50.30	50.70	50.90	Head circumference	48.80	49.10	50.30	50.90	51.40
					6 YEARS					
17.50	17.90	18.90	20.40	21.80	Weight	15.70	16.90	18.50	19.50	20.80
106.60	109.20	114.10	116.80	118.30	Standing height	106.10	108.30	111.30	115.30	118.80
58.00	58.80	61.50	63.10	63.70	Sitting height	56.10	58.30	61.00	53.00	64.40
52.50	53.30	54.50	56.00	56.50	Chest circumference	51.60	52.20	53.70	55.00	56.40
					7 YEARS					
18.40	20.10	21.00	23.00	24.90	Weight	17.30	18.00	20.50	22.00	25.00
112.80	114.50	119.20	123.20	125.30	Standing height	112.10	114.20	118.40	120.00	122.40
61.50	62.70	65.00	66.70	68.90	Sitting height	60.80	62.00	63.50	65.20	67.00
53.60	54.70	56.20	58.10	59.00	Chest circumference	52.30	53.30	56.20	57.20	58.50
					8 YEARS					
20.10	21.60	23.90	25.40	27.40	Weight	18.90	20.90	22.80	25.40	23.20
118.80	119.20	124.50	128.10	132.50	Standing height	118.00	122.20	124.80	127.10	130.90
64.00	65.10	67.00	68.30	69.90	Sitting height	63.30	65.00	66.80	68.30	69.90
54.30	56.00	58.00	60.80	62.00	Chest circumference	53.10	54.60	56.30	58.90	61.90

Contd.

					9 YEARS					
21.40	23.30	25.50	27.30	29.80	Weight	21.10	23.00	24.00	26.80	28.40
122.40	125.20	130.00	134.00	137.30	Standing height	120.30	123.90	127.00	134.70	39.30
53.70	67.10	68.50	70.30	71.40	Sitting height	63.10	65.30	68.30	70.50	73.90
57.10	58.50	60.00	61.40	63.90	Chest circumference	54.60	57.20	59.00	61.00	62.40
					10 YEARS					
22.90	24.30	27.50	26.10	35.70	Weight	20.90	23.80	27.80	30.30	34.30
127.60	132.10	134.00	138.00	143.70	Standing height	128.20	131.50	135.30	137.60	140.30
67.10	68.20	70.50	72.40	73.90	Sitting height	65.70	68.20	70.00	72.00	74.00
57.00	58.30	62.00	63.80	64.90	Chest circumference	57.00	58.60	60.70	64.00	65.00
					11 YEARS					
25.60	28.30	31.00	33.30	34.90	Weight	25.60	28.50	31.00	33.90	35.70
133.00	137.00	140.00	100.40	145.60	Standing height	133.10	135.50	139.50	143.30	147.20
68.10	71.30	73.00	74.00	75.90	Sitting height	67.20	70.10	74.00	75.50	76.90
59.00	60.80	63.00	64.90	67.90	Chest circumference	58.30	59.60	63.00	64.90	66.90
					12 YEAR					
27.70	31.00	34.30	38.50	41.50	Weight	29.60	31.40	34.80	39.60	47.00
134.70	138.50	144.00	151.10	154.90	Standing height	137.20	143.50	146.00	149.90	154.30
72.10	73.00	74.90	77.50	79.90	Sitting height	69.80	75.00	76.50	78.70	82.90
61.70	64.60	66.00	69.40	72.90	Chest circumference	60.00	61.10	65.40	68.00	73.80
					13 YEARS					
32.80	36.70	41.50	46.10	48.10	Weight	33.10	35.50	42.50	46.20	49.60
146.10	148.30	153.50	158.70	162.20	Standing height	145.10	148.50	152.80	155.80	159.90
76.10	78.00	79.80	81.40	82.90	Sitting height	75.10	78.20	79.70	80.90	83.80
65.10	68.00	70.50	74.00	76.90	Chest circumference	64.00	65.40	68.70	72.50	74.20
					14 YEARS					
36.70	40.70	44.00	49.00	53.50	Weight	36.40	41.40	46.00	47.70	52.30
151.10	153.30	156.30	163.50	172.70	Standing height	148.30	151.10	153.00	158.00	160.90
78.00	78.20	80.10	83.70	85.90	Sitting height	77.10	77.60	80.00	82.70	84.00
67.00	71.00	73.50	70.90	78.00	Chest circumference	64.00	66.40	70.00	73.00	75.30
					15 YEARS					
39.70	43.20	48.40	53.40	55.30	Weight	40.20	44.10	46.30	48.50	50.20
153.50	159.00	164.80	170.50	172.00	Standing height	149.20	151.00	156.50	160.70	164.70
80.00	84.00	85.00	87.00	89.90	Sitting height	80.00	81.20	82.20	82.70	84.00
70.50	72.60	74.50	77.40	83.60	Chest circumference	66.00	66.60	70.70	75.71	77.10

Age independent anthropometric indices. Some anthropometric indices do not require consideration of age. The labile tissues like subcutaneous fat and muscles, which reflect the energy and protein stores of the body are depleted earlier in malnutrition. Thus the weight of the child is reduced in acute malnutrition. The static tissues like skeleton are not affected appreciably in the early stages of malnutrition. Thus the height and the head circumference of the child are altered only late in the course of nutritional deprivation. If the ratio between the labile tissues and the static tissues is obtained and compared with the normal, it may be possible to detect acute malnutrition. Some common indices used in clinical practice are:

Index	Normal	Severely malnourished
$\frac{\text{Weight Kg.}}{(\text{Height cm})^{1.6}} \times 100$	0.88-0.97	0.79
$\frac{\text{Weight in Kg}}{(\text{Height cm})^{2}} \times 100$	0.15-0.16	0.14
$\frac{\text{Mid-arm circumference cm}}{\text{Head circumference cm}}$	0.32-0.33	0.25

Quac stick is a rod with two sets of markings, one indicates the height and the other shows the expected mid-arm circumference of a normal child for the corresponding height. The midarm circumference of the child is obtained and the stick is placed behind the standing child. If the height of the child is more than the height expected for the measured mid-arm circumference of the child, the child is considered to be malnourished.

Shakirs tape for mid-arm circumference. This is a plastic tape with coloured zones green (more than 13.5 cm), corresponding to the mid-arm circumference for normal, yellow (between 12.5 and 13.5 cm) borderline and red (less than 12.5 cm) wasted arms. This is an extremely simple method of detecting protein energy malnutrition in the community.

Bangle test. A bangle with an inner diameter of 4 cm is slipped up the arm. If it crosses the elbow, the child is considered malnourished. Though simple, it is not as sensitive because the width of the arm depends on the thickness of bones besides the muscles.

Biochemical criteria for early diagnosis of protein malnutrition have been reviewed in the Committee Report on the Assessment of Protein Nutritional Status (Am. J. Clin Nutr 2-807, 1970). These are not of practical utility in field studies.

(d)Nutrition supplementation. The objective of nutritional supplementation programe should be to (i) treat and rehabilitate severely malnourished subjects, (ii) improve the general health and well being of children, increase the resistance to infectious illnesses and thereby decrease morbidity, (iii) accelerate the physical growth and mental development of children and (iv) improve the academic performance and learning abilities of children.

Integrated Health Package

Infections like malaria, measles and diarrhea are widely prevalent in poor countries. These have adverse effect on the nutritional status of children and often precipitate acute

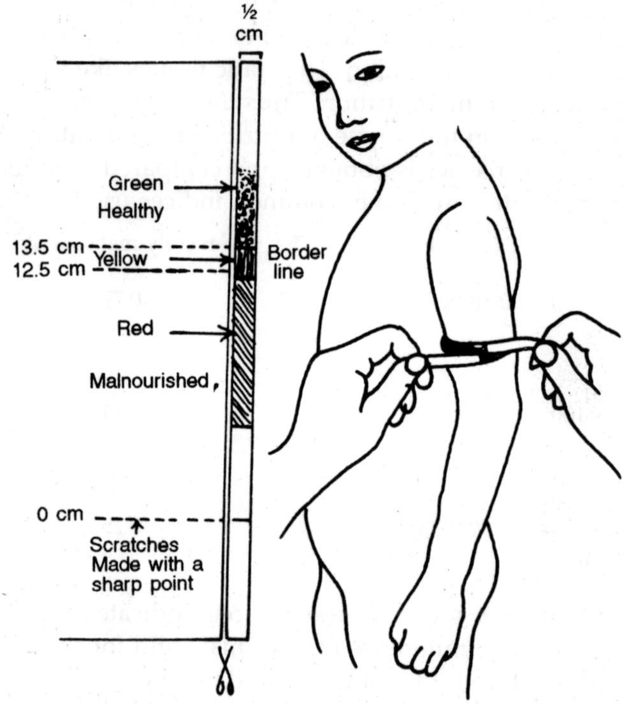

Fig 20. 8 Assessment of malnutrition in the community by measuring mid-arm circumference (Adapted from circular on International Year of the child issued by Institute of Child Health, London. With permission from Dr. D. Morley.)

malnutrition. Health package should include preventive immunisation, chemoprophylaxis, oral hydration in cases of diarrhea, periodic deworming early diagnosis and prompt treatment of common infections.

The Supplementary Feeding Programs

Preschool children, especially those under 3 years old and pregnant and lactating women suffer most often from the hazards of malnutrition. Therefore, most of the supplementary feeding programms cater to their needs. It should be recognised that not all of them need nutritional supplementation. It is necessary to define the most needy among them.

Types of Supplementary Feeding Programmes

Supplementary feeding programs may be organised in two ways *viz*. On the spot feeding 'or' delivery of carry home food packets. Both approaches have merits and limitations. On the spot feeding is often intended as a nutritional supplement, but evidence has accumulated to show that the families reduce the diet of the beneficiary to a similar extent as the supplements received. Therefore, it often becomes a substitute diet rather than a nutrition supplement. The food recipes tend to become monotonous for the liking of beneficiaries if there is less flexibility in their choice.

Distribution of carry home food packets is administratively more convenient and relatively chapter. The food is almost invariably shared by the beneficiary with other family members. Intended benefits may not be obvious in the short run. Some observers feel that there should be no serious objection to sharing by other family members because other members of the family also need some assistance.

Major limitation of the supplementary feeding programs are their high administrative cost and likelihood of inducing a cultural of dependence rather than that of self-reliance. The programs are often not self-sustaining in nature. As soon as the assistance is phased out, the original nutrition problems recur. *Several program for improving the nutritional status of children and pregnant, lactating women* were developed by the Government of India during last two decades. Some of these are described below.

Table 20.10

Protein content and calories in 100 gm of common articles of food.

Item	*Calories*	*Protein (g)*
Wheat flour	350	12.0
Rice	350	7.5
Barley	335	9.0-11.3
Tapioca dry	360	0.6
Corn flour	360	8.6
Lentils dried	350	25
Peas, dried	340	25
Bengal gram (chick pea) without husk	340	25
Red kidney beans	350	21-23
Soya beans	330	35
Groundnuts	560	27
Fresh corn	80-90	3.7-4.3
Potatoes	80-100	1.6-2.00
Milk skimmed power	360	38
Sugar	385	-
Milk, cow	65	3.2
Milk, water buffalo	115	4.3
Mutton	109	19
Eggs	160	12.8

The Mid-Day Meal Program for School Children

On the recommendation of National School Health Committee the Government of India started a scheme for providing mid-day meals to school children in the year 1962-63. The Government of India pays for 40 per cent of the expenditure. The responsibility for implementation lies with the states. Andhra Pradesh and Tamilnadu Governments have expanded this program widely in their states.

In this program the school going children are provided a mid-day meal, usually prepared from Balahar. Sukhadi, indigenous tapioca, ground nut mix extracted snacks, soya fortified bread, panjeeri or other local foods. The anticipated benefits of the program include better school performance of the children, through regular attendance and reduction in the school drop out rate.

The Special Nutrition Programme (SNP)

The SNP is a crash nutrition program for providing supplementary nutrition to children (0 to 3 years) living in the tribal areas and in urban slums. The program was started in the year 1970-71 by the department of Social Welfare and is implemented through the state governments. The entire expenditure is provided by the Governments of India. The program was later extended to include 3 to 6 years old children, pregnant mothers in the last trimester of pregnancy and lactating women.

Guidelines about nutrition supplements are given, but flexibility is permitted provided the cost of supplements is within the approved limit. Supplements are provided for 250 to 300 days. The food is distributed through feeding centres, at maternal and child health clinics and balwadis. These usually cover 100 to 200 beneficiaries within a radius of one mile.

The Vitamin A Prophylaxis Programme

In this program all children in the age group 1 to 6 years in the target area receive 200,000 I.U. of Vit. A in an oily base, orally twice a year. The Vit A doses are administered by the personnel of the Family Planning Department. The programme was extended at the national level in 1969. Evaluation in 1971-72 showed that vit A deficiency signs were significantly less, the programme was well accepted and there was 90 to 65 per cent coverage in the first and second rounds respectively.

The Anemia Prophylaxis Programme

Ferrous sulphate and folic acid tablets are distributed to the pregnant women through MCH centers in rural tribal and urban areas. Department of Health is responsible for implementation.

Applied Nutrition Programme and Integrated Rural Development Programme

Applied Nutrition Programme comprised a set of coordinated educational activities by the department of agriculture, health, education and other interested agencies with the aim of raising the levels of nutrition of local population, particularly of mothers and children in rural areas.

The Department of Rural Development of the Ministry of Agriculture was the implementing agency. The main aim was to raise the nutritional status of the population as a whole but of children and pregnant/lactating women in particular, through extension methods of education and demonstration at community level. The inputs for food and livestock production were substantially supported by UNICEF. The programme was started in 1953-54. Three major components of the programme were (i) production of protective foods, (ii) training of village workers in extension work, health education, food production and (iii) organising of feeding schemes. The possible areas of work included the following:

Health Sector. Nutritional surveillance, preventive immunisation, periodic deworming, training of health personnel in nutrition, food hygiene, nutrition rehabilitation centres, supplementary feeding for the vulnerable groups and nutrition education of public.

Education Sector. Mid-day meal programme, food and nutrition education in school curricula, training of teachers and parents in principles of nutrition, production of food and planning of home budget.

Food Production. Live stock production, dairy, poultry farming, fisheries, increased food production through intensive agricultural practices, increased production of vegetable and fruit, extension education, improved seed marketing, development of hybrid and high yielding varieties of crops.

Community Development. Homecraft and cottage industries relating to food through women's groups, youth clubs and community centers, development of cooperatives.

Transport and Communication. Better management of transport and marketing of food surpluses.

During 1978-79, 35 per cent of 1966 blocks in 20 states and 4 union territories had an operating applied nutrition programme. The programme has been since discontinued.

As a new strategy. *Integrated Rural Development programme* has been initiated in 22 blocks with the assistance from UNICEF from the year 1978. ANP activities are being coordinated with child health, provision of drinking water supply and *income generating scheme* for women and underemployed rural population. Youth are trained in economically productive craft and activities. The projects concentrate on economically under privileged segments.

Integrated Child Development Services (ICDS)

The programme aims at promotion of physical growth, mental and social development of the young child and reduction of avoidable morbidity and mortality through a package of health and education inputs. This programme is based on a report of an expert group appointed by the Ministry of Education and Social Welfare in 1971.

Contents of the Project

(i) Non-formal education of the preschool child (3 to 6 years old).

(ii) Supplementary feeding (0 to 6 years old).

(iii) Immunization of children.

(iv) Health surveillance and essential health care of preschool children.

(v) Functional literacy of the women.

The scheme was started in 1975.

The Department of social welfare is the implementing agency. It works in close coordination with Ministry of Health and also with the departments of Food and Agriculture and Community Development. It has been amply supported by UNICEF, Each ICDS projects is supervised by the Child Development Project Officer, 5 supervisors or mukhya sevikas and approximately 100 anganwadi workers and an equal number of helpers. The Ministry of Health is expected to reinforce the staffing pattern in the ICDS projects, so as to provide in all, at least 3 doctors, 4 lady health visitors, 20 auxiliary nurse midwives or female multipurpose health workers in the concerned primary health center. The staffing pattern differs in tribal and urban area projects.

The local point for delivery of the package of health, nutrition and education services is Anganwadi. Anganwadi teacher and helpers coordinate with the health team to deliver health services to preschool children under their jurisdiction. The Anganwadi workers also provide nonformal education to the 3-6 years age group children who assemble in the anganwadi for 3 to 4 hours every day. The preschool children receive supplementary feeding almost at the same scak as under SNP.

The health package consists of health check up, DPT and BCG vaccination. Oral polio vaccination was made optional. Typhoid vaccine is given to older children. There is provision for curative services by the health personnel when they visit the village oral rehydration in cases of diarrhea and referral services.

Functional literacy includes talks on health, nutrition and mother craft.

The programme is being monitored continuously.

Programme is well conceived. Some difficulties were observed. Attention of the anganwadi worker is mainly focused on 3-6 years old and under 3 years old children receive less attention. In the initial planning, *"At Risk"* approach was not adopted, but this is being gradually introduced. The anganwadi teachers were not well trained for the anticipated jobs. Lacunae are being filled by continuing education. Administrative costs are high. Programme is included in the 20 point programme of the Prime Minister of India and is being extended to 1000 blocks in the 7th Five Year Plan 1985-90.

Food for Work Programme (FFW)

Food for Work Programme was an offshoot and a form of Fmployment Guarantee Schemes. It was expected to bring nutritional improvement in the worker's families by providing employment and paying a part of wages in the form of food grain. In addition to its nutrition and employment goals, the FFW programme also stabilised the prices of foodgrain and provides minimum support price for grain to farmers.

FFW programme could be used effectively to create substantial community assets—ranging from digging of wells and protected tanks for drinking water, making of irrigation bunds and field channels for the small and marginal farmers, soil conservation, afforestation, raising common pastures, constructing schools, community centers, rural houses, roads and bridges.

The work provided under this programme should not relate to uneconomic chores such as stone breaking and making kutcha roads. FFW schemes should be used to improve the rural infrastructure to improve the quality of life and to develop economic enterprises for the rural poor. It may be possible to associate health and nutrition education and demonstration components in FFW. Integrated Rural Development Programme incorporates some of these ideas.

Accidents

Infants and young children try to explore new substances and articles by mouthing these. They should be kept away from household poisons and sharp pointed objects. Mothers should be educated about the potential dangerous situations in the household. The child should be protected from *accidental falls, injuries and burns*. Mothers should be requested to keep stoves in the kitchen at a higher level. Kerosene should not be stored in cups, tumblers, aerated water or beer bottles. Fused bulbs and empty bottles should not be used as improvised kerosene lamps.

In the rural areas, use of insecticides and fungicides for protecting food grain is common. The people should be taught about their proper use.

For details of accident prevention, see chapter on prevention of handicaps.

School Health Programmes

Health care should be a continuing process throughout life. Gains made by good health care during a period of life may be lost due to neglect later in life. In most countries of the third world, morbidity and mortality rates among children are much higher in the preschool years than during the school years. However, school-age children also suffer impairment and disabilities during these crucial years, which prevent development of their optimal growth potential and acquisition of competences for becoming useful and productive members of the society. Although health is generally regarded as a highly personal affair, it no longer remains so, it if endangers the health of others and causes concern to the society. During school years, the child's health and welfare need to be protected from the effects of overcrowding, contact with persons suffering from contagious illnesses, unhealthy environment, contaminated water and food supplies.

School-health programmes involve health problems that affect children between the ages of 5 to 18 years and which are caused by (i) school personnel, (ii) originate from the school or (iii) from the school going children to other children. A brief outline of goals, objectives and functions of school health programmes is given below:

Broad Goal of the school health programme is to help the children remain in good health and achieve their optimum for normal growth and development. To achieve the broad goals of school health programmes, following objectives should be aimed at.

Objectives of School Health Programme

(a) to provide healthful environments in the school.

(b) to increase health consciousness of school children, health education on personal hygiene, good food habits and need for physical fitness.

(c) to identify early signs of ill health, provide appropriate and timely health interventions and promote good health of children by continued surveillance throughout the period they are in school and attempt to rehabilitate children with emotional, educational or physical handicaps in the society.

(d) to prevent communicable diseases by prophylactic immunisation, chemoprophylaxis and improvement of environmental sanitation.

Common Health Problems of School Children

1. Malnutrition
2. Infectious diseases
3. Prasitic infestations including pediculosis.
4. Skin ailments especially scabies and impetigo
5. Common eye defects, errors of refraction, conjunctivities and trachoma.
6. Otitis media
7. Dental caries.

Components of School Health Programme

1. Healthful School Environment

(i) *Physical facility*

(a) Adequate sanitation.

(b) Good ventilation.

(c) Proper lighting arrangement in class rooms.

(d) Proper type of furniture to ensure good posture of students.

(e) Supply of clean potable drinking water.

(f) Arrangements for cheap nutritious food in school canteens.

(g) Clean privies and toilet facilities.

(ii) *Play and Recreation.* To ensure adequate space for playgrounds for children and gymnasium. If financial resources are available, a swimming pool or access to a swimming pool with modern sanitary and safety installations should be arranged. This is possible only in urban areas.

(iii) *Prevention of Accidents and Injuries.* School health programme officer should work with traffic authorities for control of unrestricted traffic of automobiles and heavy goods carriers in the school neighbourhood. Special school transport should be provided for children commuting from long distances. Arrangements should be made for training of school children in road safety regulations.

(iv) *Consultation with School Authorities.* The school health officer should communicate with the governing body of school, the headmaster and other teachers for all matters regarding health and safety of children.

2. Health Education

(a) Health education may be imparted directly to children or

(b) Indirectly through training of teachers and training of parents.

(c) The school health officer should consult with school authorities in preparation of school curriculum on health education and also.

(d) Motivate children to transmit the health education learnt by them in the school to their families and neighbours.

3.School Health Services

(i) Health Appraisal. Periodic medical examination of children including periodic record of weight and height; checking of refractive errors and examination of teeth for dental caries.

(ii) Referral of sick or high risk children to appropriate health agency for any remedial action for any health defects observed in the child.

(iii) Follow up of children to ensure compliance of advised health interventions.

(iv) Preventive immunisation of the unimmunised children.

(v) Examination of the teaching and other staff for any communicable diseases.

(vi) *Facilities for emergency medical care of children and first aid,* if needed in the school premises.

21

Requirement of Paediatricians by 2000 A.D.

INTRODUCTION

In India, the problem of providing adequate medical and health care to its population has always been a matter of serious concern for policy makers and planners in the formulation of health and medical development programmes during the different five-years plan periods. As a result much has been achieved during the last 35 years and a large infrastructure of hospitals, dispensaries, primary health centres, sub-centres has been built up. Medical manpower being an important resource to man these institutions, the need for expansion of training facilities during five-year plans was well realised. As a result, the number of medical colleges increased from 28 in 1950-51 to 106 in 1981-82 leading to increase, in admission capacity from 2675 to 11641 and of out-turn from 1557 to 12170 during the same period. Due to increase in the out-turn, the stock of doctors increased from 59,000 in 1951 to 2,22,800 in 1981 and the doctor-population ratio was reduced from one doctor for every 6069 persons in 1951 to one doctor for every 3016 persons in 1981.

Another note worthy development during the five-year plans has been the trend towards specialisation. The result was that the number of institutions imparting postgraduate education increased from 79 in 1966 to 98 in 1981 leading to increase in admissions and out-turn of medical postgraduates in various specialities during the period. This has increased the proportion of postgraduate out-turn to graduate out-turn over the period of time and recent estimates show that nearly 60 per cent of medical students graduating every year qualify as specialists with degree or diploma in one or the other medical speciality.

Despite the impressive progress made in development of infrastructure and medical manpower during the last three decades, the position in rural areas with respect to the health service facilities is still far from satisfactory. Vast segments of rural population have little or no access to the government health facilities providing the basic speciality services. In order to bridge the gap the Government has accepted the Alma Atta Declaration of Health For All by 2000 A.D. and has developed a strategy with more emphasis on the provision of primary health care, through the network of Village Health Guides, Trained Dais. Multipurpose Workers and supervisors located at the level of villages, sub-centre, and primary health centres and community health centres. In addition, the services in four basic specialities namely, Medicine, Surgery, Obstertrics and Gynaecology and Paediatrics will be provided through the community health centres, sub-divisional centres and district health centres (Appendix-I).

With this new strategy, the demand for generalist and specialist medical manpower is likely to increase in the subsequent plans to achieve the goal of Health For All by 2000 A.D. This raises the question as to how far this demand for generalists and specialists can be met with the expected supply by the end of the century. It involves taking proper stock of the manpower available and likely to be available over a period of time as well as suitable allocation of the manpower taking into account the anticipated requirements.

Keeping in view the recommended model of Health Services, to achieve the goal of Health For All by 2000 A.D., Mathur[1] made an attempt to estimate the likely imbalances between supply and demand in the generalists doctors using the secondary data. The study conducted by him indicates that the likely supply of doctors by 2000 A.D. will be 3,91,000 whereas the requirement of doctors will be of the magnitude varying from 4,50,000 to 5,84,000. This broadly indicates that there will be shortage of general duty doctors.

So far, no attempt has been made to examine the likely imbalances in demand and supply of specialist medical manpower in the context of goal of Health For All by 2000 A.D. Hence, in this paper, an attempt has been made to indicate the broad dimensions of the problems of imbalances rather than the precise estimates of demand and supply of specialist category of medical manpower namely, paediatricians, so as to facilitate decision concerning expansion of otherwise of training facilities for paediatricians. This specific category of medical manpower has been selected for the study as the children in the age-group 0-14 years constitute about 40 per cent of the population and also on account of the importance given to the vulnerable group of population, namely children below the age of five years by the Working Group on Health For All[2] in relation to reduction in the mortalities including infant mortality in this age group.

OBJECTIVES

The specific objectives to which this paper addresses itself are:

(i) to estimate the current stock of paediatricians in the country.

(ii) to estimate the future supply and availability of paediatricians by 2000 A.D.

(iii) to estimate the future requirement of paediatricians by 2000 A.D. in phased manner.

(iv) to estimate the gap between supply and demand of paediatricians by 2000 A.D. in phased manner.

METHODOLOGY

The sophisticated methods for estimating supply of and demand for a particular category of personnel can be successfully applied only if detailed information needed for such methods is available. The medical manpower statistics like any other category of health statistics are unfortunately inadequate and suffer form a number of limitations, such as accuracy and completeness.

Data are not available on number of doctors classified in terms of their sex area of specialisation and functional field of their employment, etc. One needs a consistent set of data for a number of years showing the detailed break-up of doctors by different characteristics. Since any effort to collect primary data on the subject requires considerable amount of resources, an attempt has been made in this study to correct, update, suitably shift and synthesise the data collected from secondary sources in the earlier study[3] and the same has been utilised for estimation of supply and demand for paediatricians by 2000 A.D. in a phased manner.

Limitations of the Study

The material utilised and methodologies adopted for estimation of demand and supply of paediatric manpower have in- built limitations which need to be highlighted as the knowledge of these limitations becomes relevant for the use of the estimates based on such data.

(1) The study is based on secondary data which have their own limitations in terms of accuracy, completness, and availability of detailed characteristics of manpower under study.

(2) The demand for paediatricians is estimated only for government health organisations where as the other organised sectors such as railways, defence, public undertakings, private organisations have been excluded because of non-availability of data. Inclusion of the demand of other than government sector would increase total demand for paediatricians.

(3) Each methodology adopted has its limitations due to number of assumptions made and validity of these assumptions need to be examined on occassions but the same has not been done due to non-availability of information.

(4) The paper is based on earlier study conducted in 1982 and hence need updating of the estimates.

(5) Therefore, the paper looks into only the quantitative aspects of mismatches between demand and supply of paediatricians.

(6) Non-availability of clear outline of development of integrated and comprehensive medical and health services in the country over long period of time has been a problem in estimating demand.

FINDINGS

Current Stock and Supply of Paediatricians by 2000 A.D.

The Medical Council of India provides the information about the current stock of medical graduates registered with them. Similarly, some of the medical specialities do have the professional associations with whom the specialists register themselves after acquiring postgraduate degree or diploma in the subject. The data provided by these associations about the number of specialists registered with them indicating the stock at a particular point of time has its own limitations as all those who acquire postgraduate qualification do not necessarily register with the association. Secondly, these are not updated for retirement, mortality and migration. Though the magnitude of this under or over registration is not known, knowledge of these limitations becomes relevant for the use of the estimates based on such data.

The Indian Academy of Paediatricians had 1718 Postgraduate paediatric doctors registered with them in 1977. The available out-turn data of 56 postgraduate medical institutions indicated that 175 postgraduate degrees and 229 postgraduate diplomas in paediatrics were awarded to doctors in 1977-78[4]. Thus, 404 qualified paediatricians were added to the stock of 1718 increasing it to 2122 paediatricians during 1977-78.

As regards to the supply aspects, the number of institutions providing postgraduate degree and diploma in paediatrics increased to 58 in 1978-79 with admission capacity of 312 student every year[5]. Because of the non-availability of data with respect to the admissions and out-turn of postgraduates in paediatrics for later years, the supply of paediatricians for future year has been estimated with assumption that their was no increase in the admission capacity and the future number of paediatricians qualifying every year are maintained at the level of admission capacity as on 1978-79.

The stock of paediatricians in 1977-78 is adjusted for their mortality (0.7%) and retirement (0.3%)[6] and also the out-turn data have been adjusted for mortality using age-specific mortality rate of 3.25 per 1000 in the age-group 20-30 years. So far as the migration is concerned, it is assumed that in - migration and out-migration of paediatricians will have no significant effect since the difference between the two was observed to be less than 0.5 per cent[7] of the paediatricians in the country.

TABLE 1

Estimated Supply of Paediatricians by 2000 A.D. in Phased Manner.

Year	*Available from stock in 1977-78*	*Survival from out-turn during 1978-2000*	*Total estimated supply*
Sixth Five Year Plan Period			
1982-83	2018	1550	3568
1983-84	1998	1857	3855
1984-85	1978	2163	4141
Later Period			
1989-90	1881	3378	5259
1994-95	1789	4868	6657
1999-2000	1701	6333	8034

Definitions adopted

Stock: The term stock includes the work force and those unemployed but seeking employment. It excludes the retired paediatricians.

Supply: The term supply includes the manpower supply to be available for services at some future time.

Thus, it is estimated that by the end of Sixth Five Year Plan there will be 4141 paediatricians in the country and this stock will increase to 5259 by 1990, then to 6657 by 1995 and finally there will be 8034 paediatricians by the end of this century.

Requirement of Paediatricians by 2000 A.D.

There is no universally accepted method for assessing future requirement of manpower and hence the component approach has been utilised to estimate the requirement of paediatricians. The broad areas of consumption of services of paediatricians, namely, medical care, teaching and other programmes/schemes of the Government of India have been considered. As this approach requires a clear outline of the development of integrated and comprehensive medical health services in the country over a long period of time the recommendation for development programmes proposed by different working groups under Health For All by 2000 A.D. and the information available from plan documents[8] and other sources have been utilised to estimate the requirement of paediatricians by the year 2000 A.D. This demand has been phased out planwise as has been done while estimating supply of paediatricians.

Medical Care: The specialists medical care is provided by hospitals and by private practitioners in urban areas whereas in rural areas it is available on referral basis only in some blocks where the primary health centres (PHC's) have been upgraded into 30 beded rural hospitals. There are 357 such rural hospitals in the country (1982).

Rural Health programmes in Sixth Five Year Plan and the Report of the Working Group on Health For All by 2000 A.D. envisages the establishment of the Community Health Centre (CHC) for a population of 1,00,000 or one community development block to provide specialist services in Medicine, Surgery, and others in rural areas by 2000 A.D. The Community Health Centres will be established either as new CHCs or by converting existing rural hospitals into Community Health Centres. Thus, the Sixth Five Year Plan has envisaged increase in number of rural hospitals (CHCs) to 430 1982-83, to 472 in 1983-84 and to 514 by the end of the Sixth Plan period (1984-85). Whereas, in the context of Health For All by 2000 A.D. it is envisaged to achieve a target of 5500 CHCs by 2000 A.D. in a phased manner, namely 1800 CHCs during 1980-85, 2250 CHCs during 1985-90, 1020 CHCs during 1990-95 and backlog, if any, during 1995-2000. (Table 2).

On the other hand, in the urban areas, there are 6805 hospitals (1982) providing specialist services for the community. These hospitals of varying sizes, of which 107 are attached with medical colleges, are owned by Government, local bodies, voluntary organisations. These number of hospitals have increased by one per cent during last six years (1976-82) but neither the sixth plan nor the report of working group on health for all by 2000 A.D. have envisaged any increased in number of hospitals.

TABLE 2

Estimated Requirement of Paediatricians for Medical Care in Various Plan Periods till 2000 A.D.

Year	*No. of paediatricians for Hospitals Non-teaching staff.*	*No. of paediatricians for Community Health Centres*	*Total No. of paediatricians*
Sixth Five Year Plan Period			
1982-83	476	430	906
1983-84	481	472	953
1984-85	486	514	1000
Report Health For All			
1980-85	486	2230	2716
1985-90	511	4480	4991
1990-95	536	5500	6036
1995-2000	561	If any backlog	6061

Requirement/demand: The term demand includes the work force and the new employment opportunities generated during the year.

Thus, it is assumed that most of the demand for paediatricians will be created by CHCs and hospitals of different sizes and the same have been estimated excluding the hospitals attached with medical colleges. This is mainly because the teachers in medical colleges provide services in the attached hospital and they have been considered separately in later section.

In order to estimate the demand for paediatricians in the hospitals of different sizes, the staffing norms recommended by Jain Committee[9] and those by Anand[10] were utilised which indicated that the hospitals with bed strength more than 200 should have one paediatrician to provide medical care services to the children below 12 years of age. Taking into account the above norms and the distribution of non-teaching hospitals by their bed strength (Appendix II) the demand for paediatricians in those hospitals is estimated to be 471 in 1982. To estimate the demand for future years it is assumed that the annual one per cent increase in the number of hospitals with bed strength more than 200 observed during 1976-82 will continue in future years.

Thus, taking into consideration the requirements of hospitals and targets set by Government of India for establishment of CHCs, it is estimated that by the end of sixth five year plan (1984-85) there will be the demand for 1000 paediatricians whereas this will increase to 2716 with the establishment of 1800 new CHCs during 1985-90 and then to 6061 by the end of the century.

Teachers: The medical council of India[11] has recommended 135 teachers for every 100 admissions in MBBS course for staffing various department of the medical colleges of which three teachers should belong to paediatrics department. However, for medical colleges having more than 100 admissions per year it is recommended that the number of teaching staff will have to be in the ratio of 1:10 students for every 50 additional admissions over 100. But it does not indicate the speciality to which this additional teaching staff to be allocated.

For the postgraduate training in paediatrics it is recommended that these institutions should have minimum four teachers of that speciality or the student teacher ratio should be such that the number of postgraduate teachers to the number of postgraduate degree students admitted per year be maintained at 1:1 whereas for diploma students it should be 2 students per postgraduate teacher per year.

In order to estimate demand of teachers in paediatrics based on the above recommendations, the 106 medical colleges have been classified by their admission capacity for MBBS course and availability of postgraduate facilities (Appendix III). The admission capacity in 58 institutions providing postgraduate degree and diploma courses in paediatrics was 255 and 57 respectively during 1978-79. As the Sixth Plan as well as the working Group of Health For All by 2000 A.D. do not envisage any further expansion of medical education, the demand of teachers in paediatrics will remain same as at present. Thus, on the basis of the norms recommended by Medical Council of India in relation to authorised admission capacity the demand for paediatricians has been estimated as 452 during 1982-83 which will continue till 2000 A.D.

Post-Partum Programmes: During the previous plan periods, number of organisations for implementation of family planning programme have been established. Among many of them post-partum programme is the one which was established in 59 institutions in 1969-70 and we have 554 institutions in the country, under this programme after 10 years of its inception (1981-82) of these 554 centres, 192 belong to type A where more than 3000 obstetrics and abortion cases are done every year, 100 belong to type-B with more than 1500 and less than 3000 cases and remaining 253 belong to type-C with less than 1500 cases[12] per year.

The Government of India has recommended additional staff for these centres under post-partum programme. These recommendations include a post of lecturer in paediatrics for teaching hospitals under this programme. With this the demand for paediatricians under this programme will continue as in 1983 which is 101 paediatricians. Further, this programme will be extended to 300 sub-divisional hospitals during Sixth Plan Period. No further expansion of this programme is envisaged by the Working Group on Health For All by 2000 A.D. Hence, the demand of 101 paediatricians under this programme will continue till 2000 A.D.

School Health Programme: In the School Health Programme it is envisaged to provide specialist services, as per the requirement, once a month at PHC level. This depends on the morbidity conditions identified by medical officers during routine weekly medical examination. These specialists services are bound to include the paediatric services and thus create the requirement of specialists medical manpower, namely, paediatricians. Due to paucity of data about medical examinations of children and morbidity conditions experienced by the school children it is not possible to estimate the demand for paediatricians under this programme.

Taking into account the estimates of demand for paediatricians for each of the programme, namely, medical care, teaching, post-partum programme, school health programme, it is estimated that by the end of Sixth Plan (1984-85) demand exists for 1553 paediatricians. The demand will increase to 3269 during 1984-85 with the new strategies developed to achieve goal of Health For All by 2000 A.D. The further increase in requirement will be of magnitude of 5544 during 1985-90 and 6614 by the end of the century. (Table 3)

TABLE 3

Estimated Demand for Paediatricians in various Plan periods till 2000 A.D.

Year	*Demand in*			
	Medical care	*Teaching*	*Post-partum programme*	*Total*
Sixth Five Year Plan				
1982-83	906	452	101	1459
1983-84	953	452	101	1506
1984-85	1000	452	101	1553
Report Health For All				
1984-85	2716	452	101	3269
1989-90	4091	452	101	5544
1994-95	6036	452	101	6539
1994-2000	6061	452	101	6614

These estimates however suffer from limitations as these do not take into account the requirements of health services under the Railways. Labour and Employment and Defence in the organised sector on one hand and voluntary and private organisation on the other hand.

Imbalances between Supply and Demand for Paediatricians.

The estimates derived for current stock and demand and then the future supply and requirement for paediatricians indicate that till the end of Sixth Five Year Plan there will be a surplus of paediatricians by more than 2000. (Table 4).

TABLE 4

Comparative Statement of Estimates of Supply, Demand and Surplus or Shortages of Paediatricians in different plan period.

Year	*Supply of paediatricians*	*Demand for paediatricians*	*Surplus/shortages of paediatricians*
Sixth Five Year Plan			
1982-83	3568	1459	2109
1983-84	3855	1506	2349
1984-85	4141	1553	2588
Report Health For All			
1980-85	4141	3269	872
1985-90	5259	5544	-285
1990-95	6657	6589	68
1995-2000	8034	6614	1420

The surplus decreases with the rural development programme of providing the Community Health Centre to every 1,00,000 population or Community Development Block envisaged by the Working Group on Health For All by 2000 A.D. as the requirement of paediatricians increase in the initial plan period of 1980-85 and 1985-90 to the magnitude of 1800 and 2250 respectively. Because of this, the surplus of paediatricians may reduce to 872 during 1980-85 and then there is likely to be a shortage of paediatricians to the tune of 285 during 1985-90. After this period again there is expected to be a balance in demand and supply during 1990-95 and then surplus during 1995-2000.

It may be pointed out that in supply projections it has been assumed that there will not be any increase in the existing intake capacity upto 2000 A.D. and will remain at the level of 1978-79. But in the event of increase in the number of medical colleges from 56 in 1978-79 to 77 in 1981 for providing postgraduate degree or diploma in paediatrics, there has been increase in admission capacity leading to increase in out-turn of paediatricians by 36 per cent. This has increased the supply of this category of medical manpower. On the other hand, increase in admission capacity has increased the demand for teachers in paediatrics which is estimated to be about 20 per cent during 1978-79 to 1982-83. Secondly, even if we take into account the marginal requirement of paediatricians in the School Health Programme and also in the organised Public Sector such as Railways, Labour and Employment, Defence, etc. and in the private sector the country will be in a position to meet the requirement with the present pattern of supply.

CONCLUSIONS

The analysis of the data with regard to supply of and demand for paediatricians in the context of the goal of Health For All by the year 2000 A.D. has not brought out any shortages of serious nature. Even if the paediatric manpower situation is viewed in the context of the paediatric problems current and likely to come up in future in terms of morbidity and mortality pattern amongst children, morbidity conditions requiring paediatric services, it will not create any serious imbalances in demand and supply of paediatricians except during short period of time. But any changes which may come in the existing structural framework of health services and that contemplated during the next 17 to 18 years in the goal of Health For All by the year 2000., may influence the requirement of paediatric manpower and hence one has to revise the estimates on such occasions and preferably every 5 years.

With the developments contemplated, the services of the paediatric specialist will be available to the community at the institutional level from CHC to the higher level and for quite sometime the responsibility for tackling paediatric problem in rural areas will remain with the auxiliaries and paramedical manpower at the grassroot level supported by physicians at the intermediatory level, namely, Primary Health Centre. These categories of manpower need short-term orientation training in tackling the immediate and basic health problems of children below 12 years of age and referring the complicated cases to appropriate health facilities.

To motivate this specialist medical manpower to move into the rural areas and provide services through Community Health Centres, tehsil hospital policy decision needs to be taken for incentives as have been adopted by some of the states in the country.

Lastly, it may be stated that very often mismatches in health manpower are viewed as unemployment problems—current as well as future. This paper provides only warning to the Health Planners and Administrators about the situation and points out, that a balance between manpower planning, production and management aspects need to be given due importance for improving the employment status of paediatricians.

APPENDIX I

Recommended Model of Health Services

For each District

District Health Centre with specialised curative services and public health experts.

|

|

For each sub-Division/Approximate 5 lakh population

A sub-Divisional Health Centre with epidemiological wing attached to it.

|

For each Block/one lakh population

A Community Health Centre with specialised medical care services in Gynae, Paediatrics, Surgery and Medicines (out of the 4 non-specialised doctors, one may be drawn from any of the locally accepted traditional systems of medicine and one should be a public health man).

|

For 30,000 population (or 15,000-20,000 in the case of hilly, tribal sparsely populated or desert areas).

A Primary Health Centre (PHC) Fully equipped to render preventive, promotive and curative services. The staffing pattern is given in Annexure IIIA.

|

For 5000 population (2,500 population in the case of hilly, tribal sparsely populated or desert areas).

One Sub-Centre having one MPW (F), MPW (M) and one part-time attendant.

For each village/1000 population (or 500 population in the case of hilly and tribal areas or sparsely populated or desert areas).

|

One Health Volunteer preferably Female, Ex-Servicemen, School Teacher, Village Vaidya or Village Dai etc.

Report of the Working Group on Health For All by 2000 A.D. Ministry of Health and Family Welfare (March 1981) Government of India.

APPENDIX II

Distribution of Hospitals according to Size and Type in 1982
(Teaching and Non-teaching)

No. of beds	*No. of Hospitals attached to Medical Colleges*	*No. of Non-teaching Hospitals*	*Total number of Hospitals*
1	2	3	4
–25	-	33219	33219
26-50	-	1476	1476
51-75	-	435	435
76-100	1	382	383
101-200	-	610	610
201-300	4	225	229
301-400	7	89	96
401-500	8	56	64
501-600	10	30	40
601-700	14	29	43
700+	63	42	105
Total	107	6698	6805

Sources: (i) Health Statistics of India, 1982, Central Bureau of Health Intelligence, DGHS, Ministry of Health and Family Welfare, Government of India, New Delhi, 1982.

(ii) Directory of Hospitals, Central Bureau of Health Intelligence, DGHS, Ministry of Health and Family Welfare, Government of India, 1975.

APPENDIX III

Distribution of Medical Colleges by Their Admission Capacity in MBBS Course

Admission capacity	*Total No.*	*No. of medical colleges and Institutions*	
		With postgraduate in paediatrics	*No postgraduation in paediatrics*
1	2	3	4
-100	63	19	44
101-150	27	17	10
151-200	14	13	1
201-250	2	1	1
Total	106	50	56
PG Institution	12	8	-
Total	-	58	56

Sources: (i) Health Statistics of India, 1978, Central Bureau of Health Intelligence, DGHS, Ministry of Health and Family Welfare (1978).

(ii) The Directory of post graduate Medical Degree and Diplomas in India, 1975, Central Bureau of Health Intelligence, DGHS, Ministry of Health and Family Welfare, Government of India, New Delhi.

REFERENCES

1. Mathur, P.N. (1982): "Medical Manpower Requirement" - Paper presented at C.C. Roy Centenary Celebration and the Conference on Medical Education and Health Care held at New Delhi, 2-5 March.
2. Report of the Working Group on Health For All by 2000 A.D. Government of India, Ministry of Health and Family Welfare (1981).
3. Kataria, M. Et al., "A supply and demand for Specialist Medical Manpower in India, 1983-84", National Institute of Health and Family Welfare, New Delhi.
4. Health Statistics of India (1979): Central Bureau of Health Intelligence, DGHS, Ministry of Health and Family Welfare, Government of India.
5. Health Statistics of India, 1981 - Central Bureau of Health Intelligence, DGHS, Government of India, Ministry of Health and Family Welfare.
6. Agarwal, S.P. (1969): "Manpower Supply - Concept and Methodology" Meenakshi Prakashan, Meerut.
7. Health Statics of India, 1977.

8. Sixth Five Year Plan Document, Planning Commission, Government of India.

9. Report of the Study Group on Hospitals (Joint Committee Report), Government of India, Ministry of Health and Family Welfare, and Ministry of Urban Development, 1968.

10. Anand, T.R. *Et. al*, "Guide to Staffing Pattern for Hospitals", NIMAE Research Report No.38.

11. Recommendations on Minimum Standard Requirements for a Medical College and Recommendation on Postgraduate Medical Education; Medical Council of India, New Delhi, 1976 and 1977.

12. Family Welfare Programme in India, Year-Book 1981-82, Government of India, Ministry of Health and Family Welfare, Department of Family Welfare, New Delhi..

13. Report of the Working Group on Health For All by 2000 A.D. Ministry of Health and Family Welfare (March 1981), Government of India.

22

Role Structure and Job Satisfaction Among Allied Health Professionals in Hospitals

The modern hospital as a complex organisation consists of a differentiated structure and varied interacting units. Allied health professionals form one such sub-structure of the hospital. The task of the health care delivery system is closely dependent upon the role structure of allied health professionals. With the ever-increasing specialization and compartmentalization of the health care systems, these allied health professionals through their defined tasks and functions have assumed a significant place in the attainment of goals in the modern hospital. It is through them that the doctors arrive at the correct diagnosis of the patient's disease and illness and initiate the treatment and recovery and rehabilitation process of the patients. The modern health care system depends to a very large extent upon the active participation and functional involvement of the allied health professionals in the administration of health care delivery system, that is in modern hospitals.

RESEARCH- SETTING AND METHOD

The present study has been conducted at the 'Sir Sunder Lal Hospital' Varanasi, which is a part of the Institute of Medical Sciences, Banaras Hindu University. This hospital is public-cum-academic institution where the doctors and the allied health professionals perform the twin functions of imparting health care delivery to the patients as well as providing academic instructions to the medical students. The organisational structure of the hospital functions along two lines of authority, one the administrative personnel and the other the medical professionals and allied health professionals. The group of allied health professional consists of the Nurse, Compounder, Social Worker, Technical Staff and Non-technical Staff. The year in which the study was conducted, the hospital had 250 members in the allied health professionals category. Following the stratified random sampling, one hundred informants were selected for the present study. Among these 30 were nurses, 20 were compounders, 10 were social workers, 15 were members of technical staff and 25 belonged to the non-technical staff.

The date for the present study were collected through an interview schedule and informal discussions with the respondents.

RESULTS AND DISCUSSION

Motivating Factors in Job Selection

Every person, who joins a profession or enters into an occupation, is motivated by certain factors. These factors differ according to the nature of the occupation and also according to the particular socio-psychological circumstances of the individual. At the occupational level economic gain, security, high social prestige and power attached to the particular occupation may serve as important inducing factors for selecting that particular occupation. At the socio-phychological level the interest, aptitude and skill of the individual, his family and social background and his level of aspiration may, in varying degrees, serve as important motivating factors for selecting a particular occupation.

Keeping the above points in view, the allied health professionals were asked to state the most important factor which was responsible for the selection of their present job. Table 1 shows that 38 per cent respondents joined medical profession in order to nurse the ailing persons, whereas 25.2 per cent respondents did so because of their special interest in the profession. For another 22 per cent respondents the main reason for entering this profession was economic gain and security; 4 per cent respondents were in this profession because of its prestige value and 7 per cent jointed it because the profession afforded them, an opportunity to acquaint themselves with respectable members of the society. Only 4 per cent of the respondents entered in the profession for the occupational security it provided.

A further examination of the motivating factors that induces people to select this job reveals that most of the nurses and the non-technical staff (60 percent and 40 percent respectively) joined the medical profession because of there keen desire to serve the ailing persons. In the case of compounders and social workers economic gain (50 per cent and 60 per cent respectively) was perceived as the most important reason. In the case of the technical staff, 40 per cent of the respondents entered the profession because of their interest in the field.

Thus, most of the respondents in the sample seem to be motivated by altruistic and humanistic factors in the selection of the jobs. Economic security and gain were not considered to be as important as their desire to be of some nelp to the patient of their interest in the subject of medical sciences.

Job Satisfaction

Allied health professionals in India are generally accorded less recognition for their services and are lowly paid employees of the hospital. Because of the specialised nature of their job and also because of the stilted organisational structure of the hospitals they have few opportunities of promotions. The hospital expects them to carry out the instructions of the doctors and perform other ancillary duties. The patients treat the doctors as experts while the allied health professionals are viewed as the junior functionaries of the hospital. Bureaucratic hurdles, tremendous work load and the uneasy interpersonal relations in the hospital create further problems of adjustment for them. All these factors go a long way in influencing the job satisfaction of the allied health professionals and often belie the expectations.

To estimate the degree of job satisfaction of the allied health professionals, they were asked to state if they enjoyed their work in the hospital. Table 2 shows that the majority of respondents (68 per cent) were satisfied with their job positions because it gave them a chance to serve the ailing humanity; 3 per cent of the respondents enjoyed their work because it provided them with a better status and prestige in the society. There were 11 per cent respondents who enjoyed their jobs because of the technical skill required. Only 18 per cent of the respondents performed their roles as a matter of routine because they had lost interest in their jobs. It seems that the high expectations they had before entering the job were fulfilled in their work places.

A breakdown of the data shows that in each category of the allied health professionals service orientation is the most important factor responsible for job satisfaction. However, this is more so in the case of the technical (73.3 per cent) and the non-technical staff (92.0 per cent) than in the other groups of allied health professionals.

Thus, it may be observed that at the altruistic level service orientation is the most important factor responsible for the job satisfaction of the allied health professionals. Benefit-orientation and consideration of pecuniary gains are less important factors as compared to the inclination to serve the patients. At the level of ideals, the allied health professionals seems to draw gratification from serving the ailing patients but at the level of actuality the position is entirely different as is evident from their responses on the reasons for being discontented with their jobs.

Reasons for Discontent

Many situations develop within the hospital to stir up irritation and discontent. Such situations adversely affect the performance of the Allied health professionals which ultimately leads to dissatisfaction with their jobs. To inquire into this aspect the respondents were asked to state the main causes for their discontent with their jobs. Table 3 indicates that 60 per cent of the respondents were dissatisfied because of a lack of appreciation of their initiatives and innovative ideas in the hospital. For some, the dissatisfaction was because of the malfunctioning in the bureaucratic set up of the hospital. Among these there were 22 per cent respondents who were dissatisfied with the excessive bureaucratic control exercised by the supervisors over the subordinates and 18 per cent of the respondents were dissatisfied because of disputes and tensions among the hospital employees.

A further distribution of the data reveals that in every group a major source of discontent was the lack of recognition of individual aptitude and initiative by the hospital administration. Members of the non-technical staff (76 per cent) social workers (7.0 per cent) and members of technical staff (60.0 per cent) showed more grievance on this count than the other groups of Allied health professionals. Bureaucratic control was stated as source of discontentment by 33.3 per cent of the nurses and by 30 per cent of the compounders. Around 20 per cent of the nurses and 15 per cent of the compounders were dissatisfied because the disputes and tensions among the hospital personnel.

Thus, it may be said that the reasons for dissatisfaction of the respondents were mainly related to the non-recognition of individual aptitude and initiative. It seems that the superiors in the hospital follow a strict routine and there was, therefore, almost no appreciation of their special talents and skill.

Extent of Communication with the Patients

The communication between the allied health professionals and patients may be "business like" that is limited to the job at hand or it may involve social talk. Free flowing and spontaneous communication between the allied health professionals and patients not only circumvent, the blocked channels but it also softens the rigidity of authority structure and stratification in the hospital organisation. Informal communication or private understanding with the allied health professional aids and abets the goal of patient care. It also contributes to the reversal of the depersonalization process of the patients in the hospital.

The informal talks between the allied health professionals and the patients is an important way to promote closer social interaction. Moreover, it adds to the confidence of the patients in the treatment process and in the therapeutic agents of the hospital. Routine contact with the patients and lack of interest in the social situation of the patients sometimes adversely affect the healing process in the hospital. In the Indian situation where impersonal and closely defined relationship is generally not acclaimed, the talk of the allied health professionals with the patients, if remains confined to the administration of therapy, is likely to affect the adjustment of patient in the hospital environment as also his treatment. Therefore, the allied health professionals were asked to mention the type of talk they generally indulged in with the patients. Table 4 shows that 56 per cent respondents talked only about the disease and pattern of treatment of the patients. But there were others who in addition to disease and treatment talked also of social and personal matters. Among these 27 per cent respondents talked about the socio-economic condition of the family and 17 per cent about the personal life of the patients as well.

The breakdown of data shows that 65 per cent of the compounders , 56 per cent of the nurses and 93.3 per cent of the technical staff talked only about the disease of the patients. With regard to the interest displayed in the socio-economic condition and personal life of the patients it was found that a higher proportion of the non-technical staff (44.0 and 32.0 per cent respectively) had shown interest than the nurses and compounders.

Though the talk of most allied health professionals was confined to the disease of the patients yet there was a significant proportion of the respondents who had shown a keen interest in the social situation of the patients and their talks with them stretched beyond medical matters.

Difficulties in Communicating

In the Indian situation the process of communication between the allied health professionals and patients is a problematic one. The patients are generally illiterate, ignorant and poor, whereas the doctors and the allied health professionals are literate and experts in this field. This leads to status-gap and thereby improper communication. Moreover, the diversity in languages and dialects in different regions of India makes the task of health professionals far more difficult, especially when they are working in regions other than their own. In such circumstances they neither understand the problem of the patients properly nor are they able to successfully communicate their advice to the patients. This problem of improper communication is much more acute in the north Indian hospitals where most of the working nurses are from south India with a very poor command of the north Indian dialects. Thus illiteracy, ignorance, poverty and language barriers among the patients, as opposed to the knowledge and professional excellence of the health professionals, create a hiatus between the patients and the allied health professionals in the hospital. Therefore, to explore and identify the problems of this communication process the respondents were asked to state the difficulties they experienced while communicating with the patients. Table 5 indicates that there were 29 per cent respondents who experienced difficulty in communicating with the patients on account of the language barrier. 35 per cent respondents identified illiteracy of the patients as a major impediment in communicating; another 21 per cent respondents found the patients non-cooperative and unresponsive to their advice. There were 15 per cent respondents who stated that their heavy work load in the hospital inhibited a smooth interaction and close rapport with the patients.

The breakdown of data shows that the nurses experienced difficulties in communicating with the patients mostly because of the language barrier (43.3 per cent) or illiteracy of the patients (33.3 per cent). Compounders were of the opinion that illiteracy and non-cooperation of the patients (35 per cent in each case) were the major hurdles in communicating with the patients. Social workers (40 per cent) expressed the view that the heavy work load was a barrier in communicating with patients.

Thus, it is clear that the communication between allied health professionals and patients in the hospital is hampered mainly because of the illiteracy of the patients and the lack of comprehension of the local dialects by the allied health professionals. The nurses, who are mainly from the south Indian States, experience much difficulty because of difference in language and dialect.

Equity in Treatment

For a fair and equal treatment of the patients it is necessary that the allied health professionals remain unbiased in their attitude towards patients while treating them. It is expected that they should not give any special benefits to their relatives and acquaintances while ignoring the needs of the other patients. If these professionals give preferential treatment to their relatives it means they are not objective and impersonal in their dealings with the patients. However, in the Indian situation the demands of social structure is too heavy. A person has to be more considerate to his own kith and kin. The hospital personnel are often put in a dilemma. To work according to rules would mean betraying one's loyalty towards one's group as has been culturally prescribed. While to flout the rules to meet the needs of close relatives goes counter to the norms of the hospital organisation. Keeping these conflict-situations in view the allied health professionals were asked. "Suppose one day a very close relative of your comes to the hospital. Will you or will you not attend to his medical needs first and assist him in getting medical facilities on the priority basis". Table 6 indicates that 18 per cent respondents stated that they would provide their relatives medicine and other hospital facilities on a priority basis. While 14 per cent of the respondents were completely against giving priority to close relatives. But a majority of the respondents (68 per cent) voted neither in favour or against the motion. They would give priority to their close relations only when circumstances permitted them to do, they stated.

The distribution of data according to the designation of the respondents points out that 70 per cent of the nurses and 60 per cent of the compounders were of the opinion that they would give preferential treatment to their relatives only if the circumstances were favourable. Twenty five per cent of the compounders and 20 per cent of the nurses were in favour of providing preferential treatment to their relatives patients.

Thus, it is clear that a majority of allied health professionals are in favour of attending to the medical needs of their needs of their relatives first. However, they would also like to maintain a balance between their job requirements and discipline within the hospitals and the demands of their relative patients.

Outside the kin group, the loyalty of an individual in the Indian society extends to his caste, class and region. The allied health professionals in their day to day dealing with the patients and their attendants are often approached for sympathy, attention and consideration on the basis of common bonds such as caste, creed and region. To yield to such demands may not be in consonance with the formal organisational matrix of the hospital. Yet such demands are fulfilled to keep up a good relationship with fellow caste and class members.

To delve into impersonal attitude of the allied health professionals, they were further asked whether in dealing with patients they were influenced by the patient's caste, class and region. Table 7 shows that a majority of the respondents (57 per cent) were totally against preferential treatment on the basis of caste and class of the patients. However, 27. per cent respondents admitted that they could give preferential treatment to the patients on the basis of the caste or class positions, if the situation so demanded. Sixteen per cent respondents were found to be ambivalent in their attitude on this subject.

Data further reveal that 50 per cent of the nurses, 45 per cent of the compounders, 70 per cent of the social workers, 66 per cent members of the technical personnel and 64 per cent members of the non-technical staff were against giving preferential treatment to patients on the basis of caste and class. There were 32 per cent non-technical staff members who stated that under compelling circumstances they could favour the patients on the basis of caste and class.

Thus, it is clear that inspite of the fact that a majority of respondents were against giving favours to patients on the grounds of caste or class, yet a significant proportion of them could provide such favours if the situation so demanded.

Final Comments

The foregoing discussion on the data indicates the following broad trends:

(a) The allied health professionals chose their job on humanitarian grounds and not so much for monetary gains. Most of them joined this profession either to nurse the ailing or because of their keen interest in participating in the health care system. Economic gain and job security were found to be less important motivating factors.

(b) The humanitarian factor has been found to be the major contributing factor in the job satisfaction of the allied health professionals. Most of them enjoyed their jobs because it provided them with a chance to serve the ailing humanity.

(c) The reason for their dissatisfaction with their jobs is the non-recognition of their initiatives and individual efforts by their superiors. Dispute and tension among personnel and excessive bureaucratic control have been found to be then other sources of discontent.

(d) The interaction between the patient and the allied health professional has been found to be problematic. Most of the allied health professionals confine their talks with the patient to disease and medicine. Some of them touch upon personal matters and the socio-economic conditions of the patients. Language barriers, illiteracy of the patients, the non-cooperative attitude of the patient and excessive work loads were found to be the major barriers in the process of smooth communication with the patient.

(e) It has been further observed that among the different strata of the allied health professionals in the hospital, the level of job satisfaction, source of discontent and role conflict due to social structural factors also differ depending upon the status they possess and the task they have to perform in the hospital.

(f) In the Indian situation the demands of society weigh very heavily upon the shoulder of every functionary working in a complex organisation. Their task performance is influenced by factors such as Kin caste class considerations. In the present study the allied health personnels have been found to favour close relatives and members of their caste and class when they visit the hospital. Thus the humanitarian impulses of the allied health personnels coupled with their lack of an inpersonal attitude makes the task of job performance of the allied health professionals incongruent with the formal and impersonal authority structure of the hospital organisation.

REFERENCES

1. Banton, Michael, *Roles-An introduction to the Study of Social Relations'*, Tavistock Publications, London.
2. Cartwright, A., Human Relations and Hospital Care', Routledge and Kegan Paul, London, 1964.
3. Robinson, G.A. *Hospital Administration*, Worths, London, 1966.
4. Srivastava, A.L., *Human Relations in Social Organisation*, Chugh Publications, Allahabad, 1979.

Table 1: Motivating Factors in Job Selectior.

Designation	*Total*	*a*	*b*	*c*	*d*	*e*	*f*
Nurse	30 (100.00)	5 (16.66)	- -	5 (6.67)	2 (60.00)	6.67 60.00)	18 (60)
Compounder	20 (100.00)	10 (50.00)	- -	4 (20.00)	- -	- -	6 (30.00)
Social Worker	10 (100.00)	6 (60.00)	- -	2 (20.00)	1 (10.00)	- -	1 (10.00)
Technical Staff	15 (100.00)	1 (6.67)	2 (13.33)	6 (40.00)	1 (6.67)	2 (12.33)	3 (20.00)
Non-Technical Staff	25 (100.00)	- -	2 (8.00)	8 (32.00)	- -	5 (20.00)	10 (40.00)
Total	100 (100.00)	22 (22.00)	4 (4.00)	25 (25.00)	4 (4.00)	7 (7.00)	38 (38.00)

Note: Figures with the parenthesis indicate percentage
a = Economic gain
b = Prestige in the society
c = Keen interest in the medical sciences
d = security
e = Acquaintance with the respectable members of the society.
f = Nursing

Table 2: Job Satisfaction

Designation	*Total*	*a*	*b*	*c*	*d*
Nurse	30 (100.00)	9 (30.00)	1 (3.33)	3 (10.00)	17 (56.67)
Compounder	20 (100.00)	4 (20.00)	1 (5.00)	2 (10.00)	13 (65.00)
Social Worker	10 (100.00)	3 (30.00)	- -	3 (30.00)	4 (40.00)
Technical Staff	15 (100.00)	1 (6.66)	1 (6.66)	2 (13.33)	11 (73.33)
Non-Technical Staff	25 (100.00)	1 4.00	- -	1 (4.00)	23 (92.00)
Total	100 (100.00)	18 (918.00)	3 (3.00)	11 (11.00)	68 (68.00)

Note: Figures with the parenthesis indicate percentages.
a = Do the job because they are in this profession otherwise they are not motivated by any interest in it.
b = Do this because it accords status and prestige in the society.
c = Do the job because they enjoy it and because of the technical skill required in this job.
d = Do the job because they enjoy it and because it provides them with a chance in serve the ailing humanity.

Table 3: Reasons for Dissatisfaction with the job

Designation	*Total*	*a*	*b*	*c*
Nurse	30 (100.00)	6 (20.00)	10 (33.33)	14 (46.67)
Compounder	20 (100.00)	3 (15.00)	6 (30.00)	11 (55.00)
Social Worker	10 (100.00)	1 (10.00)	2 (20.00)	7 (70.00)
Technical Staff	15 (100.00)	4 (26.66)	2 (13.33)	9 (60.00)
Non-Technical Staff	25 (100.00)	4 (16.00)	2 (8.00)	11 (76.00)
Total	100 (100.00)	18 (18.00)	22 (22.00)	60 (60.00)

Note: Figures within the parenthesis indicate percentages.
a = dispute and tension among personnel.
b = excessive bureaucratic control of the superiors over the subordinates.
c = lack of appreciation of individual initiative and efforts.

Table 4: Nature of Communication with the Patients

Designation	*Total*	*About disease and treatment pattern*	*About socio-economic conditions of the family*	*About personal life*
Nurse	30 (100.00)	17 (56.66)	7 (23.33)	6 (20.00)
Compounder	20 (100.00)	13 (65.00)	4 (20.00)	3 (15.00)
Social worker	10 (100.00)	6 (60.00)	4 (40.00)	- -
Technical staff	15 (100.00)	14 (93.33)	1 (6.67)	- -
Non-Tech. Staff	25 (100.00)	6 (24.00)	11 (44.00)	8 (32.00)
Total	100 (100.00)	56 (56.00)	27 (27.00)	17 (17.00)

Table 5: Difficulties in Communicating with the patients

Designation	*Total*	*Language barriers*	*Illiteracy of the patients*	*Non-cooperation of the patient*	*Excessive work loads*
Nurse	30 (100.00)	13 (43.33)	10 (33.33)	6 (20.00)	1 (3.33)
Compounder	20 (100.00)	5 (25.00)	7 (35.00)	7 (35.00)	1 (5.00)
Social worker	10 (100.00)	1 (10.00)	2 (20.00)	3 (30.00)	4 (40.00)
Technical staff	15 (100.00)	3 (20.00)	4 (26.66)	2 (13.33)	6 (40.00)
Non-Tech. Staff	25 (100.00)	7 (28.00)	12 (48.00)	3 (12.00)	3 (12.00)
Total	100 (100.00)	29 (29.00)	35 (35.00)	21 (21.00)	15 (15.00)

Table 6: Attitude or Favouring Close Relatives

Designation	*Total*	*Yes*	*No*	*It depends upon the circumstances*
Nurse	30 (100.00)	6 (20.00)	3 (10.00)	21 (70.00)
Compounder	20 (100.00)	5 (25.00)	3 (15.00)	12 (60.00)
Social worker	10 (100.00)	-	2 (20.00)	8 (80.00)
Technical staff	15 (100.00)	2 (13.33)	3 (20.00)	10 (66.67)
Non-Tech. Staff	25 (100.00)	5 (20.00)	3 (12.00)	17 (68.00)
Total	100 (100.00)	18 (18.00)	14 (14.00)	68 (68.00)

Table 7: Attitude on favouring patients on the basis of caste and class

Designation	*Total*	*Yes (when necessary)*	*No*	*Unsure*
Nurse	30 (100.00)	9 (30.00)	15 (50.00)	6 (50.00)
Compounder	20 (100.00)	5 (25.00)	9 (45.00)	6 (30.00)
Social worker	10 (100.00)	3 (30.00)	7 (70.00)	-
Technical staff	15 (100.00)	2 (13.33)	10 (66.66)	3 (20.00)
Non-Tech. Staff	25 (100.00)	8 (32.00)	16 (64.00)	1 (4.00)
Total	100 (100.00)	27 (27.00)	57 (57.00)	16 (16.00)

23

Health Services in Tribal Areas

Adivasis,* about 51.6 million and constituting about 7.76 per cent of the country's population in about 427 recognised scheduled tribal groups, inhabit mostly forests (*vanavasis*) or hills (*girijans*) in varying ecological and geoclimatic conditions in different concentrations in different regions** of the country, excepting Punjab, Haryana and Jammu and Kashmir. They vary in number, the most important are the Gonds of Madhya Pradesh, Maharashtra and Andhra Pradesh, the Bhils of Rajasthan, Gujarat, Maharashtra and M.P., and the Santhals of Bihar, Orissa and West Bengal. The smallest tribal community is the Andamanese. They are characterised by their individual, cultural, religious, social and economic lineage through which they have been able to maintain their separate entity as distinct from other population groups and even their fellow tribesmen. In a strict sense, they are biological isolates, with characteristic social, cultural, economic, nutrition, genetic factors, and health seeking behaviour.

Statewise growth rate varied from 17.3 per cent in Bihar, through 18.8 per cent H.P., to 30 per cent in Assam, Gujarat, Manipur and Nagaland; 20-25 per cent in other States. Tribewise growth rate varied from 35.27 per cent among Bhils to 14.5 per cent among Mundas. Smaller tribal groups show a highly distorted population growth. Some tribal groups of Andaman and Nicobar islands show a declining trend (Verma, 1977). Occupationally there has been a slight reduction in percentage of tribals engaged in agriculture to non-agricultural activities.

Because of economic, social and educational tardiness for historical reasons, they are under special privileges and protection under the Directive Principles of the Article 46 of the Indian Constitution, which also provides safeguards against social and economic exploitation.

A number of studies have being conducted by the National Institute of Health and Family Welfare, P.G. Institute of Medical Education and Research, Chandigarh, National Institute of Mental Health and Neuro Sciences, Bangalore, ICMR and a few universities on social-cultural aspects including health of tribal life.

In spite of education, economic and welfare programmes accounting for 50, 28 and 22 per cent respectively of total expenditure till the end of the 6th Plan period and reduced coverage of Primary Health Centres (PHCs) from 30,000 to 20,000 and sub-centres from 5,000 to 3,000, literacy rate among male is 16.35, and among female it is 8.04 per cent, and health status remained poor. In a recent study of 2 blocks in an eastern State, Singh *et al.* reports: "illiteracy rate is 80.8 per cent (67% in males, 95% in females) 57.15 per cent of people under poverty line; less than 8 per cent children immunized, and 44 per cent of children severely malnourished; average number of children to tribal women is about 6, higher by 2 than the national average; and tribal women marry at 15 years of age".

Basu, in an indepth study of various genetic traits among 4 tribal groups, Muria, Maria, Halba and Bhaitra in Jagdalpur and Konta tehsils of Baster district, reported equally unflattering socio-cultural-economic situation and moderately high prevalence of genetic and genetico-environmental disorders:

(i) Low frequency of Rh-negative gene;

(ii) Sickle cell trait varying from 8 to 18 per cent;

(iii) G-6-PD deficiency 10-19 per cent;

(iv) Thalassaemia about 2 per cent and

(v) Other abnormal conditions.

Health-seeking behaviour: Tribal people seek relief from illness, first from *Sirhas,* who are supposed to be in touch, with spirits/gods/goddesses, who, after diagnosing the cause, resurrect them from wrath; next, they use herbal medicines; and PHC or modern medical practitioner is the last resort. Individuals who were cured by PHCs have not been able to perpetuate benefits on modern medical care. Maternal care during pregnancy is poor; services of ANMs, LHVs are utilized only in difficult labour cases. Placental cord is cut with an arrow in a male child, or with a knife in a female child. *Kasa pani,* a specially prepared concoction, stated to recover the lost energy and to act as a sort of anti-infective, is given to the mother on the third day after child birth.

Child care is poor. Neonates and infants are the worst sufferers. Breast-fed infants do not receive any supplementary food which is given after the child attains one year of age.

In short, failure to understand cultural background is the main reason for the failure of most health and welfare programmes.

Bardhan *et al.* in a study among Bhils in M.P., reported that a Bhil considers himself sick when he is completely bed-ridden and is unable to work for his everyday living. He expects a quick and sure treatment. He does not believe in free treatment; free things are not of any worth. A private doctor or quack, who fits into the tribal belief system, is successful. Bhils have very scant or no appreciation of preventive or promotive health care.

Basic cleanliness among Bhils is totally lacking. They do not take baths for weeks together. They use stones and do not wash hands after defecation. Evil spirits account for most of their sickness. The only way they can fight and keep them away from inflicting illness is to keep bodies even more dirty and foul smelling as compared to spirits. When sick, he goes to *Barua* (magico-religious healer) and asks him to examine *(parakh-Baba-parakh)* who performs in one place and one stroke of time - diagnosis, treatment and follow up. He does not ask question. He makes the diagnosis which spirit has been offended, and when, where and how the person can be rehabilitated by undoing the wrong and propitiating the relevant spirit. A somewhat similar expectation is expected by them when they approach a doctor in PHC.

Moreover, the treatment is frequently participative, involving the sick person and sometimes his family as well as the whole community. This provides great psychological support and satisfaction to the ill person. People want quick, sure and one time treatment. Revisits mean incompetence of the doctor or ineffectiveness of treatment. The second visit will invariably be to private practitioners of modern medicine. Barriers in acceptance of PHC services include language, interaction pattern (patients' reluctance in responding to doctor's querry causing annoyance in doctors), keeping them at a distance (because of low personal hygiene) and closure of PHCs and sub-centres on weekly *haat or mela* days, and when they need services.

To sum up: (a) Socio-economic development appears to have bypassed the majority of tribal population and (b) while disease pattern may be the same among tribals and non-tribals, some of genetic and genetico-environmental disorders add to the morbidity and mortality among tribals; and there is a need to understand health-seeking behaviour of local tribals to be served and to modify health and welfare programmes.

II

Poverty and illiteracy are two correlates of low health status. It is also true that health is not guaranteed by economic developemnt. Some countries with a lower GNP have better health status indicators than others with a higher GNP.

The economic theory has gone profound modification in the last 2-3 decades. It is no longer an article of faith that social progress should be result of economic growth and investment of savings. Changes of economic factors are casually inter-related with what happens to all other factors in the social change.

"Health programmes can be evaluated in terms of better ability of members of the society to produce, invest and consume. Same programmes facilitate exploitation of natural resources and contribute to the environment... returns from health, education, nutrition and other social sciences... all investments in human beings... contribute directly to economic growth..." (Horwitz).

The debate has contributed to the modification of lending policies of international banks and capital exporting countries in programmes with health and nutrition as objectives — to reduce malnutrition, illiteracy, infant mortality, and to raise life expectancy in developing countries. Essential to the accomplishment of this objective is an increase in the productivity of small scale agriculture. This goal should be a part of social agenda—translated into integrated rural development projects. (Horwitz)

Moreover, resources below requirements in every sector is a trait of under-development and health is no exception. Under the circumstances, aspirations have to be met by giving them equal right to available health care services — a goal to be reached. Largest allocation of resources had to be given to those problem areas that affect largest number of people and which can be solved or reduced by providing well-proven techniques at minimum cost.

This would mean thinking and acting in terms — not of disease but also of health - promotion of health and prevention and cure of prevailing diseases. These are 'do able' GOBI-FFF (growth monitoring, ORT, breast-feeding, immunization, family spacing, food supplements, and female education) *plus* also other primary problems such as malaria, iodine deficiency, ARI, personal hygiene, food hygiene and water supply as recommended by UNICEF.

Development has to be health-focused and equity-based, necessarily rooted locally in the natural and cultural environment of the population concerned, and the locus of control at grass-root.

HIGH FERTILITY AND MORTALITY LEVELS OF TRIBAL WOMEN AND THEIR CHILDREN

Whereas high fertility levels usually reflect poor health and social conditions and need to decide number and timing of birth, high mortality levels bring the importance of recognition of high prevalence of consanguinity, Rh-negative gene, thalassaemia, G-6-PD deficiency and other genetic and genetico-environmental disorders, food habits, health-seeking bahaviour in addition to usual factors.

UNDERUTILIZATION OF HEALTH SERVICES

Till mid-1987, 1636 PHCs and 11721 sub-centres have been established. Number of programmes such as immunization, provision of safe drinking water, educational efforts on sanitation and hygiene and lately ICDs scheme, have been undertaken on a priority basis but they are underutilised. Underutilization reflects inability of the formal system to compete with the informal system, which is capable to catering to perceived needs of the people within their cultural, social, and economic context and saves them the trouble of dealing with the formal system.

CERTAIN FACTORS TO BE CONSIDERED IN HEALTH SERVICES

(i) Health is not the same for all people. Different people understand differently what health is for them, according to their culture, history and environmental, social, and economic organisations. That understanding also evolves within dynamic context of their society and expressed through their health-seeking behaviour. General indicators, such as infant mortality, life expectancy, literacy may not have the same meaning for all, at all times. Some less easily quantifiable indicators, such as sustainability of development, rate of political participation, position of women in society, cultural survival, are also informative and relevant (Borrini).

(ii) *Health is an individual and collective responsibility.* Health arises within a complex web of human, and social and ecological relationships. It does not exist separately from a healthy natural ecosystem, nor from peace, justice, collective intelligence and caring. Responsibility for ill health can often be traced back to political and economic violence and exploitation, inappropriate technologies, prejudicial policies and lack of social and human support — intersectoral action (Borrini).

(iii) Health status of disadvantaged groups is an index of socio-economic development of a country in modern times and specifically of HFA 2000 to which India is committed. Moreover, welfare of tribals is one of the special responsibilities of the Government of India. This political will needs to be supported by moral commitment of the elites particularly of those in power, matched by meaningful action.

(iv) Response by increasing number of institutions, councils, commissions and health centres is not enough — they constitute an item of statistics of national progress. It is a great deal more difficult to make them work and contribute adequately and appropriately to health in the community. Unless we face up to the gap between what we think are needs and what are felt to be needs at the grass-roots level, much of our planning is an idle exercise.

(v) Historically, many countries, whenever they had decided to solve problems of communities, less advanced and of which cultures and habits etc. are different and less known, have made special arrangements to run programmes or to monitor them or both. India is no exception. The Council for Tribal and Rural Development is an instance.

III

Judged by performance, functioning of PHCs needs to be modified—particularly in respect of approach—health services contacting people at risk instead of waiting for patients contacting; in involving community particularly traditional tribal healers; in putting greater emphasis promotive and preventive work over curative; in using proper technology in proposed interventions and adapting them to local conditions to meet the needs of health seeking behaviour of the people so that they become acceptable to the community served: and in providing nutritional supplement. In these efforts, ICDS scheme is of great help. Priority has been accorded for location of new ICDS projects in tribal development block. An 'Anganwadi Worker' (AWW) is a great ally in health work. She begins with a survey of households, enrols beneficiaries (pregnant and lactating mothers in the first 6 months after birth and children <6 years), carries out health checks and ensures regular flow of prescribed services to her target groups, arranges referral and maintains and updates household survey register, individual health and nutrition records, birth and death records and other vital statistics. She, so to speaks personfies integration of social welfare and health care activities. Her activities are monitored by HW(F), ANM, Mukhya, Sevikas and PHC doctor.

COMMUNITY PARTICIPATION

Normally, community participation* which is necessary in identification of health problems and in finding appropriate and cost effective solutions, becomes essential because of tribals' peculiar socio-cultural and health-seeking behaviour in respect of small communities within which health development takes place and all individuals live in shared natural, social, and cultural environment and together experience various needs.

Health is a community responsibility. To be able to formulate and control health promoting change, the community needs to be made aware of itself and its potential power.

Gatherings and community discussions of health problems and needs facilitate this process and help people understand' and support one another. Such meetings should be promoted, with particular attention to participation particularly of tribal leaders and healers, and teachers, and concerns of the most vulnerable groups (women and children), by health workers directly or indirectly through women's organisations, local leaders, unions or rural development personnel. Actions should develop from local decision-making because it can express the wealth of experience and concerns of the local people and be meaningful to them. Small projects can be developed with locally available resources to the extent possible and less dependence on less easily available inputs and consequently with less chance of failure and be less environmentally upsetting. Formation of a small committee, empowered to formulate and control projects will not only meet the needs of the community but will also help in cultural survival and sustaining local eco-system, which are also health needs by themselves.

In these efforts, HWs(F), VI Gs, trained *dais* and AWWs have an important role to play through home visits and through discussions of problems and needs with family members and others. Health services attempt, so to speak, to become a part of socio-cultural pattern through community participation.

LINKING OF INFORMAL AND FORMAL HEALTH SYSTEMS

The tribal informal health system appears to consist of traditional indigenous magico-religious system and herbal system. Practitioners of the former system are differently called, *Sirhas Barna* or *Syan*, with their own system of diagnosis and treatment, and the latter, practitioners of herbal medicine. Often these medicine men are not just healers, they advise about health, welfare including spiritual welfare, problems of living, what crops to plant and so forth. They fulfil two roles - cure and care, and that is, what is the special value of the informal system and gives it an edge over modern medical practitioners. The spectrum of traditional health care is large and the coverage complete. Much of their successes is attributable to the nutriting provided by, and holistic approach of traditional healers, who take into consideration internal, external, and supernatural causes of illness. They enjoy considerable social prestige, and have a broad and deep understanding of human nature and village affairs, are accessible and can provide continuity of care with a sufficient supply of medicaments. He is usually the first person consulted in illness and often the last. He gives at least some form of care where often none is available or if available, not accessible or 'closed' from government health services which work on fixed time basis.

There is a lot we can learn from them, particularly herbal medicine practitioners, but it is a question of selecting the good and safe practices. There is much we still have to find out about plants and concoctions used. As such indigenous systems cannot be ignored without causing more harm to people in general and tribals in particular. It is more profitable to link formal and informal systems and to recognise traditional practitioners and to upgrade their skill.

INTERVENTIONS

Interventions that will be necessary to meet objectives and targets must be adapted to local conditions, equity, efficacy and acceptability. Interventions or mix of interventions have to represent a trade off between acceptability and efficacy if a programme is to be effective. What is efficient to achieve equity, may not be efficient to achieve health. The mix of interventions must also be matched to persons who perform services. If adequate effectiveness is incompatible with feasibility, one has to think of changing target levels or objectives.

Interventions depend on results of survey undertaken problems and needs and their priority (if possible, approved by the local committee or the government), setting goals, fixing indicators, etc., and identifying and effective mix, adapting them to local conditions, and classifying them on the basis of application to be made at home, community, first health facility, and first referral levels. Interventions should be more promotive and preventive rather than curative.

Mothers and children, malnutrition, control of infectious diseases, water hygiene measures, deserve highest priority throughout the country including tribal areas where newly found genetic and genetico-environmental disorders, particularly those that affect health of mothers and children, also deserve priority. Achieving effectiveness in integrated MCH-FP programme requires that necessary tasks, such as screening of high risk mothers and children, ante-natal care, management and basic care of newborn, basic child care including monitoring of growth, prevention of main causes of child mortality, intense health education on limitation of family, child spacing, water hygiene, breast-feeding, weaning food, ORT, and on immunization, be carried out mostly through home visits.

This demands also maintenance of standard of services provided by field workers through supervision of PHC doctors and other supervisors giving continuing education. Equity and effectiveness demand organisation of referral services so that everybody needing services beyond the first health facility and first referral level gets higher services according to the need.

Similarly, if the tribal culture expects "quack, sure and one treatment for illness", PHC doctor should make the most of the initial contact to the extent possible and train HWs accordingly.

STUDIES

The PHC programmes are largely based on educated guesses. Most of the issues that adversely affect the programme, such as supervision, skills, shortage of drugs, transport bottleneck, etc., could be addressed through relatively simple studies that do not interfere with on-going services delivery and should be a part of every PHC programme.

HEALTH PERSONNEL

The VLGs, AWWs and HWs form the corner-stone in the health care services but often many NLGs and AWWs, particularly VLGs, are chosen out of political expediency with no real thought for the needs of the community and no chance for it to choose, though their selection by the community is supposed to be the corner-stone of the system. As a consequence, conflicts have often arisen between what the community wants and what VLGs, having had a little outside training, believe what should be. To ensure that they remain of the people' and continue to give preventive and promotive care and to cope with minor emergencies, to educate the people and to maintain good relations with other formal and informal health workers, they need continuing education in order to maintain minimum standards of care through supervision. Supervision creates self-confidence in field workers and enhances status in the community, since doctors' visits guarantee that standards are high. HWs, particularly HW(Fs) should make her 'medical presence' felt by the community through treatment of minor illnesses. With the HW(F) (ANM) living in the village (of the sub-centre), HS(F) residing in an intermediate location within easy calling distance of her HWs(F), and PHC doctor at PHC, round-the-clock cover for all high risk cases should not be difficult. All that is needed, ideally, is a sort of emergency flying squad — a doctor with bag on a jeep — to bring more expert care to the patient's bedside.

Formal health workers should be from tribal areas to the extent possible.* They need be disabused of the feeling that their posting in tribal areas is a sort of punishment; on the contrary, that should be taken as a challenge—an opportunity to demonstrate their ability to adapt their skills and technology to difficult local situations.

Medical officers should be carefully selected on the basis of their empathy towards disadvantaged people, possession of an inquiring mind, ability to probe into problems and needs of tribals and to adapt their skills and technology to difficult situations, and above all, ability to take decisions and implement them without being always dependent on his/her superiors. They certainly deserve incentives not only in the provision of quarters and better basic facilities but some substantial recognition for their services rendered.

NEED FOR A STEERING BODY

Tribal health is a special public health problem and needs to be looked into more deeply. Increase in the volume and service to improve coverage is not so much a problem as the need for a carefully devised information system providing prompt compilation of data and rapid feedback for purposes of internal management and periodic reporting of progress. Some action-oriented study on a small basis (PHC) is necessary, so that newer knowledge evolving out of the study can be ploughed back into services and evaluated. The process of adaptation is evolutionary and requires a trial and demonstration area. The PHC doctors may need some guidance and some small additional inputs. State Government officials are too busy or their hands may be tied by rules and regulations. The Council for Tribal and Rural Development should have some part to play.

ACKNOWLEDGEMENT

I am grateful to Dr. S.K. Basu and Dr. A. Bardhan for their instructive briefing.

REFERENCES

* Often referred to as Adimjati, Janjatis, Anusuchit Janjati, etc.

** (1) Seven regions are: (1) South Central (M.P., Southern Orissa and Eastern belt of A.P.) mainly inhabited by Gonds; (2) Central Northern (Chota Nagpur tribal belt of Bihar, eastern M.P., Northern Orissa, Western tribal region of W.B.) dominated by Santhal, Oraon, Munda, etc.; (3) Western Tribal (southern tribal belt of Rajasthan, eastern tribal of Gujarat, Western belt of M.P., northern Maharashtra, Dadra, Nagar Haveli and Daman) predominantly Bhils, Gamit, Dhodias and Warli); (4) Eastern tribal (hilly areas of Assam, Meghalaya, Arunachal Pradesh, Sikkim, N.W. Bengal and plains of Assam and Tripura) Bhotias, Naga, Khasi Moro, Miri, Mompas, etc.; (5) N. Western (hills of West UP and North HP) Lahaulis,

Jaunsaris and Kinnauras; (6) Southern Tribal (T.N., Karnataka and Kerala) Soliga, Kurumba, Malyali and (7) Oceanic (Andaman and Nicobar and Lakshdweep) Jarwas, Onges, Great Andamanese and Sentineles (Sharma, 1978).

* Properly interpreted, community participation means the harnessing of community knowledge and culture, community enthusiasm, community resources, and community labour, towards improved planning and implementation of health programmes. It is in itself an educational process (Feodell *et al.*).

* Even in the UK National Health Services, interpreters are not very helpful except in translating doctors' instructions. Much better are patients' advocates (*BMJ*, 295, 28.11.87, 1365).

Bardhan, A., D.C. Dubey and S.K. Sinha, *An exploration in utilisation of modern health practices of the Bhils*. Mimeographed. NIH and F.W., New Delhi.

Basu, S.K., "Genetic Socio-cultural and health care among tribal groups of Jagdalpur and Konta tehsils of Bastar district", *Anthropology Development and Nation Building*, (ed.) A.K. Kalia and K.S. Singh. Concept Publishing Co., New Delhi.

Borrini Grazia, "Health through People's Empowerment", *Ifda dossier*, 55, 9-12.

Fendell, N.R.E. and Tiwari, I.C., "Trends in primary health Care", *WHF*, 2(1), 149-52.

Horwitz Abraham, "Changing concepts of Health Services: New Opportunities for Nutrition Promotion", *Bull. PAHO*, 17(1), 61-76.

Jindal A., Kshatriya G.K. and Basu, S.K., "Genetico-environmental Studies Among the Tribal Populations of India: Consideration of Approaches for Promotion of Health", *Population Genetics and Health Care Issues and Future Strategies Proceedings of the Workshop on Population Genetics and Health Care*, March 1982. NIH and FW, New Delhi.

Singh, A.K., *et al.*, *The myth of healthy tribal Social Change*, 17 (1), 3-23 (1987).

Sharma, B.D. (1978), "Tribal Development in India". Paper X, *Int. Cong, Entmo and Anthropol Science*, 1978.

Verma, I.C. (1978). Action oriented Research in Primative Tribal Communities of Andaman Island —The Onges. Interim Report submitted to Ministry of Health and Family Welfare, New Delhi. (quoted by Jindal *et. al.*)

UNICEF, *The State of the World's Children*, 1981.

Annexure–I

Table No. 1: Targets for Major Schemes under Control of Communicable Diseases Programme during Eighth Plan 1992-97

Sl. No.	*Name of the Scheme*	*Index*	*Current Position*	*Target Set for VIII Plan*
1	2	3	4	5
1.	Malaria control Programme	(a) Annual parasite Index	2.27 (1991)	(0.5 By 2000 AD)
2.	National Leprosy Eradication	(a) Cases detected	9.19 Lakhs (1990-92)	6.24 Lakhs
		(b) Cases put on treatment	9.11 Lakhs (1990-92)	6.24 Lakhs
		(c) Cases discharged	15.48 Lakhs (1990-92)	11.86 Lakhs
3.	Control of Blindness	(a) % of Blindness	1.4%	0.4%
4.	T.B Control Programme	(a) Total No. of cases detected as % to total estimated cases	42%	50%
		(b) Disease arrested cases	66%	70%
5.	Fitaria Control Programme	Population under Protection. As on 31.12.1991	43.43 million	50 million

Source: Respective Programme Officers.

Table No. 2 of Medical Practitioners Registered with Medical Council of India alongwith Ratio

Year	*Medical Practitioners Registered with Medical Council of India (00)*	*Medical Practitioners per 10,0000 population*
1951	618	17
1961	837	21
1971	1511	27
1981	2687	39
1982	2715	38
1983	2842	39
1984	2965	40
1985	3082	41
1986	3203	41
1987	3318	42
1988	3556	44
1989 (P)	3686	46
1990 (P)	3819	46
1991 (P)	3940	47

Source: Medical Council of India, Doctors Registered with various State Medical Councils

Table No. 3: Number of Doctors Possessing Recognised Medical Qualifications (Under I.M.C. Act) and Registered with State Medical Councils from the Year 1986 to 1991

As on 31st Dec.

Sl. No.	Name of State Medical Council	1986	1987	1988	1989	1990	1991
1	2	3	4	5	6	7	8
1.	Andhra Medical Council	16516	17108	17639	18236	18898	19174
2.	Assam Medical Council	8912	9149	9428	9746	10099	10497
3.	Gujarat Medical Council	18417	19173	19806	20701	21576	21812
4.	Bihar Medical Council	22902	23450	24137	24872	25689	26374
5.	Jammu & Kashmir Medical Council	3442	3622	3676	3937	4087	4307
6.	Karnataka Medical Council	25518	26722	39355	40872	42399	44183
7.	Bhopal Medical Council	7867	8526	9147	9852	10542	11187
8.	Maharashtra Medical Council	39397	41035	42730	44684	46858	49365
9.	Orissa Medical Council	9478	9866	10081	10426	10746	11089
10.	Punjab Medical Council	24128	24615	25130	25598	26178	26636
11.	Rajasthan Medical Council	11059	11613	12243	12912	13475	14046
12.	Tamil Nadu Medical Council	38673	40023	41465	43074	44769	45588
13.	Uttar Pradesh Medical Council	28514	29376	30348	31336	32369	33178
14.	West Bengal Medical Council	37751	38738	39510	40210	40920	41727
15.	Travancore Medical Council (Cochin)	14900	15568	16455	164455(P)	16455(P)	16455(P)
16.	Hyderabad Medical Council	11780	12153	12469	12805	13199	13757
17.	Haryana Medical Council	256	319	437	523	523(P)	523(P)
18.	Medical Council of India Delhi	794	830	1639	2412	3196	4170
	TOTAL:	320304	331886	355695	368651	381978	394068

Source: Medical Council of India

(P) = Provisional

Table No.4: Number of Dentists Registered with Dental Council of India (1951-1991)

Year	*Dentists Registered*
1	2
1951	3290
1956	3003
1961	3582
1966	4374
1971	5512
1975	6559
1976	6759
1977	6614
1978	7411
1979	7518
1980	8487
1981	8648
1982	8656
1983	8801
1984	8725
1985	9598
1986	9725
1987	9750
1988	9796
1989	10475
1990	11011
1991	10751

Source: Dental Council of India

Table No. 5: Number of Recognised Training Centres for Different Courses in the State Nursing Councils and Board of Examinations during the Year 1990

Sl. No.	*Name of the State Nursing Council and Board of Examination*	*Number of Recognised Training Centres for different courses in*				
		General Nursing		*Mid Wifery*	*A.N.M/ H.W.*	*Health Visitor/ Health Supervisor*
		Men	*Women*			
1	*2*	*3*	*4*	*5*	*6*	*7*
1.	Andhra Pradesh	0	74	74	144	0
2.	Assam	4	20	20	20	1
3.	Bihar	0	21	14	35	1
4.	Gujarat	7	21	20	4	0
5.	Haryana	1	6	4	9	1
6.	Himachal Pradesh	0	4	4	8	1
7.	Kerala	0	61	61	31	3
8.	Mahakoshal	0	17	16	37	0
9.	Maharashtra	0	46	41	34	0
10.	Madras	0	25	22	18	3
11.	Karnataka	0	30	31	21	4
12.	Orissa	0	5	5	19	1
13.	Punjab	3	26	3	13	1
14.	Rajasthan	16	3	8	17	2
15.	Uttar Pradesh	0	24	14	48	4
16.	West Bengal	0	28	0	21	6
17.	Mid India Board	4	8	8	4	0
18.	South India Board	4	20	20	8	0
19.	A.F.M.S. Examination Board	0	8	16	0	0
20.	Tripura	0	1	0	3	1
	Grand Total:	39	448	381	494	29

Source: Indian Nursing Council.

ANM=Auxiliary Nursing Midwives..

H.W.=Health Worker

Table No. 6: Number of Registered General Nursing Midwifery, Auxiliary Nurse Midwives and Health visitors as on 31.12.1990

Sl. No.	*Name of the State Nursing Council & Examination Boards*	*Gen. Nursing Midwifery*		*Auxiliary Nurse-mid-Wives/health Workers*	*Health Visitor*
		Men	*Women*		
1	2	3	4	5	6
1.	Andhra Pradesh	495	14982	15860	1227
2.	Assam	158	2112	2054	46
3.	Bihar	54	8829	7501	1510
4.	Gujarat	873	23418	8573	1276
5.	Haryana	124	3259	3882	162
6.	Himachal Pradesh	212	1312	2055	274
7.	Karnataka	*	23401*	20707	3787
8.	Kerala	333	22414	6738	674
9.	Mahakoshal	2386	55813	15454	574
10.	Maharashtra	1639	36645	10861	551
11.	Madras	2287	31368	7210	1478
12.	Orissa	4381	11449	882	110
13.	Punjab	1293	22179	10447	1963
14.	Rajasthan	*	9819*	10424	322
15.	Uttar Pradesh	638	12190	10849	2734
16.	West Bengal	746	16426	16934	1204
17.	Mid India Board	NON-REGISTERING BODY			
18.	South India Board	NON-REGISTERING BODY			
19.	A.F.M.S. Examination Board	NON-REGISTERING BODY			
	Grand Total:		3,11,235	1,50,431	17,892

Note:

A.F.M.S. Armed Forces Medical Services.

* Sex-Wise Break-up not available.

Source: Indian Nursing Council.

Table No. 7: Village Health guides Training Programme and the Member of PHC's covered for the Training

Sl. No.	State/UT	PHC's (funct-ioning as on 1.4.80) to be covered under HG Scheme	PHCs covered	Total No. of VGHs Trained			No. of VGHs Actually working			Period upto which informa-tion Eelates to
				Male	Female	Total	Male	Female	Total	
1	2	3	4	5	6	7	8	9	10	11
1.	Andhra Pradesh	420	420	33122	2502	35624	28698	5636	34334	31-03-87
2.	Arunachal Pradesh $	—	—	—	—	—	—	—	—	—
3.	Assam	146	146	8171	11936	20107	0	11306	11306	31-03-90
4.	Bihar	587	100	NR	NR	11180*	NR	NR	10431*	31-03-85
5.	Goa, Daman & Diu	15	15	426	458	884	0	0	0	31-03-91
6.	Gujarat	251	251	21267	6993	28260	0	6993	6993	31-03-90
7.	Haryana	89	89	9981	299	10280	0	270	270	30-06-90
8.	Himachal Pradesh	77	77	4976	615	5591	3305	362	3667	31-12-90
9.	Jammu & Kashmir $	—	—	—	—	—	—	—	—	—
10.	Karnataka	269	191	12681	2447	15128	12681	2447	15128	31-12-90
11.	Kerala $	—	—	—	—	—	—	—	—	—
12.	Madhya Pradesh	465	448	36000	1000	37000	32546	1147	33693	30-09-89
13.	Maharashtra	428	428	17182	29672	46854	15029	27483	42512	31-12-90
14.	Manipur	25	25	1118	600	1718	1107	590	1697	30-06-88
15.	Meghalaya	22	22	899	1401	2300	137	1159	1296	31-03-87
16.	Mizoram	12	12	585	232	817	400	175	575	31-03-91
17.	Nagaland	14	14	349	199	548	349	199	548	31-12-90
18.	Orissa	314	314	18627	4670	23297	16530	4487	21017	30-09-90
19.	Punjab	129	129	1196	10461	11657	1196	10461	11657	31-03-90
20.	Rajasthan	232	232	20941	9018	29959	6289	2693	8982	30-09-89
21.	Sikkim	15	11	257	88	345	180	60	240	30-09-90
22.	Tamil Nadu $	—	—	—	—	—	—	—	—	—
23.	Tripura	27	27	1118	813	1931	1050	787	1837	30-09-90
24.	Uttar Pradesh	907	907	89071	1040	90111	NR	NR	90111*	31-03-90

Contd..

1	2	3	4	5	6	7	8	9	10	11
25.	West Bengal	335	335	31754	9478	41232	30905	9328	40233	31-12-89
26.	A & N Islands	2	2	209	137	346	98	108	206	31-03-91
27.	Chandigarh	0	1	20	24	44	20	22	42	31-12-90
28.	Dadra & Nagar Haveli	2	2	68	4	72	18	1	19	30-06-90
29.	Delhi	8	3	89	38	127	0	0	0	30-09-87
30.	Lakshadweep	7	7	11	31	42	2	18	20	31-12-90
31.	Pondicherry	12	12	150	120	270	120	80	200	31-12-90
	Total:	4810	4220	310268	94276	415724	150660	85812	337014	—

Note:1. NR = Information not received

2. $ = Alternative Health Guide Scheme is functioning in these States/UTS.

3. * = Separate Male & Female Break-up is not available.

(Figures are provisional)

Source: Rural health Statistics- March, 1992

Table No. 8: Number of ANM/HW(F) and LHV/HA(F) Training Schools and their Annual Admission Capacity (AAC)

Sl. No.	*State/UT*	*ANM/HW(F) Schools*			*Total Annual Admission Capacity*	*LHV/HA(F) Promotional Schools*	*Total Annual Admission Capacity*	*Period upto which Information relates to*
		Govt.	*Voluntary*	*Total*				
1	2	3	4	5	6	7	8	9
1.	Andhra Pradesh	10	78	88	3395	3	110	31-03-87
2.	Arunachal Pradesh	1	0	1	24	0	0	31-03-91
3.	Assam	18	4	22	1105	1	40	31-12-91
4.	Bihar	31	2	33	2450	2	380	31-03-85
5.	Goa	1	0	1	20@	0	0	31-12-91
6.	Gujarat	19	2	21	995	2	100	30-12-91
7.	Haryana	9	0	9	456	1	120	30-09-91
8.	Himachal Pradesh	7	1	8	450	1	30	31-12-90
9.	Jammu & Kashmir	14	2	16	360	NR	NR	31-03-85
10.	Karnataka	19	2	21	605	4	120	31-12-91
11.	Kerala	13	18	31	1066	3	120	31-12-91
12.	Madhya Pradesh	36@@	1	37	780uc	2	300	30-09-89
13.	Maharashtra	22	0	22	1289	5	225	31-12-91
14.	Manipur	3	0	3	90	1	35	31-03-91
15.	Meghalaya	2	0	2	60	0	0	31-03-87
16.	Mizoram	1	0	1	40	0	0	31-03-92
17.	Nagaland	3	0	3	80	0	0	30-09-91
18.	Orissa	19	0	19	760	1	60	31-12-90
19.	Punjab	6	4	10	400	1	35	31-03-91
20.	Rajasthan	27	0	27	1620	3	180	31-12-89
21.	Sikkim	1	0	1	40	1	5	30-06-91

Contd..

1	2	3	4	5	6	7	8	9
22.	Tamil Nadu	9	5	14	667	3	200	30-06-90
23.	Tripura	3	0	3	100	1	20	30-09-91
24.	Uttar Pradesh	46	3	49	1292	4	228	30-09-91
25.	West Bengal *	24	2	26	1709	6	540	31-12-91
26.	A & N Islands	1	0	1	25	0	0	30-09-91
27.	Chandigarh	0	0	0	0	0	0	30-09-91
28.	Dadra & Nagar Haveli	0	0	0	0	0	0	30-06-91
29.	Daman & Diu	0	0	0	0	0	0	30-09-91
30.	Delhi	2	0	2	80	1	30	31-03-86
31.	Lakshadweep	0	0	0	0	0	0	31-12-91
32.	Pondicherry	0	0	0	0	0	0	31-12-91
	Total:	347	124	471	19908	46	2873	—

Note:NR = Information not received

@ = Includes 4 males candidates

*= 4 Non Stipendary institution as per Q.P.R. for Quarter ending June, 88 No. of 10 Vol. Schools have been reduced by Maharashtra, QPR June

@@ = At present only 15 MPW(F) Training centres are functioning, other 21 training schools are giving refresher course to trained ANM/MPW(F)

UC = Under Clarification (Figures are provisional)

Source: Rural Health Statistics - March, 1992.

Table No. 9: Number of Dais Trained during 1974 to 31-3-1992

Sl. No.	*State/UT*	*Estimates No. of Untrained Dais*	*Dais Trained as on 1-4-91 since 1974*	*Target 1991-92*	*Dais Trained during 1991-92 (Apr. 91- Mar. 92)*	*Total Dais trained as on 31-3-92*	*Period upto which information relates*
1	2	3	4	5	6	7	8
1.	Andhra Pradesh	3045	44835	1000	NR	44835**	31-03-87
2.	Arunachal Pradesh @	0	440	0	0	440	31-03-91
3.	Assam	1409	13979	250	250	14229	31-12-91
4.	Bihar	NR	56029	500	NR	56029	31-03-85
5.	Goa	0	178	0	0	178	31-12-91
6.	Gujarat	5853	28362	750	783	29145	31-12-91
7.	Haryana	500	12114	250	121	12235	31-12-91
8.	Himachal Pradesh	NR	9418	50	NR	9418	31-12-90
9.	Jammu & Kashmir	NR	4244	500	NR	4244	31-03-85
10.	Karnataka	6634	41092	1750	1297	42389	31-12-91
11.	Kerala $	0	2906	0	0	2906	30-06-91
12.	Madhya Pradesh	NR	43395	1000	NR	43395	30-09-89
13.	Maharashtra	5000	39690	500	132	39822	31-12-91
14.	Manipur	NR	1276	25	NR	1276	31-03-91
15.	Meghalaya	0	1137	0	NR	1137	31-03-87
16.	Mizoram	54	935	5	30	965	31-03-92
17.	Nagaland	0	0	0	NR	0	31-03-91
18.	Orissa	40000	35341	750	NR	35341	30-12-90
19.	Punjab	600	22267	100	NR	22267	31-03-91
20.	Rajasthan	7856	19929	300	NR	19929	31-03-90
21.	Sikkim	NR	254	0	0	254	30-06-91
22.	Tamil Nadu	8545	37226	250	NR	37226	30-06-91
23.	Tripura	NA	1451	50	5	1456	31-12-91
24.	Uttar Pradesh	28477	144816	900	0	144816	31-09-91
25.	West Bengal	10500	34200	1000	NR	34200	31-12-89
26.	A & N Islands	150	144	25	7	151	31-12-91

Contd..

1	2	3	4	5	6	7	8
27.	Chandigarh	90	401	20	26	427	31-12-91
28.	Dadra & Nagar Haveli	50	238	0	0	238	30-06-91
29.	Daman & Diu *	0	0	0	0	0	30-09-91
30.	Delhi	NR	180	20	NR	180	31-03-91
31.	Lakshadweep	0	21	0	0	21	31-12-91
32.	Pondicherry	15	407	5	0	407	31-12-91
	Total:	118778	596905	10000	2651	599556	—

Note: NR = Information not received

$ Dais Training Programme has since been stopped from 1980 onwards in Kerala State

@ No system of traditional dais is practised in Arunachal Pradesh

** Figures taken from status report on Primary Health care received in meeting held in January, 1988

* Information included in Goa

The No. of trained dais prior to 1974 was 43,500 which is not

Included in the above statement, revised figures received from Maharashtra, Karnataka & Gujarat

Source: Rural Health Statistics - March, 1992.

Table No. 10: Number of Doctors in Government Agencies and Average Population served in different States/UTs - 1991

Sl. No.	State/UTS	Doctors engaged under Govt. Agency	Population served per Govt. Doctor	Period to which data relates
1	2	3	4	5
1.	Andhra Pradesh	1059	1:61471	31-12-91
2.	Arunachal Pradesh	233	1:3536	31-12-90
3.	Assam	2660	1:8750	31-12-91
4.	Bihar	NA	+	31-12-91
5.	Goa	540	1:2166	31-12-91
6.	Gujarat	3645	1:11404	31-12-91
7.	Haryana	NA	1:11705	-
8.	Himachal Pradesh	NA	1:5350	-
9.	Jammu & Kashmir	NA	+	31-12-91
10.	Karnataka	3397	1:13536	31-12-91
11.	Kerala	4163	1:7213	31-12-91
12.	Madhya Pradesh	NA	+	31-12-91
13.	Maharashtra	NA	+	31-12-91
14.	Manipur	684	1:2675	31-12-91
15.	Meghalaya	322	1:5357	31-12-90
16.	Mizoram	146	1:5000	31-12-91
17.	Nagaland	202	1:5401	31-12-89
18.	Orissa	4965	1:64178	31-12-91
19.	Punjab	3462	1:5642	31-12-91
20.	Rajasthan	NA	+	31-12-91
21.	Sikkim	101	1:4297	31-12-89
22.	Tamil Nadu	3189	1:17879	31-12-91
23.	Tripura	672	1:3822	31-12-90
24.	Uttar Pradesh	8630	1:15438	31-12-91

Contd..

1	2	3	4	5
25.	West Bengal	NA	+	31-12-91
26.	A & N Islands	122	1:3448	31-12-91
27.	Chandigarh	864	1:913	31-12-91
28.	Dadra & Nagar Haveli	12	1:11000	31-12-90
29.	Daman & Diu	19	1:5346	31-12-91
30.	Delhi	NA	1:6233	—
31.	Lakshadweep	28	1:1714	31-12-91
32.	Pondicherry	350	1:2174	31-12-91
	Total:	39466	—	—

Note:+= Not Available, Ratio has been worked out with the Annual estimates of Population of the year to which the data relates.

Government Agency includes Central/State Government Hospital, Public Sector undertaking hospital etc.

Source: Directorate of Health Services.

Table No. 11: Subjectwise Distribution of Indian Doctors trained Abroad Registrants (As on 31-12-1991)

Subject	Country of Training															
	USA		CANADA		UK		W.GERMANY		OEC		ANZ		OTHER		TOTAL	
	T	R	T	R	T	R	T	R	T	R	T	R	T	R	T	R
Gen. Medicine	244	135	31	16	676	412	20	8	134	86	5	0	84	36	1194	693
Surgery	153	83	34	15	1265	656	8	2	31	17	14	3	115	56	1620	832
Medicine & Surgery	4	1	2	2	23	4	0	0	10	7	1	0	20	7	60	21
Public Health	10	4	1	1	29	0	0	0	1	1	0	0	4	1	45	7
Dentistry	28	17	3	1	20	6	4	1	3	1	1	0	6	4	65	30
Veternary Science	179	70	19	6	40	21	13	6	25	4	6	2	18	10	300	119
Anesthesialogy	22	11	6	2	177	67	5	2	5	1	6	0	52	26	273	109
Paediatrics	145	85	19	6	188	77	4	2	9	4	5	2	54	19	424	195
Ophthalmology	16	10	12	6	213	95	3	1	12	4	4	1	40	21	300	138
Obst. & Gyanecology	53	21	14	4	557	244	8	4	13	5	1	0	81	45	727	323
Physiology	20	10	5	2	8	2	2	2	1	0	0	0	6	2	42	18
Psychiatry	17	6	6	3	56	12	0	0	0	0	0	0	7	4	86	25
Radiology	19	11	1	0	48	20	0	0	1	1	0	0	8	3	77	35
TB-Chest	6	1	1	0	34	15	1	0	0	0	0	0	9	4	51	20
Pathology	35	19	3	2	28	12	4	1	1	0	2	0	18	9	91	43
Cardiology	11	6	1	0	24	9	0	0	4	4	1	0	4	3	45	22
Others	96	39	17	8	242	95	9	4	22	8	1	0	100	51	487	205
Total:	1058	529	175	74	3628	1747	81	33	272	143	47	8	626	301	5887	2835

T: Total, R: Reported Return, W. Ger: West Germany, OEC: Other European Countries, ANZ: Australia and New Zealand.

Table No. 12: Medical Experts Serving on Foreign Assignments in various Developing Countries during 1991

Sl. No.	*Name of the Country*	*Bilateral Assignment*	*ITEC Assignment*	*Total*
1.	Bahrain	2	-	2
2.	Ethiopia	-	1	1
3.	Iran	1	-	1
4.	Kuwait	2	-	2
5.	Libya	5	-	5
6.	Malaysia	7	-	7
7.	Oman	9	-	9
8.	Saudi Arabia	9	-	9
9.	Yemen	2	-	2
	Total:	37	1	38

Note: ITEC-Indian Technical Economic Cooperation

Table No. 13: Health Manpower Working in Rural Areas Medical Specialists Working at Upgraded PHCs/CHCs

Sl. No.	State/U.T	Surgeons			OBST & Gynaes			Physicians		
		S	P	V	S	P	V	S	P	V
1	2	3	4	5	6	7	8	9	10	11
1.	Andhra Pradesh	0	0	0	0	0	0	0	0	0
2.	Arunachal Pradesh	7	7	0	7	7	0	4	4	0
3.	Assam	8	4	4	8	6	2	8*	2*	6
4.	Bihar	NR	NR	NR	NR	NR	NR	NR	NR	NR
5.	Goa	4	2	2	4	2	2	1	1	0
6.	Gujarat	164	67	97	38	19	19	0	0	0
7.	Haryana	114	84	30	21	9	12	21	5	16
8.	Himachal Pradesh	15	13	0	6	6	0	15	15	0
9.	Jammu & Kashmir	4	1	3	4	1	3	4	1	3
10.	Karnataka	66	59	7	45	37	8	70	68	2
11.	Kerala	NR	NR	NR	NR	NR	NR	NR	NR	NR
12.	Madhya Pradesh	86	49	37	97	56	41	86	52	34
13.	Maharashtra	NR	NR	NR	NR	NR	NR	NR	NR	NR
14.	Manipur	9	4	5	9	0	9	9	1	8
15.	Meghalaya	0	0	0	0	0	0	2	0	2
16.	Mizoram	1	0	1	1	0	1	0	0	0
17.	Nagaland	3	0	3	3	0	3	3	0	3
18.	Orissa	140	140	0	66	66	0	0	0	0
19.	Punjab	58	50	8	58	48	10	58	52	6
20.	Rajasthan	NR	NR	NR	NR	NR	NR	NR	NR	NR
21.	Sikkim	1	1	0	1	0	1	1	1	0
22.	Tamil Nadu	30	30	0	30	30	0	147	147	0
23.	Tripura	0	0	0	0	0	0	0	0	0
24.	Uttar Pradesh	142	96	46	144	26	118	6	4	2
25.	West Bengal	70	42	28	80	41	39	80	39	41
26.	A & N Islands	0	0	0	0	0	0	0	0	0
27.	Chandigarh	1	1	0	1	1	0	4	4	0
28.	Dadra & Nagar Haveli	0	0	0	0	0	0	0	0	0
29.	Daman & Diu	0	0	0	0	0	0	0	0	0
30.	Delhi	0	0	0	0	0	0	0	0	0
31.	Lakshadweep	0	0	0	0	0	0	0	0	0
32.	Pondicherry	0	0	0	0	0	0	3	3	0
	Total:	923	652	271	623	355	268	522	399	123

Contd..

Table No. 13 Contd..

Sl. No.	State/U.T.	Paediatricians			Total Specialists			Period up to which information relates to
		S	P	V	S	P	V	
1	2	12	13	14	15	16	17	18
1.	Andhra Pradesh	0	0	0	0	0	0	31-03-87
2.	Arunachal Pradesh	5	5	0	23	23	0	31-03-91
3.	Assam	NR*	NR*	NR	24	12	12	31-12-88
4.	Bihar	NR	NR	NR	NR	NR	NR	31-03-85
5.	Goa	1	1	0	10	6	4	31-12-91
6.	Gujarat	38	10	28	240	96	144	31-12-91
7.	Haryana	21	2	19	177	100	77	31-12-91
8.	Himachal Pradesh	6	6	0	42	42	0	30-09-90
9.	Jammu & Kashmir	4	1	3	16	4	12	31-03-89
10.	Karnataka	33	27	6	214	191	23	31-12-91
11.	Kerala	NR	NR	NR	146	146	0	31-12-91
12.	Madhya Pradesh	97	42	55	366	190	167	30-09-89
13.	Maharashtra	NR	NR	NR	305	169	136	31-12-91
14.	Manipur	NA	2	0	27	7	20	31-03-91
15.	Meghalaya	0	0	0	2	0	2	31-12-91
16.	Mizoram	1	1	0	3	1	2	31-03-92
17.	Nagaland	3	0	3	12	0	12	31-03-91
18.	Orissa	66	42	24	272	248	24	31-12-90
19.	Punjab	NR	NR	NR	174	150	24	31-03-91
20.	Rajasthan	NR	NR	NR	425	415	10	31-12-89
21.	Sikkim	1	0	1	4	2	2	30-06-91
22.	Tamil Nadu	0	0	0	207	207	0	31-06-91
23.	Tripura	0	0	0	0	0	0	31-12-91
24.	Uttar Pradesh	142	123	19	434	249	185	30-09-91
25.	West Bengal	80	11	69	320	133	187	31-12-89
26.	A & N Islands	0	0	0	0	0	0	31-12-91
27.	Chandigarh	1	1	0	7	7	0	31-12-91
28.	Dadra & Nagar Haveli	0	0	0	0	0	0	30-06-91
29.	Daman & Diu	0	0	0	0	0	0	30-09-91
30.	Delhi	1	0	1	1	0	1	30-09-87
31.	Lakshadweep	0	0	0	0	0	0	31-12-91
32.	Pondicherry	0	0	0	3	3	0	31-12-91
	Total:	500	274	226	3454	2410	1044	

Note: NA=Not available.
NR=Information not received
S=Number Sanctioned, P=Number in Position, V=Vacant Posts
*=Including Paediatricians as separate figures are not available (Figures are Provisional)

Source: Rural Health Statistics - March, 1992.

Table No. 14: Health Man power employed in Rural areas Medical Officers at PHCs

Sl. No.	*State/UT*	*Doctors at PHCs*			*Period upto which information relates to*
		S	*P*	*V*	
1	*2*	*3*	*4*	*5*	*6*
1.	Andhra Pradesh	1916	1555	361	31-03-87
2.	Arunachal Pradesh	24	24	0	31-03-91
3.	Assam	584	584	0	30-09-89
4.	Bihar	2121	2121	0	31-03-85
5.	Goa	53	43	10	31-12-91
6.	Gujarat	1026	911	115	31-12-91
7.	Haryana	645	491	154	31-12-91
8.	Himachal Pradesh	264	249	15	31-12-90
9.	Jammu & Kashmir	158	158	0	31-03-85
10.	Karnataka	1290	1104	186	31-12-91
11.	Kerala	1189	1189	0	31-12-91
12.	Madhya Pradesh	1647	1347	300	30-09-89
13.	Maharashtra	3254*	2741*	513	31-12-91
14.	Manipur	119	102	17	31-03-91
15.	Meghalaya	86	74	12	31-12-91
16.	Mizoram	22	24	2(2+)	31-12-91
17.	Nagaland	29	29	0	31-03-91
18.	Orissa	488	418	70	31-12-90
19.	Punjab	1706	1615	91	31-03-90
20.	Rajasthan	961	953	8	31-12-89
21.	Sikkim	34	21	13	30-06-91
22.	Tamil Nadu	2609*	2609*	o	30-06-91
23.	Tripura	161	106	55	31-12-91
24.	Uttar Pradesh	3787	2263	1524	30-09-91
25.	West Bengal	1413	1203	210	31-12-89
26.	A & N Islands	29	23	6	31-12-91
27.	Chandigarh	7	7	0	31-12-91
28.	Dadra & Nagar Haveli	7	4	3	30-06-91
29.	Daman & Diu	1	1	0	30-09-91
30.	Delhi	6	6	0	30-09-87
31.	Lakshadweep	9	9	0	31-12-91
32.	Pondicherry	29	29	0	31-12-91
	Total:	25674	22013	3661	

Note: S=Number Sanctioned, P=Number in Position, V=Vacant Posts
*=Figures includes MOs at allopathic disp. and ISM disp. (Figures are provisional)
Source: Rural Health Statistics - March, 1992.

Table No. 15: Health manpower working in Rural Areas - Parmedical

Sl. No. States/UTs	Block Extension Educators			Health Assistants (Male)			Health Assistants (Female)/LHVs			Health Workers (Male)		
	S	P	V	S	P	V	S	P	V	S	P	V
1 2	3	4	5	6	7	8	9	10	11	12	13	14
1.Andhra Pradesh	416	416	0	1610	1610	0	1872	1732	140	8050	7095	955
2.Arunachal Pradesh	0	0	0	5	5	0	14	14	0	179	179	0
3.Assam	153	153	0	793	793	0	557	310	247	0	0	0
4.Bihar	888	888	0	NR	NR	NR	1583	1248	335	1761	1761	0
5.Goa	13	12	1	33	26	7	25	25	0	173	151	22
6.Gujarat	138	69	69	1780	1543	237	1044	903	141	5280	4461	819
7.Haryana	90	72	18	505	484	21	629	404	225	2616	2121	795
8.Himachal Pradesh	81	81	0	376	366	10	364	306	58	1225	1225	0
9.Jammu & Kashmir	82	78	4	316	316	0	NR	67&	NR	381	377	4
10.Karnataka	482	298	184	862	689	183	2091	1910	181	5945	4958	887
11.Kerala	178	154	24	1171	1039	132	1094	1772	678+	5094$	3896	1198
12.Madhya Pradesh	465	440	25	1613	1613	0	1886	1367	519	9736	9328	408
13.Maharashtra	@	@	@	3996	3390	606	4652	4156	496	8096	7349	747
14.Manipur	NR	NR	NR	68	68	0	78	66	12	326	326	0
15.Meghalaya	23*	23*	0*	39	22	17	40	40	0	0	0	0
16.Mizoram	14	14	0	61	61	0	70	70	0	301	301	0
17.Nagaland	15	15	0	28	28	0	31	31	0	238	238	0
18.Orissa	329	329	0	170	170	0	914	859	55	798	708	90
19.Punjab	132	128	4	644	617	27	773	746	27	2852	2435	417
20.Rajasthan	232	232	0	928	928	0	820	658	162	3761	3420	341
21.Sikkim	12	12	0	0	0	0	12	12	0	0@	0@	0
22.Tamil Nadu	382	334	48	4418	4120	298	2245	1947	292	4561	3852	619
23.Tripura	19	18	1	154	89	65	10	31	21+	562	442	120
24.Uttar Pradesh	1026	1026	0	0	0	0	1418	1418	0	0	0	0
25.West Bengal	341	317	24	1689	1689	0	1689	947	742	10134	9120	1014
26.A & N Islands	6*	6*	0*	0	0	0	19	16	3	46	46	0
27.Chandigarh	1	1	0	4	4	0	2	2	0	8	8	0
28.Dadra & Nagar Haveli	4	3	1	0	0	0	8	7	1	21	8	13
29.Daman & Diu	0	0	0	0	0	0	0	0	0	14	11	3
30.Delhi	3	3	0	48	41	7	52	48	4	200	192	8
31.Lakshadweep	0	0	0	0	0	0	1	1	0	0	0	0
32.Pondicherry	3	3	0	29	29	0	20	20	0	0	0	0
Total:	5528	5125	403	21340	19740	1600	24013	21233&	2947	72658	64008	8650

Contd.

Sl. No. States/UTs	Health Workers (Female/ANM) S	P	V	Pharmacists S	P	V	Lab. Technicians S	P	V	Nurse-Midwise S	P	V	Period upto which information relates to
1 2	15	16	17	18	19	20	21	22	23	24	25	26	27
1.Andhra Pradesh	7027	6277	750	957	506	451	851	480	371	610	480	130	31-03-87
2.Arunachal Pradesh	179	179	0	30	30	0	9	9	0	9	9	0	31-03-91
3.Assam	4037	4037	0	1802	950	132	306	255	51	35&	38	3+	31-12-91
4.Bihar	10041	7541	2500	1249	1249	0	636	636	0	NR	NR	NR	31-03-85
5.Goa	197	192	5	10	10	0	22	21	1	15	14	1	31-12-91
6.Gujarat	7389	6947	442	1259	558	701	836	653	183	2450	1301	1149	31-12-91
7.Haryana	2628	2505	123	494	404	90	574	464	110	2415	2293	122	31-12-91
8.Himachal Pradesh	1705	1593	112	464	437	27	528	484	44	528	484	44	30-09-90
9.Jammu & Kashmir	696	381	315	72	72	0	43	43	0	214	214	0	31-03-85
10.Karnataka	8656	8053	603	1835	1497	338	981	498	483	465*	317	148	30-09-90
11.Kerala	5094	5094	0	847	847	0	215	215	0	445	420	25	31-12-91
12.Madhya Pradesh	11916	11148	768	465	435	30	505	470	35	NR	NR	NR	30-09-89
13.Maharashtra	11397	10852	545	2515	2181	334	1537	1409	128	2129	1806	323	31-12-91
14.Manipur	488	442	46	78	75	3	19	9	10	89	89	0	31-03-91
15.Meghalaya	451	436	15	78	40	38	41	21	20	74	59	15	31-12-91
16.Mizoram	318	318	0	48**	39	9	18	10	8	0	0	0	31-12-91
17.Nagaland	238	162	76	31	31	0	31	26	5	20	20	0	31-05-91
18.Orissa	6241	6241	0	310	248	62	108	108	0	394	386	8	31-12-90
19.Punjab	2852	2852	0	633	615	18	432	400	32	868	859	9	31-03-91
20.Rajasthan	7841	6860	981	2375	2355	20	898	685	213	NR	NR	NR	31-12-89
21.Sikkim	144	144	0	0	0	0	20	20	0	0	0	0	30-06-91
22.Tamil Nadu	8681	8505	176	1503	1503	0	587	587	0	175	175	0	30-06-91
23.Tripura	405	400	5	47	57	10+	25	38	13+	125	125	0	31-12-91
24.Uttar Pradesh	23029	23029	0	927	927	0	899	869	30	259	259	0	30-06-91
25.West Bengal	10134	8126	2008	1252	1163	89	439	374	65	3544	3004	540	31-12-89
26.A & N Islands	106	106	0	22	22	0	21	21	0	88	80	8	31-12-91
27.Chandigarh	14	14	0	2	2	0	6	6	0	2	2	0	31-12-91
28.Dadra & Nagar Haveli	39	28	11	4	3	1	4	4	0	0	0	0	30-06-91
29.Daman & Diu	0	0	0	1	0	0	2	2	0	0	0	0	30-09-91
30.Delhi	102	89	13	12	11	1	30	28	2	17	16	1	30-09-87
31.Lakshadweep	9	9	0	9	9	0	7	7	0	16	15	1	31-12-91
32.Pondicherry	95	95	0	10	10	0	23	23	0	14	14	0	31-12-91
Total:	132189	121765	10424	18621	16287	2334	10653	8875	1778	15000	12479	2521	

Note: NR=Note received

@=Post of BEEs do not exist in Maharashtra.

&=Total includes 6 posts in position in J&K for which coresponding sanctioned posts are not known.

+=Exceeding the no. sanctioned.

*=Bee figures are of 31-12-87 for Meghalaya and A & N Islands 30-09-90

Source: Rural Health Statistics - March, 1992

(Figures are Provisional)

Table No. 16: Number of Medical Graduates (including Post-graduates) on the live Register of Employment exchanges in each State/Union Territory during 1986-90

Sl. No.	State/UTs	Number as on				
		30-6-86	30-6-87	30-6-88	30-6-89	30-6-90
1	2	3	4	5	6	7
1.	Andhra Pradesh	1894	4727	3329	2914	2661
2.	Arunachal Pradesh	0	0	1	1	0
3.	Assam	138	191	108	102	190
4.	Bihar	1514	1564	1133	1513	1283
5.	Goa	110	180	163	220	228
6.	Gujarat	785	663	600	613	513
7.	Haryana	405	563	709	896	963
8.	Himachal Pradesh	113	317	187	161	220
9.	Jammu & Kashmir	10	0	2	42	23
10.	Karnataka	1078	994	759	817	863
11.	Kerala	1492	1568	1309	1624	2079
12.	Madhya Pradesh	1133	1421	1077	744	760
13.	Maharashtra	3844	4319	3868	3847	3951
14.	Manipur	45	96	113	126	99
15.	Meghalaya	5	5	1	0	4
16.	Mizoram	4	5	4	6	3
17.	Nagaland	0	0	0	0	0
18.	Orissa	528	737	1057	1097	1083
19.	Punjab	732	288	233	243	323
20.	Rajasthan	673	885	1115	1876	1831
21.	Sikkim	0	0	0	0	0
22.	Tamil Nadu	2419	2499	2394	2068	3729
23.	Tripura	17	17	17	17	11
24.	Uttar Pradesh	1814	1853	1579	1309	1285
25.	West Bengal	2145	2690	2675	2798	3443
26.	A & N Islands	1	1	1	6	9
27.	Chandigarh	606	790	669	697	721
28.	Dadra & Nagar Haveli	0	0	7	7	7
29.	Daman & Diu**	0	0	0	0	0
30.	Delhi	3873	4383	4176	3965	3738
31.	Lakshadweep	7	7	7	7	7
32.	Pondicherry	228	266	306	369	420
	Total:	25613	31029	27599	28085	30447

Note: 1. *= No employment exchange is functioning in this state.
2. **=Data are not maintained.

Source: Directorate General of Employment & Training.

Table 17: Number of Pharmacists and Nurses (General) on the live register of Employment Exchanges in Each State/U.T. as on 31-12-1988

Sl. No.	*State/UTs*	*Pharmacists*	*Nurses*
1	*2*	*3*	*4*
1.	Andhra Pradesh	3373	1430
2.	Arunachal Pradesh	0	0
3.	Assam	276	177
4.	Bihar	3089	653
5.	Goa	135	108
6.	Gujarat	681	91
7.	Haryana	840	258
8.	Himachal Pradesh	426	57
9.	Jammu & Kashmir	103	18
10.	Karnataka	1023	280
11.	Kerala	1893	2415
12.	Madhya Pradesh	941	647
13.	Maharashtra	2278	981
14.	Manipur	111	326
15.	Meghalaya	1	1
16.	Mizoram	0	0
17.	Nagaland	0	0
18.	Orissa	620	248
19.	Punjab	743	109
20.	Rajasthan	579	473
`21.	Sikkim *	0	0
22.	Tamil Nadu	3209	1119
23.	Tripura	74	14
24.	Uttar Pradesh	1842	311
25.	West Bengal	9752	815
26.	A & N Islands @	0	0
27.	Chandigarh	168	332
28.	Dadra & Nagar Haveli	0	0
29.	Delhi	1984	2579
30.	Daman & Diu **	0	0
31.	Lakshadweep	0	0
32.	Pondicherry	66	78
33.	Central Employment Exchanges	0	0
	Total:	34207	13520

Note: * No employment exchange is functioning in these States/Union Terriroties.
** Data are not maintained.
@ Not available

Source: Directorate General of Employment & Training, Ministry of Labour.

Table No. 18: Number of Hospitals and Beds according to Rural/Urban Areas as on 1-1-1992

Sl. No.	States/UTs	Rural		Urban		Total	
		Hospitals	Beds	Hospitals	Beds	Hospitals	Beds
1	2	3	4	5	6	7	8
1.	Andhra Pradesh (1-1-86)	322	5888	836	36672	1158	42560
2.	Arunachal Pradesh (1-1-91)	12	506	6	585	18	1091
3.	Assam (1-1-91)	151	3949	117	8712	268	12661
4.	Bihar (1-1-88)	76	2298	222	25839	298	28137
5.	Goa	43	877	69	2602	112	3479
6.	Gujarat (1-1-91)	190	7378	1595	47192	1785	54570
7.	Haryana	8	543	71	6460	79	7003
8.	Himachal Pradesh	19	446	40	3356	59	3802
9.	Jammu & Kashmir (1-1-89)	15	481	50	7751	65	8232
10.	Karnataka	25	3015	268	34409	293	37424
11.	Kerala (1-1-91)	1440	43246	597	32953	2037	76199
12.	Madhya Pradesh (1-1-91)	329	22032	73	3278	402	25310
13.	Maharashtra (1-1-91)	345	12120	1759	99300	2104	111420
14.	Manipur (1-1-91)	21	765	4	695	25	1460
15.	Meghalaya	0	0	8	1635	8	1635
16.	Mizoram	4	136	10	992	14	1128
17.	Nagaland (1-1-91)	21	321	10	793	31	1114
18.	Orissa	117	3343	165	11120	282	14463
19.	Punjab (1-4-90)	90	2795	140	12223	230	15018
20.	Rajasthan (1-1-91)	15	1042	199	18151	214	19193
21.	Sikkim (1-1-91)	0	0	5	525	5	525
22.	Tamil Nadu (1-1-90)	89	4235	319	44545	408	48780
23.	Tripura	10	275	13	1256	23	1531
24.	Uttar Pradesh (1-1-86)	83	2585	652	44693	735	47278
25.	West Bengal (1-1-91)	131	7610	282	46872	413	54482
26.	A & N Islands	4	204	4	542	8	746
27.	Chandigarh	0	0	2	1500	2	1500
28.	D & N Haveli (1-1-91)	2	62	0	0	2	62
29.	Daman & Diu	0	0	3	150	3	150
30.	Delhi	4	152	77	18320	81	18472
31.	Lakshadweep	2	70	0	0	2	70
32.	Pondicherry	0	0	10	2608	10	2608
	Total:	3568	126474	7606	515729	11174	642103

Source: Directorate of Health Services

Table No. 19: Number of Hospitals and Beds According to Ownership as on 1-1-1992

Sl. No.	States/UTs	Government		Local Bodies		Pvt. & Vol. Org.		Total		Population ** served per	
		Hosp.	Beds	Hosp.	Beds	Hosp.	Beds	Hosp.	Beds	Hosp.	Bed
1	2	3	4	5	6	7	8	9	10	11	12
1.	Andhra Pradesh (1-1-91)	317	22776	0	0	841	19784	1158	42560	55313	1505
2.	Arunachal Pradesh (1-1-91)	18	1091	0	0	0	0	18	1091	45761	755
3.	Assam (1-1-91)	141	9687	47	982	80	1992	268	12661	92973	1968
4.	Bihar (1-1-88)	242	22553	1	48	55	5536	298	28137	271362	2874
5.	Goa	16	1813	0	0	96	1666	112	3479	43327	1373*
6.	Gujarat (1-1-91)	239	20531	76	4669	1470	29370	1785	54570	22898	749
7.	Haryana	59	4771	0	0	20	2232	79	7003	207519	2341
8.	Himachal Pradesh	53	3615	0	0	6	187	59	3802	86286	1339
9.	Jammu & Kashmir (1-1-89)	15	481	0	0	50	7751	65	8232	109549	865
10.	Karnataka	209	26711	28	714	56	9999	293	37424	159294	1208
11.	Kerala	138	27030	0	0	1899	49169	2037	76199	14739	394
12.	Madhya Pradesh (1-1-91)	402	25310	0	0	0	0	402	25310	156330	2483
13.	Maharashtra (1-1-91)	693	62684	92	10955	1319	37781	2104	111420	35219	665
14.	Manipur (1-1-91)	21	1360	0	0	4	100	25	1460	70255	1203
15.	Meghalaya	4	985	0	0	4	650	8	1635	215616	1055
16.	Mizoram	11	818	0	0	3	310	14	1128	50518	627
17.	Nagaland (1-1-91)	31	1114	0	0	0	0	31	1114	35181	979
18.	Orissa	247	13051	6	111	29	1301	282	14463	111191	2168
19.	Punjab (1-4-90)	187	11133	4	103	39	3782	230	15018	85080	1303
20.	Rajasthan	214	19193	0	0	0	0	214	19193	207536	2314

Contd.

1	2	3	4	5	6	7	8	9	10	11	12
21.	Sikkim (1-1-91)	5	525	0	0	0	0	5	525	86835	827
22.	Tamil Nadu (1-1-90)	282	37935	7	479	119	10366	408	48780	133906	1120
23.	Tripura	23	1531	0	0	0	0	23	1531	110502	1647
24.	Uttar Pradesh (1-1-86)	534	34267	42	985	159	12026	735	47278	166792	2593
25.	West Bengal (1-1-91)	263	46967	21	603	129	6912	413	54482	156454	1186
26.	A & N Islands	6	717	0	0	2	29	8	746	36647	393
27.	Chandigarh	2	1500	0	0	0	0	2	1500	376500	502
28.	D & N Haveli (1-1-91)	1	50	0	0	1	12	2	62	64759	2809
29.	Daman & Diu	1	100	0	0	2	50	3	150	*	*
30.	Delhi (1-1-90)	27	9037	22	3698	32	5737	81	18472	113341	497
31.	Lakshadweep	2	70	0	0	0	0	2	70	23415	669
32.	Pondicherry	8	2462	0	0	2	146	10	2608	74589	286
	Total: (As on 1-1-92)	4411	411868	346	23347	6417	206888	11174	642103	76082	1324**

Note: * Included in Goa.

** Served per bed have been worked out on the basis of the Annual Estimates of Population as on 1st March and the period to which data relates.

Source: Directorate of Health Services.

Table No. 20: Number of Dispensaries and Beds According to Rural/Urban as on 1-1-1992

Sl. No.	States/UTs	*Rural*		*Urban*		*Total*	
		Dispensaries	*Beds*	*Dispensaries*	*Beds*	*Dispensaries*	*Beds*
1.	Andhra Pradesh (1-1-91)	137	206	45	37	182	243
2.	Arunachal Pradesh (1-1-91)	30	60	1	2	31	62
3.	Assam (1-1-91)	297	36	28	6	325	42
4.	Bihar (1-1-88)	411	0	16	96	427	96
5.	Goa	307	0	319	0	626	0
6.	Gujarat (1-1-91)	2519	1086	3746	4358	6265	5444
7.	Haryana	39	18	175	384	214	402
8.	Himachal Pradesh	190	186	23	27	213	213
9.	Jammu & Kashmir (1-1-89)	583	0	27	0	610	0
10.	Karnataka	603	345	232	238	835	583
11.	Kerala	1442	95	508	68	1950	163
12.	Madhya Pradesh (1-1-91)	152	0	126	2	278	2
13.	Maharashtra (1-1-91)	796	452	8406	1966	9202	2418
14.	Manipur (1-1-91)	49	0	3	0	52	0
15.	Meghalaya	21	0	2	0	23	0
16.	Mizoram	22	220	0	0	22	220
17.	Nagaland (1-1-91)	57	64	8	0	65	64
18.	Orissa	131	75	64	4	195	79
19.	Punjab (1-4-90)	1249	4961	224	570	1473	5531
20.	Rajasthan (1-1-91)	20	12	256	152	276	164
21.	Sikkim (1-1-91)	135	0	0	0	135	0
22.	Tamil Nadu (1-1-90)	147	138	365	140	512	278
23.	Tripura	470	0	6	0	476	0
24.	Uttar Pradesh (1-1-86)	1318	5137	432	592	1750	5729
25.	West Bengal (1-1-91)	408	0	143	0	551	0
26.	A & N Islands	2	0	5	0	7	0
27.	Chandigarh	7	0	27	0	34	0
28.	D & N Haveli (1-1-91)	5	4	0	0	5	4
29.	Daman & Diu	15	0	13	0	28	0
30.	Delhi	97	0	546	0	643	0
31.	Lakshadweep	0	0	0	0	0	0
32.	Pondicherry	11	38	15	157	26	195
	Total:	11670	13133	15761	8799	27431	21932

Source: Directorate of Health Services.

Table No. 21: Number of Dispensaries and Beds According to Ownership as on 1-1-1992

Sl. No.	States/UTs	Government		Local Bodies		Pvt. & Vol. Org.		Total	
		Disp.	Beds	Disp.	Beds	Disp.	Beds	Disp.	Beds
1.	Andhra Pradesh (1-1-91)	125	6	0	0	57	237	182	243
2.	Arunachal Pradesh (1-1-91)	31	62	0	0	0	0	31	62
3.	Assam (1-1-91)	317	0	0	0	8	42	325	42
4.	Bihar (1-1-88)	427	96	0	0	0	w	427	96
5.	Goa	32	0	0	0	594	0	626	0
6.	Gujarat (1-1-91)	179	37	283	111	5803	5296	6265	5444
7.	Haryana	170	396	3	6	41	0	214	402
8.	Himachal Pradesh	208	204	2	2	3	7	213	213
9.	Jammu & Kashmir (1-1-89)	610	0	0	0	0	0	610	0
10.	Karnataka	799	514	25	65	11	4	835	583
11.	Kerala	53	163	0	0	1897	0	1950	163
12.	Madhya Pradesh (1-1-91)	278	2	0	0	0	0	278	2
13.	Maharashtra (1-1-91)	319	352	1304	991	7579	1075	9202	2418
14.	Manipur (1-1-91)	27	0	25	0	0	0	52	0
15.	Meghalaya	23	0	0	0	0	0	23	0
16.	Mizoram	22	220	0	0	0	0	22	220
17.	Nagaland (1-1-91)	65	64	0	0	0	0	65	64
18.	Orissa	172	14	8	0	15	65	195	79
19.	Punjab (1-4-90)	1440	5513	21	6	12	12	1473	5531
20.	Rajasthan	276	164	0	0	0	0	276	164
21.	Sikkim (1-1-91)	135	0	0	0	0	0	135	0
22.	Tamil Nadu (1-1-90)	236	68	247	112	29	98	512	278
23.	Tripura	476	0	0	0	0	0	476	0
24.	Uttar Pradesh (1-1-86)	1555	5329	126	324	60	76	1750	5729
25.	West Bengal (1-1-91)	246	0	243	0	62	0	551	0
26.	A & N Islands	7	0	0	0	0	0	7	0
27.	Chandigarh	34	0	0	0	0	0	34	0
28.	D & N Haveli (1-1-91)	5	4	0	0	0	0	5	4
29.	Daman & Diu	2	0	0	0	26	0	28	0
30.	Delhi	303	0	194	0	146	0	643	0
31.	Lakshadweep	0	0	0	0	0	0	0	0
32.	Pondicherry	15	44	0	0	11	151	26	195
	Total:	8587	13378	2481	1617	16363	7063	27431	21932

Note: + Not Available.

Source: Directorate of Health Services.

Table No. 22: Number of Hospitals, No. of Hospital Beds & Number of Beds All Types Alongwith Ratio

Years (as on 31st Dec.)	*Number of hospitals*	*No. of Hospitals per 1000000 Population*	*No. of Hospital Beds*		*No. of Beds (all types)*	
			Actual	*Ratio per 100000 Population*	*Actual*	*Ratio per 100000 Population*
1951	2694	7	—	—	117178	32
1961	3054	7	—	—	230000	57
1971	3862	7	—	—	348655	64
1981	6804	10	476226	68	569495	83
1982	6897	10	486805	68	583773	82
1983	7189	10	500628	69	599074	82
1984	7369	10	514989	69	62712	86
1985	7474	10	535735	71	656850	88
1986	8067	10	555264	72	694121	91
1987	9803	12	585889	74	706471	91
1988	10840	13	598059	74	751091	95
1989	11079	13	602490	74	794712	97
1990	11571	13	629453	75	806409	97
1991	11174	13	642103	75	810548	95

* Figures are provisional.

Source: Directorate of Health Services.

Table No. 23: Establishment of Primary Health Centres and Subcentres in India Since First Five Years Plan

Period	*PHCs*	*Sub-Centres*
1st Five Year Plan	725	
2nd Five Year Plan	2565	
3rd Five Year Plan	4631	
Inter-Plan Period 3 Years		
As on 31.03.1967	4793	17521
As on 31.03.1968	4946	21539
As on 31.03.1969	4919	22826
4th Five Year Plan		
As on 31.03.1970	5015	23527
As on 31.03.1971	5112	28489
As on 31.03.1972	5183	28167
As on 31.03.1973	5248	31034
As on 31.03.1974	5283	33509
5th Five Year Plan		
As on 31.03.1975	5293	33616
As on 31.03.1976	5328	34088
As on 31.03.1977	5380	38110
As on 31.03.1978	5400	38115
As on 31.03.1979	5423	40124
As on 31.03.1980	5484	47112
6th Five Year Plan		
As on 31.03.1981	5740	51405
As on 31.03.1982	5851	57975
As on 31.03.1983	5959	65643
As on 31.03.1984	6375	77236
As on 31.03.1985	7284	84590
7th Five Year Plan		
As on 31.03.1986	12934*	92483
As on 31.03.1987	14281*	101549
As on 31.03.1988	16449	109644
As on 31.03.1989	18811	120767
As on 31.03.1990	20536	130390
As on 31.03.1991	21641	130960
As on 31.03.1992	22441	131318

Note: * = Includes Subsidiary Health Centres also.
Source: Rural Health Statistics, March, 1992.

Table No. 24: Primary Health Centres-Progress of Establishment

Sl. No.	State/UT	No. funct-ioning as on 1-4-85	7th Plan target (1985-1990)	1985-90		No. Funct-ioning as on 1-4-90	1990-91		No. funct-ioning as on 1-4-91	1991-92		No. funct-ioning as on 1-4-92
				Target	Achiev-ement		Target	Achiev-ement		Target	Achiev-ement	
1	2	3	4	5	6	7	8	9	10	11	12	13
1.	Andhra Pradesh	555	1150	700	728	1283	60	0	1283	0	NR	1283
2.	Arunachal Pradesh	0	28	27	28	28	3	4	32	4	1	33
3.	Assam	237	200	220	203	440	2	2	442	50	37	479
4.	Bihar	796	1500	1452	1205	2001	191	493	2494	0	0	2494
5.	Goa	13	7	7	7	20	0	0	20	2	1	21
6.	Gujarat	310	690	655	396	706	0	170$	876	0	35	911
7.	Haryana	163	231*	231	203	366	0	29	395	0	0	395
8.	Himachal Pradesh	117	110*	81	84	201	25	0	201	5	2	203
9.	Jammu & Kashmir	123	200	228	143	266	50	15&	281	20	0	281
10.	Karnataka	365	774*	774	768	1133	50	0	1133	50	40	1173
11.	Kerala	199	800*	835	687	886	25	25	911	80	0	911
12.	Madhya Pradesh	680	731	801	501	1181	120	1	1182	290	NR	1182
13.	Maharashtra	1539	261	462	107	1646	100	1	1647	0	3	1650
14.	Manipur	31	37*	39	37	68	9	0	68	2	2	70
15.	Meghalaya	32	33*	40	39	71	10	8	79	6	2	81
16.	Mizoram	19	18	18	16	35	0	0	35	3	3	38
17.	Nagaland	21	14*	15	12	33	2	0	33	2	NR	33
18.	Orissa	484	500	528	440	924	100	100	1024	40	5	1029
19.	Punjab	1706	330	195	330	2036	52	0	2036	12	12	2048
20.	Rajasthan	448	702	568	600	1048	250	275	1323	50	50	1373
21.	Sikkim	18	2	4	2	20	1	2	22	1	1	23

Contd.

1	2	3	4	5	6	7	8	9	10	11	12	13
22.	Tamil Nadu	436	1057	1045	950	1386	107	43	429	0	NR	1429
23.	Tripura	32	15	34	17	49	15	0	49	0	1	50
24.	Uttar Pradesh	1169	2500	2586	1934	3103	169	535	3638	154	NR	3638
25.	West Bengal	1172	488	429	372	1544	50	0	1544	20	NR	1544
26.	A & N Islands	6	5	7	10	16	2	2	18	1	1	19
27.	Chandigarh	0	0	0	0	0	0	0	0	0	0	0
28.	Dadra & Nagar Haveli	3	3	5	2	5	0,	0	5	0	0	5
29.	Daman & Diu	2	0	2	2	4	1	0	4	0	NR	4
30.	Delhi	8	0	0	0	8	0	0	8	0	0	8
31.	Lakshadweep	7	0	0	0	7	0	0	7	0	0	7
32.	Pondicherry	14	6	4	8	22	2	2	24	3	2	26
	Total:	10705	12392	11992	9831	20536	1396	1707	22243	795	198	22441

Notes:

All figures upto 31.3.88 regarding establishment of PHCs during 1985-88 are provided by Planning Commission

* = Revised target as arrived at working group discussion on Annual Plan 1989-90.

$ = Reported information as on 1-4-91. Therefore, 170 PHCs were probably established during 1990-91, against the previous years targets.

Source: Rural Health Statistics - March, 1992.

Table No. 24 : Sub-Centres - Progress of Establishment

Sl. No.	State/UT	No. functioning as on 1-4-85	7th Plan target (1985-1990)	1985-90		No. Functioning as on 1-4-90	1990-91		No. functioning as on 1-4-91	1991-92		No. functioning as on 1-4-92
				Target	Achievement		Target	Achievement		Target	Achievement	
1	2	3	4	5	6	7	8	9	10	11	12	13
1.	Andhra Pradesh	6129	4000	4035	1765	7894	0	0	7894	0	NR	7894
2.	Arunachal Pradesh	55	135	137	100	155	0	18	173	0	11	184
3.	Assam	1711	3421	3400	3399	5110	0	0	5110	0	NR	5110
4.	Bihar	8299	6500	6550	6500	14799	0	0	14799	0	0	14799
5.	Goa	135	10	10	10	145	0	0	145	0	2	147
6.	Gujarat	4869	1787	1500	1564	6433	0	300	7134	0	150	7284
7.	Haryana	1591	776	761	708	2299	0	0	2299	0	0	2299
8.	Himachal Pradesh	952	560	315	550	1502	0	0	1502	0	0	1502
9.	Jammu & Kashmir	609	1367	1466	851	1460	0	120*	1580	0	0	1580
10.	Karnataka	4964	2061*	866	2829	7793	0	0	7793	0	0	7793
11.	Kerala	2270	2824*	2820	2824	5094	0	0	5094	0	NR	5094
12.	Madhya Pradesh	6615	5385	4666	5295	11910	0	0	11910	0	NR	11910
13.	Maharashtra	6391	4419	4722	2857	9248	0	116	9364	0	13	9377
14.	Manipur	301	119	112	119	420	0	0	420	0	0	420
15.	Meghalaya	217	230	316	98	315	0	27	342	0	14	356
16.	Mizoram	162	58	58	58	220	0	0	220	0	12	232
17.	Nagaland	133	124	126	68	201	0	0	201	0	NR	201
18.	Orissa	4127	1800	1800	1299	5426	0	0	5426	0	0	5426
19.	Punjab	2603	250	250	250	2853	0	0	2853	0	0	2853
20.	Rajasthan	3790	4210	4208	4210	8000	0	96	8096	0	0	8096
21.	Sikkim	82	50	40	50	132	0	5	137	0	5	142

Contd.

1	2	3	4	5	6	7	8	9	10	11	12	13
22.	Tamil Nadu	5860	3000	1973	2821	8681	0	0	8681	0	NR	8681
23.	Tripura	230	300*	268	242	472	0	23	495	0	1	496
24.	Uttar Pradesh	15653	6559*	5559	6000	21653	0	0	20153	0	NR	20153
25.	West Bengal	6100	4600	5211	1773	7873	0	0	7873	0	NR	7873
26.	A & N Islands	31	42	50	66	97	0	0	97	0	12	109
27.	Chandigarh	12	0	0	0	12	0	0	12	0	0	12
28.	Dadra & Nagar Haveli	19	15	15	15	34	0	0	34	0	0	34
29.	Daman & Diu	14	0	3	16	30	0	0	30	0	NR	30
30.	Delhi	42	0	0	0	42	0	0	42	0	0	42
31.	Lakshadweep	14	10	0	0	14	0	0	14	0	0	14
32.	Pondicherry	73	0	0	0	73	0	3	76	0	0	76
	Total:	84053	54612	51237	46337	130390	0	708	131098	0	220	131318

Notes:

* = 7th Plan Target of Sub-centers changed by Planning Commission in Annual Plan - 1989-90 discussion.

All figures of sub-centres upto 31.3.88 provided by Planning Commission. (Figures are provisional)

No targets of sub-centres were given to States/U.T.s during 90-91.

Source: Rural Health Statistics - March, 1992.

Table No. 25 : Community Health Centres - Progress of Establishment

Sl. No.	State/UT	No. functioning 1-4-85	7th Plan target (1985-1990)	1985-90		No. Functioning 1-4-90	1990-91		No. functioning 1-4-91	1991-92		No.of functioning 1-4-92
				Target	Achievement		Target	Achievement		Target	Achievement	
1	2	3	4	5	6	7	8	9	10	11	12	13
1.	Andhra Pradesh	27	100	113	19	46	30	0	46	0	NR	46
2.	Arunachal Pradesh	0	7	6	6	6	0	0	6	2	0	6
3.	Assam	12	30	37	44	56	0	3	59	10	9	68
4.	Bihar	50	97	65	46	96	10	10	106	0	0	106
5.	Goa	3	2	2	2	5	1	0	5	2	0	5
6.	Gujarat	22	100	110	13	135	15	15	150	0	11	161
7.	Haryana	2	50	47	39	41	7	0	41	10	0	41
8.	Himachal Pradesh	28	7	6	7	35	5	0	35	3	0	35
9.	Jammu & Kashmir	19	15	13	14	33	5	2	35	2	0	35
10.	Karnataka	98	58@	66	48	146	10	0	146	10	23	169
11.	Kerala	4	100	75	50	54	0	0	54	15	NR	54
12.	Madhya Pradesh	58	100	91	114	172	20	3	175	50	NR	175
13.	Maharashtra	147	78	95	136	283	15	0	283	0	2	285
14.	Manipur	6	10	15	3	9	4	0	9	7	2	11
15.	Meghalaya	3	8	11	0	3	10	15	18	4	2	5
16.	Mizoram	1	4	3	4	5	0	0	5	1	1	6
17.	Nagaland	1	6	3	2	3	1	0	3	1	NR	3
18.	Orissa	59	92	74	25	84	25	0	84	35	8	89
19.	Punjab	10	56	44	58	68	16	0	68	16	18	86
20.	Rajasthan	76	25	100	110	186	10	0	186	15	16	217

Contd.

1	2	3	4	5	6	7	8	9	10	11	12	13
21.	Sikkim	0	2@	5	0	0	1	0	0	1	0	0
22.	Tamil Nadu	30	120	91	42	72	40	1	73	0	NR	73
23.	Tripura	3	7	9	5	8	2	0	8	0	0	8
24.	Uttar Pradesh	74	259	212	143	217	15	20	237	49	NR	237
25.	West Bengal	23	184	140	64	87	40	0	87	30	NR	87
26.	A & N Islands	0	3	3	2	2	0	0	2	1	1	3
27.	Chandigarh	1	0	0	0	1	0	0	1	0	0	1
28.	Dadra & Nagar Haveli	0	2	1	0	0	1	0	0	1	0	0
29.	Daman & Diu	0	0	0	0	0	0	0	0	0	NR	0
30.	Delhi	0	0	0	0	0	0	0	0	0	0	0
31.	Lakshadweep	1	0	4	0	1	1	0	1	2	0	1
32.	Pondicherry	1	1	1	0	1	1	1	2	1	0	2
	Total:	759	1523	1442	1096	1855	285	70	1940	268	90	2015

Note:

All figures of CHCs upto 31.3.88 regarding Estt. of CHCs during 1985-88 were provided by Planning Commission.

@=Revised targets as arrived at Annual Plan working group discussion for 1989-90.

(Figures are Provisional)

Source: Rural Health Statistics - March, 1992.

Table No. 26: Number of PHCs and Sub-centres required and in Position in Tribal areas as on 31-12-91

Sl. No.	States/UTs	PHCs			Sub-Centres		
		Required	In position	Achievement (%)	Required	In position	Achievement (%)
1.	Andhra Pradesh	137	116	84.67	915	654	71.48
2.	Arunachal Pradesh*	24	22	91.67	190	208	109.47
3.	Assam	121	74	61.16	804	445	55.35
4.	Bihar	489	208	42.54	3522	1824	51.79
5.	Goa	0	0	0	0	0	0
6.	Gujarat	294	183	62.24	2005	1632	81.40
7.	Haryana	0	0	0	0	0	0
8.	Himachal Pradesh	10	15	150.00	65	97	149.23
9.	Jammu & Kashmir	N.R.	N.R.	0	N.R.	N.R.	0
10.	Karnataka	266	307	115.41	1855	1850	99.73
11.	Kerala	55	58	105.45	369	174	47.15
12.	Madhya Pradesh	752	633	84.18	5019	4935	98.33
13.	Maharashtra	265	265	100.0	1662	1603	96.45
14.	Manipur	35	35	100.0	221	221	100.0
15.	Meghalaya *	67	45	67.16	447	235	52.57
16.	Mizoram *	35	35	100.0	220	314	142.73
17.	Nagaland *	63	65	103.17	418	213	50.96
18.	Orissa	354	349	98.59	2300	1485	64.57
19.	Punjab	0	0	0	0	0	0
20.	Rajasthan	168	158	94.05	1111	934	84.07
21.	Sikkim	1	3	300.0	10	19	190.0
22.	Tamil Nadu	12	13	108.33	70	111	158.57
23.	Tripura	30	22	73.33	200	245	122.50
24.	Uttar Pradesh	219	189	86.30	1381	1376	99.64
25.	West Bengal	107	91	85.05	712	417	58.57
26.	A & N Islands	4	2	50.00	30	25	83.33
27.	Chandigarh	0	0	0	0	0	0
28.	Dadra & Nagar Haveli *	5	5	100.0	34	34	100.0
29.	Daman & Diu	2	1	50.0	17	14	82.35
30.	Delhi	0	0	0	0	0	0
31.	Lakshadweep*	2	7	350.0	17	14	82.35
32.	Pondicherry	0	0	0	0	0	0
	Total:	3517	2901	82.49	23594	19079	80.86

Note:

* = Predominately Tribal States/UTs having no TSP.
PHCs = Primary Health Centres
N.R = Not Received.

Source: Tribal Development Planning Cell.

Table No. 27 : Number of Cancer Patients treated in Specialised Cancer Hospitals during 1990 and 1991

Sl. No.	States/UTs	No. of Hospi-tals	1990					1991				
			Total No. of Beds	Admis-sions	Disc-charges	Deaths	Number hospitals report-ed (P)	Total No. of Beds	Admis-sions	Disch-arges	Deaths	Number of Hospitals reported
1	2	3	4	5	6	7	8	9	10	11	12	13
1.	Andhra Pradesh	1	250	NR	NR	NR	NR	NR	NR	NR	NR	NR
2.	Assam	1	84	656	584	28	1	NR	NR	NR	NR	NR
3.	Bihar	1	56	NR	NR	NR	NR	NR	NR	NR	NR	NR
4.	Gujarat	1	58	NR	NR	NR	NR	58	670	639	35	1
5.	Himachal Pradesh	1	35	192	0	0	1	35	208	205	3	1
6.	Karnataka	2	369	7000	6782	242	2	384	7310	7047	227	2
7.	Kerala	1	200	2532	2208	324	1	200	2322	2014	308	1
8.	Madhya Pradesh	5	299	6636	6300	281	5	32	918	885	51	2
9.	Maharashtra	2	403	12073	11663	404	2	370	11589	11225	385	1
10.	Orissa	1	130	1627	1556	70	1	NR	NR	NR	NR	NR
11.	Tamil Nadu	4	814	12308	11914	407	4	739	11843	11448	338	3
12.	Tripura	1	50	520	500	23	1	50	584	564	20	1
13.	Uttar Pradesh	1	106	1038	961	61	1	106	1283	1209	66	1
14.	West Bengal	3	359	100	89	11	1	30	98	89	9	1
	Total:	25	3245	44682	42557	1851	20	2014	36825	35320	1442	14

Note:

NR = Information not received.

Source: Specialised Cancer Hospitals.

Table No. 28 : Number of Cancer Patients treated in specialised cancer hospitals according to various Cancer causes as per ICD (IX Revision 1975) during 1991

Sl. No.	States/UTs	Malignant Neoplasm of Liporal Cavity Phar YNX (140-149)	Malignant Neoplasm of Digective Organs & Peritoneum (150-159)	Malignant Neoplasm of Respiratory and Intrathoracic Organs (160-165)	Malignant Neoplasm of Bone, Connective tissue, Skin & Breast (170-175)	Malignant Neoplasm of Genito-Urinary Organs (179-189)	Malignant Neoplasm of Other & Un-Specified sits (190-199)	Malignant Neoplasm of Lymphatic and Haemopoietic tissue (200-208)	Benign neo plasm (210-229)	Carcinoma In Situ (230-234)	Other & Unspecified Neo-Plasm (235-239)	Grand Total
1	2	3	4	5	6	7	8	9	10	11	12	13
1.	Andhra Pradesh	NR	NR	NR	NR	NR	NR	NR	NR	NR	NR	NR
2.	Assam	NR	NR	NR	NR	NR	NR	NR	NR	NR	NR	NR
3.	Bihar	NR	NR	NR	NR	NR	NR	NR	NR	NR	NR	NR
4.	Gujarat	215	108	58	116	121	33	1	16	0	2	670
5.	Himachal Pradesh	18	22	34	12	110	4	8	0	0	0	208
6.	Karnataka	899	1112	439	980	1918	352	1004	332	19	255	7310
7.	Kerala	509	485	315	188	373	141	148	66	55	42	2322
8.	Madhya Pradesh	119	200	63	59	219	23	69	160	2	4	918
9.	Maharashtra	2298	1394	772	1806	2466	820	1710	131	0	192	11589
10.	Orissa	NR	NR	NR	NR	NR	NR	NR	NR	NR	NR	NR
11.	Tamil Nadu	1576	1614	744	1698	2421	867	1609	651	9	654	11843
12.	Tripura	198	143	46	23	80	4	74	0	5	11	584
13.	Uttar Pradesh	314	130	101	139	393	112	94	0	0	0	1283
14.	West Bengal	8	13	8	25	27	2	15	0	0	0	98
	Total:	6154	5221	2580	5046	8120	2358	4732	1356	90	1160	36825

Source: Specialised Cancer Hospitals.

Table No. 29 : Number of Patients of Mental Disorders treated in Specialised Mental Hospitals during 1990 and 1991

Sl. No.	States/UTs	No. of Mental Hospitals	1990					1991				
			Total No. of Beds	Admissions	Discharged	Deaths	No. of Hosp. Reported	Total No. of Beds	Admissions	Discharged	Deaths	No. of Hosp. Reported
1	2	3	4	5	6	7	8	9	10	11	12	13
1.	Andhra Pradesh	2	900	4177	3646	22	2	900	2611	2477	0	1
2.	Assam	1	750	1428	1404	81	1	1200	1620	1541	132	1
3.	Bihar	3	2473	6307	6290	129	2	2473	5818	5835	108	2
4.	Goa	1	272	2161	2161	7	1	278	2273	2258	14	1
5.	Gujarat	6	943	452	435	24	4	842	471	402	30	5
6.	Jammu & Kashmir	2	180	781	776	2	1	180	770	757	2	1
7.	Karnataka	2	1180	4536	4727	18	2	1180	4777	5203	18	2
8.	Kerala	3	1344	5255	5187	20	2	1344	8810	8956	57	3
9.	Madhya Pradesh	2	355	580	563	14	2	370	567	566	13	2
10.	Maharashtra	5	5990	11523	11842	321	5	6005	11321	11803	361	5
11.	Nagaland	1	25	78	67	5	1	25	NR	NR	NR	NR
12.	Orissa	1	60	1156	1152	1	1	60	1128	1131	5	1
13.	Punjab	1	811	234	240	31	1	911	195	198	14	1
14.	Rajasthan	2	410	3616	3513	17	1	410	1457	1450	8	1
15.	Tamil Nadu	1	1800	4639	4469	111	1	1800	4800	4543	94	1
16.	Uttar Pradesh	4	1499	2089	2074	47	4	1499	1136	1173	19	3
17.	West Bengal	7	1416	940	816	26	2	1066	NR	NR	NR	NR
18.	Delhi	1	578	NR	NR	NR	NR	604	642	599	33	1
	Total:	45	20571	49952	49362	876	33	21147	48396	48892	908	31

Note:

NR = Information not received.

Source: Specialised Mental Hospitals.

Table No. 30 : Number of Patients of Mental Disorder Treated in Specialised Mental Hospitals according to various causes as per I.C.D - IX during 1991

Sl. No.	States/UTs	I.C.D. Codes Number and Disease											
		Psycoses (290-299)			Neuroses (300-316)			Mental Retarted (317-319)			Grand Total (290-319)		
		M	F	T	M	F	T	M	F	T	M	F	T
1	2	3	4	5	6	7	8	9	10	11	12	13	14
1.	Andhra Pradesh	1761	642	2403	147	41	188	17	3	20	1925	686	2611
2.	Assam	1195	389	1584	22	5	27	6	3	9	1223	397	1620
3.	Bihar	4558	928	5486	261	21	282	24	26	50	4843	975	5818
4.	Goa	718	617	1335	644	287	931	4	3	7	1366	907	2273
5.	Gujarat	312	96	408	9	0	9	54	0	54	375	96	471
6.	Jammu & Kashmir	417	269	686	49	29	78	4	2	6	470	300	770
7.	Karnataka	2666	1197	3863	647	180	827	63	24	87	3376	1401	4777
8.	Kerala	5035	1815	6850	1033	467	1500	295	165	460	6363	2447	8810
9.	Madhya Pradesh	352	94	446	84	18	102	15	4	19	451	116	567
10.	Maharashtra	7892	2777	10669	468	11	479	113	60	173	8473	2848	11321
11.	Nagaland	NR	NR	NR	NR	NR	NR	NR	NR	NR	NR	NR	NR
12.	Orissa	501	347	848	131	102	233	36	11	47	668	460	1128
13.	Punjab	128	47	175	7	4	7	9	0	9	146	49	195
14.	Rajasthan	580	468	1048	205	148	353	50	6	56	835	622	1457
15.	Tamil Nadu	2388	1054	3442	1089	59	1148	167	43	210	3644	1156	4800
16.	Uttar Pradesh	698	251	949	166	10	176	11	0	11	875	261	1136
17.	West Bengal	NR	NR	NR	NR	NR	NR	NR	NR	NR	NR	NR	NR
18.	Delhi	344	164	508	10	7	17	16	4	20	440	202	642
	Total:	29545	11155	40700	4972	1389	6357	884	354	1238	35473	12923	48396

Note: NR=Not Received

Source: Specialised Mental Hospitals

Table No. 31: Reported cases and deaths due to communicable diseases in States/U.Ts in India during 1991

Sl. No.	*States/UTs*	*Diptheria*		*Poliomyelitis*		*Tetanus-Neonatal*		*Tetanus Others*		*Whooping Cough*		*Measles*		*A.R.I*	
		C	*D*	*C*	*D*	*C*	*D*	*C*	*D*	*C*	*D*	*C*	*D*	*C*	*D*
1	*2*	*3*	*4*	*5*	*6*	*7*	*8*	*9*	*10*	*11*	*12*	*13*	*14*	*15*	*16*
1.	Andhra Pradesh	5340	11	726	1	304	19	752	136	10603	7	4436	42	1145261	675
2.	Arunachal Pradesh	157	0	9	0	7	0	1	1	818	0	1293	1	34021	8
3.	Assam	119	18	41	0	168	34	253	43	5000	11	6060	1	566366	19
4.	Bihar	..	..	..	..	..	..	..	..	..	..	..	..	..	..
5.	Goa	0	0	5	0	2	1	2	0	1	0	138	0	11706	1
6.	Gujarat	615	31	354	18	241	32	565	95	1879	1	6388	96	349186	120
7.	Haryana	11	0	66	3	277	61	343	62	164	3	581	3	420037	70
8.	Himachal Pradesh	8	4	6	0	6	2	39	4	31	0	284	1	738375	150
9.	Jammu & Kashmir	1020	1	14	0	60	0	0	0	355	0	1896	0	97520	3
10.	Karnataka	489	7	163	16	319	55	675	132	2184	5	3062	23	766778	146
11.	Kerala	12	2	22	0	2	1	36	6	3460	3	12531	2	2328262	114
12.	Madhya Pradesh	302	3	2611	13	5397	169	1085	96	12513	39	3903	35	410662	1055
13.	Maharashtra	268	7	96	9	101	48	1025	278	380	0	6820	30	412191	93
14.	Manipur	0	0	0	0	0	0	0	0	1011	0	434	0	7210	0
15.	Meghalaya	22	1	9	0	4	1	7	1	1909	0	3483	1	101030	14
16.	Mizoram	0	0	0	0	4	1	7	4	285	0	711	4	12507	6
17.	Nagaland	72	0	36	0	282	2	112	0	677	0	457	5	681	0
18.	Orissa	148	13	341	17	1448	147	2674	200	10960	6	5880	14	1425513	346
19.	Punjab	12	1	61	3	150	25	241	108	112	1	195	1	210199	110
20.	Rajasthan	749	24	973	17	427	38	857	109	900	4	2072	28	172049	155
21.	Sikkim	0	0	0	0	0	0	0	0	4	0	506	0	34166	2
22.	Tamil Nadu	11	1	776	5	61	27	781	34	40	1	7334	43	185652	164
23.	Tripura	0	0	1	0	0	0	33	7	830	0	727	0	65836	2
24.	Uttar Pradesh	622	33	347	20	1214	215	789	155	15782	3	2118	1	296302	41
25.	West Bengal	2430	202	1045	11	511	169	2719	315	2055	1	5796	25	5051	99
26.	A & N Islands	0	0	0	0	3	1	1	0	16	0	330	0	48765	21
27.	Chandigarh	1	0	8	0	4	0	48	8	48	0	103	0	56128	8
28.	Dadra & Nagar Haveli	0	0	1	0	0	0	0	0	42	0	92	0	21236	1
29.	Daman & Diu	0	0	0	0	0	0	3	0	20	0	52	0	3011	3
30.	Delhi	136	41	959	48	248	53	1984	77	1441	0	1902	50	139130	210
31.	Lakshadweep	0	0	0	0	1	0	2	0	0	0	43	0	5904	0
32.	Pondicherry	0	0	0	0	0	0	2	1	0	0	28	0	55109	0
	Total:	12550	400	8670	181	11241	1101	15036	1872	73520	85	79655	401	10126044	3691

Note : ARI—Acute Respiratory Infection.

Contd.

Sl. No.	States/UTs	*Pneumoni*		*Enteric Fever*		*Viral Hepatitis*		*Dog Bites/ Rabies*		*Syphilis*		*Gonoccocal Iofection*		*Tuberculosisi*	
		C	*D*	*C*	*D*	*C*	*D*	*C*	*D*	*C*	*D*	*C*	*D*	*C*	*D*
1	2	17	18	19	20	21	22	23	24	25	26	27	28	29	30
1.	Andhra Pradesh	17940	71	45326	46	27963	94	468	95	21429	0	56171	8	209565	1105
2.	Arunachal Pradesh	331	5	2210	2	705	4	0	0	111	0	83	0	6304	31
3.	Assam	20240	53	18818	22	13142	44	422	0	374	0	768	0	19125	88
4.	Bihar	..	..	..	..	..	..	..	..	..	..	..	..	..	..
5.	Goa	120	7	65	0	101	0	2	2	3	0	0	0	6878	4
6.	Gujarat	6159	114	7675	27	4693	156	12	5	267	0	337	0	30475	228
7.	Haryana	19323	111	2779	15	906	12	172	0	162	0	110	0	32986	308
8.	Himachal Pradesh	89719	87	14428	8	2005	6	2	1	111	0	44	0	16285	227
9.	Jammu & Kashmir	10727	0	5134	0	263	0	124	0	185	0	67	0	1931	0
10.	Karnataka	10116	124	20800	38	2470	92	988	45	5990	3	10041	5	48117	560
11.	Kerala	11159	62	9483	8	7584	13	138	27	397	0	1495	0	46250	317
12.	Madhya Pradesh	42380	129	68206	806	10030	79	128	7	2413	1	2125	2	68190	313
13.	Maharashtra	9437	403	18324	130	7650	383	110	110	3034	2	1951	0	94010	1053
14.	Manipur	1881	2	1314	0	1048	0	0	0	22	0	175	0	755	8
15.	Meghalaya	2808	17	4007	2	797	2	121	0	53	0	789	1	1957	12
16.	Mizoram	1191	11	427	0	607	3	0	0	38	0	36	9	1023	59
17.	Nagaland	179	0	110	0	109	0	35	1	133	0	53	0	200	0
18.	Orissa	41789	514	55774	82	13100	161	18	9	3856	2	5179	1	47114	1541
19.	Punjab	2537	43	4276	7	1871	13	2	1	105	0	375	0	20590	167
20.	Rajasthan	31914	247	5477	74	1553	68	503	4	234	0	468	0	30550	190
21.	Sikkim	2184	10	4	0	642	4	553	0	0	0	0	0	1131	27
22.	Tamil Nadu	6613	85	11520	12	408	2	42	3	3723	0	3652	4	45949	326
23.	Tripura	2502	15	1777	3	328	2	1	1	81	0	104	0	NR	NR
24.	Uttar Pradesh	44758	181	27888	28	904	78	62	2	512	1	2245	0	44145	227
25.	West Bengal	143	65	14261	64	3152	89	276	276	794	0	731	7	31932	327
26.	A & N Islands	88	11	116	1	301	16	0	0	29	0	61	0	886	46
27.	Chandigarh	3887	107	1084	2	620	6	4	0	0	0	0	0	824	57
28.	Dadra & Nagar Haveli	190	2	35	0	69	1	0	0	23	0	4	0	158	1
29.	Daman & Diu	0	0	99	0	269	1	0	0	19	0	4	0	884	10
30.	Delhi	22675	631	9387	67	4236	120	183	31	532	0	478	0	57857	1533
31.	Lakshadweep	13	0	95	2	79	0	0	0	0	0	0	0	123	0
32.	Pondicherry	334	0	3244	2	1059	0	28	16	92	0	20	0	31853	16
	Total:	403337	3089	354143	1448	93497	1449	4394	636	44722	9	87566	37	898047	8773

Note: C=Cases, D=Deaths, NR=Not rceived

Data is provisional an not comparable due to ill-defined coverage

Source: Monthly Health conditions Reports-States/U.T.S.D.H.S.